Sleep, Health, and Society

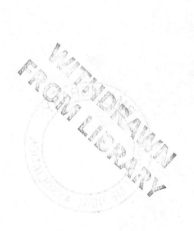

Sleep, Health and Society

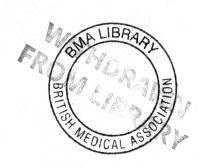

Sleep, Health, and Society
From Aetiology to Public Health

SECOND EDITION

Edited by

Francesco P. Cappuccio
Professor of Cardiovascular Medicine & Epidemiology
Health Sciences – Mental Health and Wellbeing
Warwick Medical School
University of Warwick
Coventry, UK

Michelle A. Miller
Associate Professor (Reader)
Health Sciences – Mental Health and Wellbeing
Warwick Medical School
University of Warwick
Coventry, UK

Steven W. Lockley
Associate Professor
Division of Sleep and Circadian Disorders
Brigham and Women's Hospital & Harvard Medical School
Boston, MA, USA
School of Psychological Sciences
Monash University
Melbourne VIC, Australia

Shantha M. W. Rajaratnam
Professor
School of Psychological Sciences
Monash University
Melbourne VIC, Australia

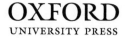

OXFORD
UNIVERSITY PRESS

OXFORD

UNIVERSITY PRESS

Great Clarendon Street, Oxford, OX2 6DP,
United Kingdom

Oxford University Press is a department of the University of Oxford.
It furthers the University's objective of excellence in research, scholarship,
and education by publishing worldwide. Oxford is a registered trade mark of
Oxford University Press in the UK and in certain other countries

First Edition published in 2010
Second Edition published in 2018

Impression: 1

Published in the United States of America by Oxford University Press
198 Madison Avenue, New York, NY 10016, United States of America

British Library Cataloguing in Publication Data
Data available

Library of Congress Control Number: 2018942143

ISBN 978-0-19-877824-0

Printed and bound by
CPI Group (UK) Ltd, Croydon, CR0 4YY

Acknowledgements

We are delighted to see the publication of the second edition of *Sleep, Health and Society*. The 'Sleep, Health & Society Programme' was established at the University of Warwick, in close collaboration with Harvard Medical School and the Brigham and Women's Hospital in Boston, in 2005. We are grateful to the late Professor Yvonne Carter (to whom we dedicate this book), Professor Ed Peile from the University of Warwick, and Paul Blake (from Cephalon), for their foresight, vision, and encouragement in the early stages of this endeavour. Since 2010—when the first edition was published—the programme has progressed and important additional collaborations have ensued globally with the welcome participation of Monash University in the editorial group of the current edition.

We don't have the space to personally acknowledge all collaborators, colleagues, and students who, over the past 12 years, have contributed to making the programme grow in popularity (as measured by the number of citations of our scientific publications and by the numerous media appearances and productions), but we are thankful for their support. The programme has established 'sleep epidemiology' as a credible discipline in the specialist research scenario, and its results have opened avenues of research and applications that go well beyond the original boundaries of neuroscience.

This second edition is structured as three sections (Sleep; Health; Society)—to highlight the wide importance of the science of sleep and wakefulness. We need to understand not only the effect of sleep on health and disease, but also its historical and social role, the public health importance of 'sleep' as a fundamental function of the body, and the effects of sleep disruption on society more widely. The number of chapters has increased, but the writing style has been simplified to allow an easy access to non-scientists and lay audience alike. Therefore, this volume is an 'evolution', rather than an extension, of our first edition.

One again we express a big thank you to Oxford University Press, and to Nicola Wilson, Caroline Smith, James Cox, and Jess White, for their expert support, and patience, during the production process.

Finally, we wish to thank the readers and those who—more and more—show interest in this fascinating topic.

Francesco P. Cappuccio
Michelle A. Miller
Steven W. Lockley
Shantha M. W. Rajaratnam
May 2018

Contents

Abbreviations

AAP	American Academy of Pediatrics	CHD	coronary heart disease
AASM	American Academy of Sleep Medicine	CI	confidence interval
		CMSC	chronic musculoskeletal complaints
ACGME	Accreditation Council for Graduate Medical Education	COPD	chronic obstructive pulmonary disease
ACR	American College of Rheumatology	CPAP	continuous positive airway pressure
AD	Alzheimer's disease	CPPC	chronic painful physical condition
ADA	Americans with Disabilities Act	CRH	corticotropin-releasing hormone
ADHD	attention deficit hyperactivity disorder	CRP	C-reactive protein
		CSF	cerebrospinal fluid
AHI	apnoea–hypopnoea index	CT	computed tomography
AMA	American Medical Association	CVD	cardiovascular disease
aMT6s	6-sulphatoxymelatonin	DLB	dementia with Lewy bodies
APAP	autotitrating positive airway pressure	DR	dorsal raphe
		DSPS	delayed sleep phase syndrome
ApoE4	apolipoprotein E4	DSWPD	delayed sleep–wake phase disorder
APPLES	Apnoea Positive Pressure Long-term Efficacy Study		
$A_{2A}R$	adenosine 2A receptor	DVLA	Driving and Vehicle Licensing Agency
ASHRAE	American Society of Heating, Refrigerating and Air-Conditioning Engineers	EDS	excessive daytime sleepiness
		EEG	electroencephalogram/ electroencephalography
ASPS	advanced sleep phase syndrome		
ASWPD	advanced sleep–wake phase disorder	EMG	electromyogram
		EOG	electrooculogram
ATP	adenosine triphosphate	EPIC-Norfolk	Norfolk cohort of European Prospective Investigation into Cancer and Nutrition
BF	basal forebrain		
BG	basal ganglia		
BMI	body mass index	ESS	Epworth Sleepiness Scale
BPAP	bi-level positive airway pressure	EWTD	European Working Time Directive
BSD	Benzodiazepine and Sedative Drugs		
		FFI	fatal familial insomnia
BZRAs	benzodiazepine receptor agonists	FIRST	Flexibility in Duty Hour Requirements for Surgical Trainees (trial)
CARDIA	Coronary Artery Risk Development in Young Adults (study)		
		FM	fibromyalgia
CBT	core body temperature	GABA	γ-aminobutyric acid
CBT-I	cognitive-behavioural therapy for insomnia	GDP	gross domestic product
		GH	growth hormone
CCT	correlated colour temperature	GPe	external globus pallidus
CDC	Centers for Disease Control and Prevention	GWASs	genome-wide association studies
		GWB	general wellbeing

HLA	human leukocyte antigen
HOS	hours of service
HPA	hypothalamic pituitary adrenal
HR	heart rate
hs-CRP	high-sensitivity C-reactive protein
ICU	intensive care unit
IL	interleukin
IOM	Institute of Medicine
ipRGCs	intrinsically photosensitive retinal ganglion cells
IQ	intelligence quotient
IVGTT	intravenous glucose tolerance test
KLS	Kleine–Levin syndrome
LC	locus coeruleus
LDL	low-density lipoprotein
LED	light-emitting diode
LH	lateral hypothalamus
LPT	lateral pontine tegmentum
LTD	long-term depression
LTP	long-term potentiation
MCH	melanin-concentrating hormone
MET	metabolic equivalent
MetS	metabolic syndrome
MMSE	Mini Mental State Exam
MSLT	multiple sleep latency test
MWT	maintenance of wakefulness test
NAcSh	shell of the nucleus accumbens
NPY	neuropeptide Y
NREM	non-rapid eye movement
NSF	National Sleep Foundation
NS-SEC	National Statistics Socio-economic Classification
OHS	obesity hypoventilation syndrome
OH&S	occupational health and safety
OR	odds ratio
OSA	obstructive sleep apnoea
OSAS	obstructive sleep apnoea syndrome

PAI	plasminogen activator inhibitor
PAP	positive airway pressure
PB	parabrachial
PD	Parkinson's disease
PLMD	periodic limb movement disorder
PNE	primary nocturnal enuresis
POA	preoptic area
PREDICT	Positive Airway Pressure in Older People: a randomised controlled trial
PSG	polysomnography
PWN	person with narcolepsy
PZ	parafacial zone
RBD	REM sleep behaviour disorder
RCT	randomized controlled trial
REM	rapid eye movement
RHT	retinohypothalamic tract
RLS	restless legs syndrome
SCN	suprachiasmatic nuclei
SES	socio-economic status
SF-12	Short Form Health Survey
SLD	sublaterodorsal nucleus
SNS	sympathetic nervous system
SWD	shift work disorder
SWS	slow-wave sleep
TLRs	Toll-like receptors
TMN	tuberomamillary nucleus
TNF-α	tumour necrosis factor-α
TSH	thyroid-stimulating hormone
UPR	unfolded protein response
vlPAG	ventrolateral periaqueductal grey area
VLPO	ventrolateral preoptic area
vPAG	ventral periaqueductal grey
VTA	ventral tegmental area
WASO	wake after sleep onset
WHO	World Health Organization

Contributors

Esther F. Afolalu, M.Sc., Ph.D.
Department of Psychology
University of Warwick
Coventry (UK)

Joseph G. Allen, B.S., M.P.H., D.Sc.
Department of Environmental Health
Harvard T. H. Chan School of
Public Health
Boston, MA (USA)

Sara Arber, Ph.D.
Department of Sociology
University of Surrey
Guildford (UK)

John Axelsson, Ph.D.
Department of Clinical Neuroscience
Karolinska Institute
Stockholm (Sweden)

Stephanie Bioulac, M.D.
Clinique du sommeil, CHU de Bordeaux
University of Bordeaux (CNRS, SANPSY,
USR 3413)
Bordeaux (France)

Donald L. Bliwise, Ph.D.
Department of Neurology
Emory University School of Medicine
Atlanta, GA (USA)

**Francesco P. Cappuccio, M.D., D.Sc.,
F.R.C.P.**
Division of Health Sciences
University of Warwick,
Warwick Medical School
University Hospitals Coventry &
Warwickshire NHS Trust
Coventry (UK)

Jose G. Cedeño Laurent, Ph.D.
Department of Environmental Health
Harvard T. H. Chan School of
Public Health
Boston, MA (USA)

Daniel A. Cohen, M.D., M.M.Sc.
Eastern Virginia Medical School
Sentara Healthcare
Norfolk, VA (USA)

Catherine Coveney, Ph.D.
School of Applied Social Sciences
De Montfort University
Leicester (UK)

Bradley A. Edwards, Ph.D.
Department of Physiology,
School of Psychological Sciences,
Monash Institute of Cognitive and
Clinical Neurosciences
Monash University
Melbourne, VIC (Australia)

A. Roger Ekirch, Ph.D.
Department of History
Virginia Tech
Blacksburg, VA (USA)

Lawrence J. Epstein, M.D.
Division of Sleep Medicine
Harvard Medical School
Division of Sleep and Circadian Disorders
Brigham and Women's Hospital
Boston, MA (USA)

Patrick M. Fuller, Ph.D.
Division of Sleep Medicine
Harvard Medical School
Department of Neurology
Beth Israel Deaconess Medical Center
Boston, MA (USA)

Jonathan Gabe, Ph.D.
School of Law
Royal Holloway, University of London
Egham (UK)

David Gozal
Herbert T. Abelson Professor of Pediatrics
University of Chicago Medicine
Comer Children's Hospital
Chicago (USA)

Garun S. Hamilton, M.B.B.S., Ph.D.,
F.R.A.C.P.
Monash Lung and Sleep, Monash Health
School of Clinical Sciences, Monash
University
Melbourne, VIC (Australia)

Pasquale F. Innominato, M.D., Ph.D.
Division of Biomedical Sciences
University of Warwick,
Warwick Medical School
Coventry (UK)
University Hospitals Birmingham NHS
Foundation Trust
Birmingham (UK)

Göran Kecklund, Ph.D.
Department of Clinical Neuroscience
Karolinska Institute
Stockholm (Sweden)

Leila Kheirandish-Gozal
Director, Clinical Sleep Research
Department of Pediatrics
University of Chicago Medicine
Chicago (USA)

Christopher P. Landrigan, M.D., M.P.H.
Division of Sleep and Circadian Disorders,
Departments of Medicine and Neurology,
Brigham and Women's Hospital &
Harvard Medical School Department of
Medicine, Children's Hospital Boston
Boston, MA (USA)

Clark J. Lee, J.D., M.P.H., C.P.H.
Center for Health & Homeland Security
University of Maryland
Baltimore, MD (USA)

Steven W. Lockley, Ph.D.
Division of Sleep and Circadian Disorders
Brigham and Women's Hospital &
Harvard Medical School, Boston,
MA (USA)
School of Psychological Sciences
Monash University, Melbourne VIC
(Australia)

Dora A. Lozsadi, M.D., DPhil., F.R.C.P.
Division of Neuroscience
St George's Hospital
London (UK)

Robert Meadows, Ph.D.
Department of Sociology
University of Surrey
Guildford (UK)

Jean-Arthur Micoulaud-Franchi, M.D.
Clinique du sommeil, CHU de Bordeaux
University of Bordeaux (CNRS, SANPSY,
USR 3413)
Bordeaux (France)

Michelle A. Miller, Ph.D.
Division of Health Sciences
University of Warwick, Warwick
Medical School
Coventry (UK)

Henry Nicholls
Narcolepsy UK
London (UK)

Matt O'Neill
Narcolepsy UK
London (UK)

Michele L. Okun, Ph.D.
Department of Psychology
University of Colorado
Colorado Springs, CO (USA)

Pierre Philip, M.D.
Clinique du sommeil, CHU de Bordeaux
University of Bordeaux (CNRS, SANPSY,
USR 3413)
Bordeaux (France)

Andrew J. K. Phillips, Ph.D.
Division of Sleep and Circadian Disorders
Brigham and Women's Hospital
Harvard Medical School
Boston, MA (USA)

Shantha M. W. Rajaratnam, Ph.D.
School of Psychological Sciences
Monash University
Melbourne, VIC (Australia)

Fatanah Ramlee, M.Sc., Ph.D.
Department of Psychology and
Counselling
Sultan Idris Education University
Perak (Malaysia)

Glenn Rosenbluth, M.D.
Department of Pediatrics
University of California, San Francisco
San Francisco, CA (USA)

Asim Roy, M.D.
Ohio Sleep Medicine Institute
Dublin, OH (USA)

Patricia Sagaspe, Ph.D.
CHU de Bordeaux, University of
Bordeaux (CNRS, SANPSY, USR 3413)
Bordeaux (France)

Mikael Sallinen, Ph.D.
Finnish Institute of Occupational Health
University of Helsinki
Helsinki (Finland)

Michael K. Scullin, Ph.D.
Department of Psychology and
Neuroscience
Baylor University
Waco, TX (USA)

John D. Spengler, Ph.D.
Department of Environmental Health
Harvard T. H. Chan School of
Public Health
Boston, MA (USA)

David Spiegel, M.D.
Center on Stress and Health
Stanford University School of Medicine
Stanford, CA (USA)

Richard G. Stevens, Ph.D.
University of Connecticut School of
Medicine
Farmington, CT (USA)

Tina Sundelin, Ph.D.
Department of Clinical Neuroscience
Karolinska Institute
Stockholm (Sweden)

Nicole K. Y. Tang, D.Phil., C.Psychol.
Department of Psychology
University of Warwick
Coventry (UK)

Anne Venner, Ph.D.
Division of Sleep Medicine
Harvard Medical School
Department of Neurology
Beth Israel Deaconess Medical Center
Boston, MA (USA)

Simon J. Williams, Ph.D.
Department of Sociology
University of Warwick
Coventry (UK)

Amy R. Wolfson, Ph.D.
Loyola University Maryland
Baltimore, MD (USA)

Terra Ziporyn, Ph.D.
Executive Director and Co-Founder
Start School Later, Inc.
Annapolis, MD (USA)

Part 1

Sleep

Chapter 1

Sleep, health, and society: The contribution of epidemiology

Francesco P. Cappuccio, Michelle A. Miller, Steven W. Lockley, and Shantha M. W. Rajaratnam

Introduction

Sleep disturbances and sleep deprivation are common in modern society. Since the beginning of the century, populations have shown a steady constant decline in sleep duration, due to changes in a variety of environmental and social conditions (e.g. less dependence on daylight for most activities, extended shift work, 24-7 round-the-clock activities). Industry—including airlines, long-distance driving, shift-work manufacturing industry and emergency services—was the first to appreciate the potential detrimental effects that sleep deprivation and disruption would have on health and wellbeing. It has taken, however, many decades to reach the current level of understanding of the wider implications for individuals and populations of a chronic and sustained sleep deprivation.

Through the application of epidemiological methods of investigation, we have learnt that sleep deprivation is associated with a variety of chronic conditions and health outcomes, detectable across the entire lifespan, from childhood to adulthood to older age. This book summarizes the epidemiological evidence linking disturbances of sleep quantity and quality to several chronic conditions, explores evidence of causality, and explores the public health implications with a view to inform a discourse on possible preventive strategies.

Textbooks of sleep medicine have traditionally focused predominantly on the physiology and patho-physiology of sleep (Kryger et al., 2005) with a view to facilitating the diagnosis of a variety of sleep-related conditions and their treatment. Mainly directed at physiologists, sleep technicians, respiratory physicians, psychiatrists, and paediatricians, these textbooks almost invariably glance at the epidemiology of sleep and at the implications for public health. The scope of *Sleep, Health and Society*, now in its second edition, is to fill a significant gap by a population-based approach to the problem of sleep-related risk and disease.

The role of epidemiology

Epidemiology differs from clinical medicine in that the unit of interest is the population, not the individual. Clinical investigations are conducted on sick people, the results relate to patients, and decisions are related to the treatment of individuals. Epidemiological research studies the sick and the well, the results relate to populations, and decisions are related to public health (Rose, 1985). Epidemiology may be defined as the *quantitative study of the distribution, frequency, determinants, and control of health problems and disease in populations* (Figure 1.1).

The purpose of epidemiology is to obtain, interpret, and use health information to promote health and reduce disease. Using this definition, it is clear that epidemiology is concerned with populations, not only death, illness, and disability in populations, but also with more positive health states and with the means to improve health.

Epidemiology is a crucial discipline for the promotion of public health. It provides a set of skills, approaches, and philosophy which allows investigators to detect causes of health problems, to establish the association between ill-health and a variety of risk factors, to test treatments and public health interventions, and to monitor changes in states of health over time. It is a discipline which describes the distribution of health and ill-health in a population (e.g. *What* is the problem and its frequency? *Who* is affected? *Where* and *when* does this health problem manifest in the population?). It also provides the tools to compare the health characteristics of populations. Epidemiology may play a role in identifying the *cause* of a health problem (e.g. a genetic trait, an infectious agent, a particular behaviour, an environmental exposure). The epidemiological approach provides a framework within which 'causation' can be hypothesized and tested. The primary objective in epidemiology is to judge whether an association between exposure and disease or health problem is, in fact, causal. A *causal association* is one in which a change in the frequency or quality of an exposure or characteristic results in a corresponding change in the frequency of a disease or outcome of interest. *Causality* is more likely if an association between exposure and disease can satisfy most of the following criteria: *strength, consistency, specificity, right time sequence, dose relationship, reversibility, biological plausibility, and coherence* (Bradford Hill, 1965). Making judgements about causality would require an assessment of the *validity* of the findings and of the *likelihood of alternative explanations* for the results. It would then require the assessment of the role of *chance*, the role of *bias*, and the role of *confounding*.

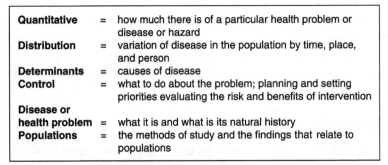

Fig. 1.1 Epidemiology definitions.
Reproduced from Cappuccio, F.P., et al., Eds. (2010) *Sleep, Health, and Society*. 1st Ed. Oxford: Oxford University Press.

Once the disease occurs, epidemiology provides a means to monitor the course and outcome (*natural history*) of the condition. It also allows us to answer questions regarding the *efficiency and effectiveness* of interventions and therapies and their impact on populations (i.e. How effective are particular interventions for controlling disease in communities? Is intervention A more effective than intervention B? What are the outcomes of these two lines of intervention?). Of course, such information needs to be placed alongside other data before a choice of interventions is made (e.g. What are the side-effects of the treatments? What are the views of consumers and patients regarding the procedure? How much does the intervention cost?). Such data may help determine where best to direct resources. Identifying health states in the population may facilitate establishing the *need for services* and the *determination of priorities*. Given limited resources, public health practitioners are always under pressure to use resources optimally and to produce the greatest return, in the form of health gain, for a given investment of time, money, materials, and personnel. Epidemiology cannot do this alone: it needs to integrate results with health services research, health economics, and other social sciences to inform wise public health decisions and promote health at a population level.

Epidemiology thus has many applications and is an essential tool for providing information about public health problems, and their magnitude and distribution, causation, prevention, prognosis, and treatment, and likely impact of interventions. Increasing our understanding of health problems and their determinants and possible solutions places us in a better position to make appropriate policy.

The book

This book follows in the footsteps of the first edition, published in 2010 (Cappuccio et al., 2010), designed to summarize for the first time the epidemiological evidence linking disturbances of sleep quantity and quality to several chronic conditions, to assess the epidemiological evidence for causality, and to explore the public health implications with a view to inform a discourse on possible preventive strategies. This second edition maintains the same focus of embracing sleep disturbances as a universal behavioural change likely to impact health and wellbeing in the short and long term across the entire lifespan, from childhood to adulthood to older age. The book is structured as 26 chapters grouped into three sections—'Sleep', 'Health', and 'Society'. While updated information is provided on previous core areas relating to sleep–wake regulation (chapters 2, 3, and 5); the genetics of sleep (chapter 6); approaches to the evaluation of sleep disorders (chapter 7); the epidemiology of sleep, cardio-metabolic, and other chronic conditions (chapters 8, 9, 10, and 12); sleep in children (chapter 14); the sociology of sleep (chapter 19); sleep and shift work (chapters 20 and 22); and sleep and the law (chapter 25), the second edition also covers important new topics based on evidence gathered over the last few years, such as sleep in relation to cognition (chapter 4), epilepsy (chapter 11), pregnancy (chapter 13), circadian rhythm and chronotypes (chapter 15), cancer (chapter 16), pain (chapter 17), drowsy driving (chapter 21), the built environment (chapter 23), and adolescents & school start times (chapter 24). Finally, the volume includes new historical perspectives of sleep in western cultures (chapter 18) and a personal account of what it is like living with narcolepsy (chapter 26). In order to pack almost twice as much into a single volume, we decided to write less about each topic and in an accessible prose to appeal to a more general readership, yet maintain scientific rigour. The aim of this new style was to create greater awareness amongst the public at large, beyond those involved in science.

The brief to authors was to take a population perspective, and to consider the extent to which their particular area of expertise translates into the population and public health arena. To maximize the take-home messages on the population and public health perspective, each chapter ends with a *Summary* of the main points for easy reference.

We hope this second edition will appeal to public health professionals; medical students; allied health professions; psychologists, general practitioners, and specialist physicians; policy makers; specialists in medical education; professionals involved in shift work; occupational health professionals; and industry, regulatory bodies, and voluntary organizations, as well as patients' groups.

Brief historical note

As clearly highlighted by William Dement (Dement, 2005), 'Interest in sleep and dreams has existed since the dawn of history' and there is a wealth of scholarly work that highlights the interests, concerns, beliefs, and roles of sleep and associated activities (e.g. dreams, nightmares) over the centuries, from prehistoric ages to our modern society. Until very recently, sleep had been considered a passive state. In MacNish's 1834 definition (MacNish, 1834), 'Sleep is the intermediate state between wakefulness and death: wakefulness being regarded as the active state of all the animal and intellectual functions, and death as that of their total suspension'. It was not until the end of the nineteenth century and well into the twentieth century that the concept that sleep could be an active and dynamic state gained credence and some scientific support through early experiments on animals and humans. The discovery, in 1930, that the electrical activity and rhythms of the human brain—recorded in an electroencephalogram (EEG)—vary significantly and constantly during wakefulness and sleep sparked an increased interest in unravelling the scientific basis of sleep. The work of Sigmund Freud and his interpretation of dreams undoubtedly contributed to creating an interest in sleep among health professionals.

After World War II we witnessed the start of the animal experimentation on sleep, leading to an understanding of some of the deep brain mechanisms underpinning sleep and wakefulness—the modern neuroscience.

With similar pace this experimentation led to an understanding of the pathology of sleep, from insomnia, narcolepsy with cataplexy, and, much later, obstructive sleep apnoea syndrome, firstly described in 1836 by Charles Dickens in the character 'Young Dropsy'—a young, obese, always sleepy boy who snored (referred to as Pickwickian syndrome). Similarly, the discipline now known as 'chronobiology', which for centuries had described the 24-hour rhythmic cycles governing the biological activities of the plant and animal kingdoms, began to be applied to the sleep–wake cycles of animals and humans.

The scientific interest, measured by the number of publications in the field of sleep research since 1945, provides a crude indication of the exponential growth of knowledge and allows us to monitor some milestone discoveries (Figure 1.2).

The first description that rapid eye movements (REMs) occur in sleep precedes the landmark study that suggested that REMs represented a 'lightening' of sleep and might indicate dreaming, owing to the close association with irregular respiration and an increase in heart rate (Aserinsky & Kleitman, 1953). A second spark in the research progress in sleep medicine was the discovery of sleep apnoea in 1965. In the early 1970s, the internal biological clock regulating the sleep–wake cycle and many other rhythmic biological activities (the suprachiasmatic nucleus or SCN) was described. This autonomous circadian pacemaker has since been intensively studied, and more recently its genetic regulation (e.g. *Clock* genes) has been described. The 1980s and 1990s were dominated by studies of the significance of excessive daytime sleepiness and the discovery and applications of continuous positive airway pressure (CPAP) for the management of obstructive sleep apnoea syndrome and its complications. Finally, at the end of the twentieth century and at the dawn of the twenty-first there was a very sharp increase in the scientific output of sleep research, with a disproportionate representation of population studies on the effect of sleep on health risks and a debate on the public health issues associated with declining trends in the quantity and quality of sleep in the modern society as potential contributing factors to, or risk markers for, ill-health and reduced safety (Ferrie et al., 2011). This was the dawn of *sleep epidemiology*.

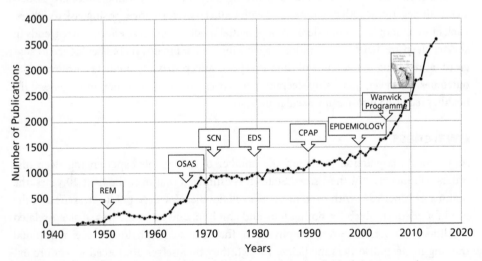

Fig. 1.2 Seventy years of sleep research: publication trends in the field of sleep research (1945–2015).
Source: data from Medline search 1945–2015 for sleep.

Sleep, health, and society

Throughout our life we spend approximately a third of our time asleep. We spend more time asleep as babies and children and then settle for a pattern of approximately 6–8 hours per night. Whilst subjective sleep duration remains constant with age, directly measured sleep patterns indicate that, with age, total sleeping time, sleep efficiency, and slow-wave sleep decline and waking after sleep onset increase. Sufficient sleep is necessary for optimal daytime performance and wellbeing, yet there is a large difference in the time people spend asleep at night, ranging from < 6 hours to > 9 hours per night. The epidemiology of sleep duration indicates that a good night's sleep equates to 6–8 hours of continuous sleep, with changes in sleep duration or continuity being associated with negative impacts on health outcomes. Adult women report sleeping consistently less than men up to the age of 50–55 years, but then the pattern reverses. There are also geographical variations in average sleeping time (whether due to environmental, genetic, or socioeconomic factors). In the Far East, people tend to sleep less at night than in Europe and in the Americas, although daytime napping seems more common. Both short sleep and long sleep have been associated with increased all-cause mortality and other outcomes from chronic disease. The secular increases in cardiovascular disease, diabetes, and obesity have been paralleled by a steady deterioration in sleeping patterns, with an increase in the proportion of short sleepers. A recent analysis of self-reported sleep hours in the USA between 1975 and 2006 did not detect any significant increase in the numbers of short sleepers (< 6 hours per night) over the 31-year period (Knutson et al, 2010). However, when the analysis was carried out by employment status, a significant 20% increase in the numbers was detected amongst full-time workers, with the excess time awake being spent predominantly in working activities. Working overtime and working shifts are associated with negative health outcomes and with reduced performance, posing risk to others. Lack of sleep should be considered as a potential mediator of these effects since trends in shorter sleep are associated with longer working hours. Finally, there is evidence to suggest that reducing the amount of time we spend asleep strongly predicts cardiovascular outcomes. However, increasing sleeping hours over time may be a marker of general ill-health, predicting non-cardiovascular mortality.

Awareness

As the world population increases, the number of individuals experiencing sleep disorders will increase. In the United States it is estimated that over the next 20 years, the number of Americans with sleep disorders will double. However, public awareness of the need for adequate sleep for both adults and children, and an awareness of sleep-related conditions, is poor. Moreover, the physicians that treat such individuals receive minimal training in sleep disorders medicine. In fact, they themselves are forced to endure excessive work schedules during their internship and residency training, which desensitizes them to sleep as a fundamental biological necessity, degrades their ability to provide quality patient care and to benefit fully from their training experience, and places them at increased risk of ill-health, injuries, and sleep-related road traffic accidents during their training. These difficult, and often conflicting, interests need to be addressed so that the medical field can provide an optimal platform for learning and patient care.

The public awareness of the importance of sleep, the need for good sleep behaviour, and awareness of sleep disorders in general is poor in both adults and children. Various professional bodies in the UK, USA, and Australia are attempting to redress the balance. However, not always is the political will in harmony with the evidence-based health needs.

Conclusions

Taken all together, these aspects bring the results of the epidemiology of sleep outside the clinical setting and well within the domain of public health. One of the main questions still to answer is whether, in these circumstances, sleep disturbances result from the associated ill-health, or are intermediate markers in the pathways of disease causation, or whether changes in sleep patterns can be causal in determining ill-health. The bi-directional relationships between sleep duration and disease and the non-linear associations remain some of the research challenges to establishing causality. A long-term intervention trial of non-drug-induced sleep extension would be necessary to test the effect of sleep duration on fatal outcomes. However, this is an unlikely scenario, since such a study would be impractical, large, lengthy, and expensive. This leaves the burden of proof to observational epidemiology to inform potential changes in public health policies. At the same time, the deleterious effects of shift work on several outcomes, such as risk of self-harm and harm to others (e.g. medical errors, road accidents, attentional failures in high-risk occupations), which are by and large mediated by excessive sleepiness and fatigue caused by sleep debt, have recently benefited from stronger evidence from randomized clinical trials and are now informing policy changes. The field of sleep epidemiology is still in its infancy, yet it has already provided a wide-ranging insight into a new and important behavioural variable to consider in the spectrum of modifiable risk factors for common diseases.

References

Aserinsky, E. & Kleitman, N. 1953. Regularly occurring periods of eye motility, and concomitant phenomena, during sleep. *Science*, **118**, pp. 273–4.

Bradford Hill, A. 1965. The environment and disease: association or causation? *Journal of the Royal Society of Medicine*, **58**, pp. 295–300.

Cappuccio, F. P., Miller, M. A. & Lockley, S. W. eds. 2010. *Sleep, Health, and Society: From aetiology to public health*. Oxford: Oxford University Press.

Dement, W. C. 2005. History of sleep physiology and medicine. In: Kryger, M. H., Roth, T. & Dement, W. C. eds. *Principles and Practice of Sleep Medicine*. 4th ed. Philadelphia, PA: Elsevier Saunders, pp. 1–12.

Ferrie, J. E., Kumari, M., Salo, P., Singh-Manoux, A. & Kivimäki, M. 2011. Sleep epidemiology—a rapidly growing field. *International Journal of Epidemiology*, **40**, pp. 1431–7.

Knutson, K. L., Van Cauter, E., Rathouz, P. J., DeLeire, T. & Lauderdale, D. S. 2010. Trends in the prevalence of short sleepers in the USA: 1975-2006. *Sleep*, **33**, pp. 37–45.

Kryger, M. H., Roth, T. & Dement, W. C. 2005. *Principles and Practice of Sleep Medicine*. 4th ed. Philadelphia, PA: Elsevier Saunders.

MacNish, R. 1834. *The Philosophy of Sleep*. New York: D. Appleton.

Rose, G. 1985. Sick individuals and sick populations. *International Journal of Epidemiology*, **14**, pp. 32–8

Chapter 2

Principles of sleep–wake regulation

Steven W. Lockley

Introduction

Given the expanding and powerful associations emerging between sleep behaviour and health, measurement of sleep should be a core component of all public health research, as necessary as knowledge about smoking, alcohol use, diet, and exercise. Sleep is an essential behaviour, more important than food in terms of survival, and it is important to understand the regulation of sleep in order to be able to measure and interpret sleep data appropriately. This chapter provides an introduction to sleep–wake regulation and outlines some of the challenges inherent in measuring sleep.

Sleep–wake regulation

Basic sleep behaviour and physiology

Sleep is a behavioural state characterized by minimal behaviour and a particular posture during which it is more difficult, but not impossible, to stimulate the individual. Sleep is therefore a state of relative, but not complete, disengagement with the environment while also being rapidly reversible, unlike coma or hibernation. The reasons for why we sleep are unclear but a number of hypotheses have been proposed, including energy conservation, tissue repair, memory consolidation, and brain thermoregulation. In humans and a small number of other mammals, sleep has been most carefully characterized by changes in brain electrophysiology. Discernible sleep 'stages' were first reported in the human electroencephalogram (EEG) in the 1930s and were formally defined by Rechtschaffen and Kales in 1968.

There are two distinct types of sleep—rapid eye movement (REM) and non-rapid eye movement (NREM) sleep—which alternate every ~ 45 minutes to form a ~ 90-minute NREM-REM sleep cycle. The proportion of NREM and REM sleep per cycle changes throughout the night, with a higher proportion of REM generally in the latter half of the night. NREM is generally associated with more stable physiology—regular breathing patterns, lower heart rate, lower temperature—whereas REM is a more active state with a more variable, but generally higher, breathing rate, heart rate, blood pressure, brain temperature, and brain blood flow (but lower core temperature). On average, about 25% of the sleep episode will consist of REM sleep. By definition, REM is usually associated with rapid eye movements, detected in an electrooculogram (EOG), and with inhibition of the skeletal muscles, recorded in an electromyogram (EMG) from the muscles under the chin. EEG brain activity is very active during REM sleep, exhibiting irregular, low-amplitude, high-frequency waves very similar to those seen during wakefulness. During NREM sleep the EEG activity is more synchronous, with higher amplitude, lower frequency ('slow') waves that gradually predominate with increasing 'depth' of sleep. NREM sleep is further divided into three sleep stages—N1, N2, N3— which reflect increasing synchrony in the EEG and increasing thresholds for arousal. Stage N3 (formerly known as Stage 3–4 sleep) has the highest proportion of 'slow-wave' or 'deep' sleep (SWS) and the time spent in this stage is correlated with the duration of prior sleep deprivation.

Two-process model of sleep–wake regulation

The two-process model of sleep regulation remains the cornerstone on which our understanding of sleep–wake timing and structure is built (Dijk & Lockley, 2002). The model proposes that two oscillatory processes, an hourglass-like homeostat and the endogenous 24-hour circadian pacemaker, interact to determine the timing, duration, and structure of sleep and the time course of daytime sleepiness and cognitive functioning.

It is well understood that it is generally easier to fall asleep at 1 a.m. than at 1 p.m. This 24-hour rhythm in sleep propensity is determined by an endogenous near-24-hour pacemaker in the suprachiasmatic nuclei (SCN) of the hypothalamus. The circadian ('about a day') pacemaker controls the timing of many rhythmic behavioural, physiological, and metabolic functions, including sleep propensity, sleep structure, temperature regulation, production of hormones such as melatonin and cortisol, cardiac and lung function, and many more (Czeisler & Klerman, 1999). The circadian pacemaker determines the 24-hour patterns of sleepiness in the two-process model—defined as *Process C*—which predicts maximum sleep propensity at ~ 6 a.m., close to habitual waketime, and minimum sleep propensity at ~ 9 p.m., prior to habitual bedtime and just before the onset of melatonin production (the 'wake maintenance zone').

Sleep duration depends on the circadian timing of sleep—there is only a narrow window of time where sleep can continue for a long duration and remain uninterrupted. Sleeping outside this circadian 'window' causes difficulties with falling asleep if sleep occurs too early, or difficulties staying asleep if the sleep opportunity is too late. The latter problem accounts for why shift-workers have trouble sleeping during the day—the circadian drive for alertness wakes them up. Regarding sleep structure, REM sleep is highly controlled by the circadian system, with a distinct rhythm peaking in the early morning. Sleeping at the wrong circadian phase will therefore reduce the amount of REM sleep.

It is also intuitively understood that it is easier to fall asleep the longer one has been awake, and easier to wake up the longer one has been asleep. This homeostatic determinant of sleep propensity is defined as *Process S* and is best represented physiologically by the amount of slow-wave activity during sleep (SWS or Stage N3), which exhibits a strong sleep-dependent decline with increasing time asleep, or measured in the EEG during wake (delta activity, 0.5–5.0 Hz). Process S predicts maximum sleep propensity at the end of the waking day just before habitual bedtime, and minimal propensity for sleep just before waketime.

Under normal circumstances, these two processes oscillate in opposition in order to maintain a long bout of consolidated wakefulness during the day and a long bout of consolidated sleep at night (Dijk & Czeisler, 1995). The gradual increase in the circadian alerting signal through the day is counteracted by the increasing homeostatic pressure for sleep with longer time awake, permitting a prolonged consolidated wake episode. Conversely, the increasing circadian drive for sleep through the night is opposed by the reduction in homeostatic drive for sleep that decreases during the sleep episode, the sleep effectively 'releasing' the sleep pressure built up during the day, permitting a prolonged sleep episode. These processes also interact such that the circadian influence on sleep structure increases with increasing time asleep; as the homeostatic sleep pressure is reduced, the relative influence of the circadian system increases (Dijk & Czeisler, 1995).

Diurnal preference

The resultant balance between these two processes determines one's diurnal preference, sometimes referred to as 'morningness-eveningness', or whether someone is a 'lark' or an 'owl'. Diurnal preference describes an individual's behavioural preference for sleep timing and for optimal daytime functioning. Questionnaires used to measure diurnal preference ask about when one prefers to go to bed, or when one prefers to complete tasks requiring attention and concentration, or simply whether one is an extreme or moderate morning or evening type. While sometimes referred to as 'chronotype', diurnal preference is not a simple measure of circadian phase, however, but rather a reflection of the interaction between the circadian and homeostatic processes—not either exclusively—or the phase relationship between the circadian and homeostatic processes. These internal phase relationships change with age, however, and so self-reported diurnal preference is therefore not specific to a particular underlying phase relationship and may be misleading if used to estimate circadian timing.

Daytime functioning

The two-process model also describes the general time course of sleepiness and performance through the day, with a general increase in sleepiness with longer time awake, and a strong circadian rhythm in sleepiness, mood, and performance. Under normal sleep–wake conditions, daytime functioning is relatively stable during the day before exhibiting a wake-dependent decline towards the end of day, although differences in the phase angle of entrainment are reflected in the different time course of sleepiness and performance exhibited by morning- and evening-types through the day. Morning types, waking later in their circadian cycle, have high alertness and performance in the morning and then decline rapidly through the day, whereas evening types, waking earlier in their circadian cycle, are more sleepy and poorer performers in the morning but do not decline as much as morning types by the end of the day.

A third process is required to explain the sub-maximal alertness experienced upon awakening. The two-process model would predict lowest sleep pressure at the end of the sleep episode and therefore maximal alertness upon waking, inconsistent with most people's experience of taking some time to get going in the morning. In the laboratory, this 'sleep inertia' takes several hours to dissipate such that it takes several hours before maximal alertness is reached. This time course has been termed *Process W* (Åkerstedt et al., 2008) and it interacts with both Process C and Process S, exhibiting a greater severity and duration when waking from an adverse circadian phase or deeper sleep.

Factors affecting sleep–wake regulation

Role of light in sleep–wake regulation

Light can affect both circadian timing (Process C) and sleepiness and performance directly (Process S and W) (Cajochen, 2007; Czeisler & Gooley, 2007). Light has a number of 'non-visual' effects on human physiology separate and apart from vision, including resetting the circadian pacemaker, suppressing pineal melatonin production, elevating morning cortisol levels, increasing night-time heart rate and core temperature levels, and acutely improving subjective and objective measures of alertness. These non-visual effects of light are determined by a range of light properties including the timing, intensity, duration, pattern, wavelength, and history of exposure (Figueiro et al., 2008; Lucas et al., 2014), and these factors may be important when interpreting light exposure 'risk'.

As described earlier (see 'Two-process model of sleep–wake regulation'), the suprachiasmatic nuclei (SCN) control 24-hour rhythms in many aspects of human physiology, metabolism, and behaviour. The endogenous period of this circadian pacemaker clock is near to, but not exactly, 24 hours, and in order to ensure that these rhythms are timed appropriately to anticipate future environmental events (e.g. food availability), environmental time cues must reset this internal clock. The 24-hour light–dark cycle is the primary environmental time signal ('*zeitgeber*'). This light information is captured exclusively by the eyes using specialized intrinsically photosensitive retinal ganglion cells (ipRGCs) and transduced directly to the SCN via a dedicated neural pathway, the retinohypothalamic tract (RHT). The ipRGCs contain the photopigment melanopsin, which is most sensitive to short-wavelength (blue) light at ~ 480 nm (Figueiro et al., 2008).

Each day the light–dark cycle resets the internal clock, which in turn synchronizes the physiology, metabolism, and behaviour controlled by the clock. Failure to receive this light–dark information, as experienced by many totally blind individuals, causes the circadian pacemaker to revert to its endogenous non-24-hour period and become desynchronized from the 24-hour light–dark cycle. Consequently, the majority of totally blind subjects experience non-24-hour sleep–wake disorder as their sleep–wake cycle, alertness, and performance patterns and other rhythms become desynchronized from the 24-hour social day (Lockley et al., 2007). Circadian misalignment also occurs in sighted subjects who are not exposed to a stable 24-hour light–dark cycle, for example in night shift-workers or after a rapid change in light–dark patterns following transmeridian travel ('jet-lag'). Exposure to a stable 24-hour light–dark cycle is therefore required to maintain normal circadian entrainment, including entrainment of the sleep–wake cycle and sleep propensity rhythms described by Process C.

Light also has a direct effect on Process S, in that light exposure can acutely enhance alertness and performance during both the day and the night (Cajochen, 2007) and reduces homeostatic sleep pressure (SWS) in night-time sleep following light exposure. Light is not required, however, to generate or maintain the phase relationships between Process C and Process S, as these relationships persist in totally blind subjects whose circadian systems cannot detect light.

Role of melatonin in sleep–wake regulation

The major biochemical correlate of the light–dark cycle is provided by the pineal hormone melatonin. Under normal light–dark conditions, melatonin is produced only during the night and provides an internal representation of the environmental photoperiod, specifically night-length ('scotoperiod'). The synthesis and timing of melatonin production requires an intact afferent signal from the SCN, and ablation of this pathway—as occurs in some people owing to spinal damage at the upper cervical level—completely abolishes melatonin production, although other circadian rhythms not requiring this projection remain intact. Ocular light exposure during the night acutely inhibits melatonin production and provides an indirect assessment of light input to the SCN via the RHT. Given the close temporal relationship between the SCN and melatonin production, the melatonin rhythm is often used as a marker of circadian phase and the melatonin suppression response as a proxy for RHT-SCN integrity and sensitivity. The specific night-time production of melatonin and the exquisite sensitivity of this hormone to light also make it a potential biomarker for assessing light exposure during the night.

The melatonin rhythm is also closely associated with sleep in diurnal animals such as humans but may not have a direct effect on sleep *in vivo*. Nocturnal animals such as rats and hamsters also produce melatonin at night during their active episode. As described previously, the human circadian sleep propensity rhythm is closely correlated with the melatonin profile, and the opening of the sleep 'gate' occurs simultaneously with the onset of melatonin release. If plasma melatonin is suppressed by light exposure at night, alertness levels simultaneously improve, suggesting that melatonin and sleepiness are directly related. These events may simply be contemporaneous, however, as individuals who do not produce melatonin (e.g. tetraplegic individuals, many people taking beta-blockers, pinealectomized patients) still exhibit circadian sleep–wake rhythms and have only minor changes in sleep timing and structure. Light exposure in the daytime will also improve alertness, at a time when melatonin is not produced, suggesting either that melatonin is not a direct mediator of alertness and/or that separate mechanisms exist during the day and night to enhance alertness by light. The presumed association between melatonin and sleep arises from the effects of exogenous melatonin treatment, which does induce sleepiness and, when taken at a time when endogenous melatonin is not produced, can improve sleep. These pharmacological effects are not necessarily an indication of endogenous melatonin function.

Sleep and circadian influences on endocrinology and metabolism

Many hormones and peptides are influenced by the circadian system, sleep, or a combination of both. Some hormones have a strongly endogenous circadian rhythm that is minimally influenced by sleep. Pineal melatonin, which has a night-time peak (~ 2 a.m.) under normal conditions, is virtually unaffected by sleep, for example, although it is strongly suppressed directly by exposure to light at night. Cortisol, which rises during sleep to a maximum shortly before habitual waketime, is also relatively unchanged during sleep or wake conditions, although waking from sleep causes a small direct elevation (Figure 2.1). Conversely, some hormones, for example growth hormone (GH), are very strongly sleep-dependent with little influence of the circadian system. GH is secreted primarily during slow-wave sleep (SWS) and has lower levels under conditions of sleep deprivation. Sleep deprivation, therefore, could dramatically reduce GH secretion. Other outcomes are influenced by both. For example, thyroid-stimulating hormone (TSH) appears to be under minimal circadian control, with only a small peak close to sleep onset under normal conditions. When assessed under circadian-rhythm conditions, however, a very different pattern emerges; TSH has a strong circadian rhythm with a night-time peak that is suppressed by sleep at night under normal conditions (Figure 2.1) (Czeisler & Klerman, 1999). Similar careful consideration is needed when examining insulin and glucose levels; while they are clearly influenced by meals, when hourly snacks are provided to spread out nutrient intake equally over 24 hours, an underlying circadian rhythm is revealed, with minimal levels during the biological night and a morning peak, particularly for insulin. The effects of partial chronic sleep deprivation and circadian desynchrony on metabolic biomarkers have also been examined, with dramatic results: in a very short space of time—a matter of days—chronic sleep deprivation or circadian desynchrony can induce a pre-diabetic or even diabetic state in initially healthy young adults (Morris et al., 2012; Van Cauter et al., 2008).

Considerations in epidemiology

Measuring sleep and circadian phase

A number of methods are available to try and measure sleep, each with their own limitations. The gold-standard method, polysomnography (PSG), is largely impractical for most population-level studies, and if used, it tends to be performed in a sleep laboratory for only one or two nights and cannot be considered representative of typical sleep in a home environment. While simply asking people about their sleep seems straightforward, as with other retrospective survey-based assessments, measurement of sleep is thwarted by recall bias, making it hard to assess exposure accurately. Even with this limitation, however, powerful relationships have still been demonstrated between sleep and disease using these methods. If patient compliance is high, daily sleep logs can provide good general information about certain aspects of sleep, such as sleep duration or sleep timing, but cannot provide any information on sleep stage. Certain disorders, for example the sleep-state misperception experienced by insomniacs or cognitive impairment, can confound subjective reports or

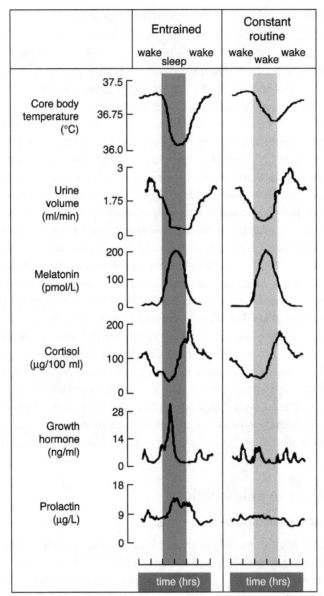

Fig. 2.1 Sleep and circadian-dependent influences on endocrine function. The figure shows the relative profiles of temperature, urine volume, and a number of common endocrine markers under normal baseline 16-h wake—8-h sleep to 16-h wake (W-S-W) conditions (left panels, sleep shown by dark shaded area) and under Constant Routine (CR) conditions where subjects remain awake in a time-free environment, under dim light and in a semi-recumbent posture with hourly snacks for 30 hours or more.

Melatonin (third panel) and cortisol (fourth panel) profiles are relatively unchanged by sleep, except that there is a small wake-dependent rise in cortisol in the morning not seen during CR conditions. There is a large sleep-dependent increase in the amplitude of core body temperature (top panel) and a lowering of the temperature minimum reached owing to the direct hypothermic reduce compliance, however. Careful consideration of the study population is necessary to decide whether sleep logs are appropriate.

There is increasing interest in developing objective methods to measure sleep that do not require PSG. Wrist actigraphy is the most common approach, which was initially available only as an expensive research tool, but has now been expanded to become a relatively inexpensive consumer product. While relatively easy to measure, rest–activity cycles present some difficulties in accurately measuring sleep and are therefore more suitable for assessing sleep patterns or stability than actual sleep time. Actimetry has also been combined with other non-invasive measures, such as heart rate, heart rate variability, oximetry, or breathing patterns, to enhance the accuracy of distinguishing sleep from wake, and introducing the possibility of measuring sleep stage. Assessments have also moved beyond the wristband to other approaches, such as sensors embedded in clothes or in a ring. Not all measures require an individual to wear a device, but rather measure data from under-bed or under-pillow sensors or from signals collected at the bedside. Attempts have also been made to scale down PSG to a headband containing only several electrodes, although the approach remains relatively impractical. With all of these methods, however, validation remains problematic. Most of the devices have not been validated against PSG, and of those that have, the studies tend to be performed in a controlled sleep laboratory environment in healthy subjects. Few, if any, have been validated against PSG in a home environment, where they are intended to be used, or in non-healthy populations which often comprise the groups in which sleep needs to be measured. Care must therefore be taken to assess the validation status if devices are to be used in large-scale epidemiological studies.

Measuring circadian phase is also difficult as, by definition, the outcome may change according to the time of day measured; consequently, multiple time points across the day and night need to be sampled. Recently, however, a number of studies have started to address this issue by developing methods to assess circadian phase from the relationships between multiple measures at the same time point—a sort of 'fingerprint of time'—or from multiple non-invasive continuous measures. If successful, and accessible, such a method could revolutionize our understanding of the role of circadian phase on both healthy physiological and disease processes, and would permit a much more accurate interpretation of test results or allow treatment timing to be scheduled according to one's circadian phase, greatly enhancing progress towards personalized medicine.

A number of proxy markers have been used to estimate circadian phase, including sleep timing and diurnal preference. These methods have some shortcomings when used

effect of sleep in addition to the circadian decline in temperature at night. Growth hormone (fifth panel), and to a lesser extent prolactin (bottom panel), have a sleep-dependent increase in levels such that production of these hormones is greatly reduced if sleep is absent (right panels).

to estimate circadian phase as there is at least a 5-hour range, and often more, in the phase relationship between sleep and circadian phase, even in normal sleepers. Sleep may also bear no relationship at all with circadian phase under extreme cases, for example in shift-workers: if only sleep data were measured without knowledge of the work pattern, then the sleep timing would clearly not be an accurate measure of circadian phase in shift-workers. Similar shortcomings exist for diurnal preference given that it is estimated largely on the basis of sleep preferences, and as such, sleep timing and diurnal preference are not considered reliable markers of circadian time.

Influences of sleep and circadian phase

The practice of using single time-point biomarkers or measurements in epidemiology brings potential confounds with respect to circadian and sleep influences. For example, a high cortisol level would be normal for a morning blood draw, but abnormal for an evening draw (Figure 2.1). While not ideal, accounting for time of day in analyses, or maintaining a fixed time of day for data collection, is at least a minimum requirement for being able to interpret markers that have any circadian component to their variation. This is a compromise position, of course, as it assumes that all individuals have the same timing in relation to their circadian rhythms. This is not the case, and there is at least a 5-hour range in circadian phase across the population, even in normally phased healthy subjects (Wright Jr et al., 2005). Systematic changes in circadian timing—for example, those that occur in adolescence or old age, or in certain sleep disorders such as insomnia or delayed sleep–wake rhythm disorder— broaden this range, potentially confounding the single time-point results.

The confound becomes more severe when dealing with a population that may have a greater degree of circadian disruption, for example in shift-workers and others who are desynchronized owing to jet-lag, or undergraduates keeping unusual schedules, as the direction and magnitude of circadian misalignment are unpredictable. For example, the melatonin metabolite 6-sulphatoxymelatonin (aMT6s) concentration in a morning void urine sample may reliably correlate with overall 24-hour production in non-shift-workers with normal circadian rhythms, but has little predictive value in shift-workers who may be advanced or delayed relative to normal. Similar confounds may exist in relation to the effects of sleep. Sleep duration in the night or nights prior to sampling may affect some biomarkers directly, and therefore knowledge of at least the previous night's sleep may be an important covariate. These factors are similarly particularly problematic if interpreting single time-point alertness, mood, or performance measures as current vigilance level is highly dependent on the interaction between the number of hours awake and the circadian phase. Large cohort numbers do not necessarily account for these confounds if the sampling is not distributed appropriately in relation to the underlying pattern. For example, sampling melatonin in the daytime will not provide information about its levels regardless of the size of the population as melatonin is only produced at night. Given that more and more aspects of our biology are being found to be circadian- or sleep-related, the design and interpretation of biomarker sampling need careful consideration to avoid misleading results.

While measuring sleep and sleep disruption is of interest in its own right, it is important to remember that sleep also gates ocular light exposure to the circadian system (Dijk & Lockley, 2002). The sleep–wake pattern determines the light–dark exposure pattern, or photoperiod, as wake is associated with light exposure and sleep occurs with the eyes closed, shutting off virtually all light input. Changes in sleep–wake patterns therefore also mean simultaneous changes in light–dark exposure, which can have substantial effects on circadian rhythms (Czeisler & Gooley, 2007). This causative relationship is sometimes ignored, with findings often associated only with sleep, not sleep or dark. This reciprocal relationship has been used proactively as a way to estimate light exposure at night from sleep duration, and relate the exposure level to disease risk (Stevens et al., 2014). In addition to light exposure at night, sleep duration may also be an important proxy biomarker for other sleep- or light-affected outcomes such as the release of melatonin, cortisol, GH, and TSH.

Conclusions

Given the wide-ranging impact of circadian rhythms and sleep on physiology, behaviour, and metabolism, it may not be surprising that alterations in clock- and sleep-related genes, and their subsequent effects on light exposure, hormone patterns, sleep, and metabolism, are associated with disease risk. Similarly, systematic alterations in behaviour, whether genetically driven or societally induced, will also impact sleep and circadian organization, with potentially important effects on medical and mental health. Epidemiology has an important role to play in understanding the contribution of sleep and circadian rhythms on the aetiology of poor health and disease and in distinguishing between the genetic or behavioural basis of disease. Epidemiologists must therefore understand how to measure sleep and circadian rhythms as accurately as possible and understand how sleep, circadian phase, or light may affect the measurement, analysis, or interpretation of other outcomes. As stated at the start of the chapter, measuring sleep should be a core component of all health research, and failure to include sleep will exclude a third of our entire lives.

Summary

- Sleep is an essential behaviour, vital to good health and wellbeing, and assessment of sleep and sleep disorders should be a core component of all public health research.
- Sleep is an active state, defined behaviourally by changes in posture and arousal threshold and defined electrophysiologically as different sleep stages by changes in the frequency and synchronization of EEG recordings.
- Sleep consists of rapid eye movement (REM) and non-REM (NREM) sleep, which alternate in a ~ 90–100 minute cycle, causing changes in breathing rate, heart rate, blood pressure, and body and brain temperature.
- Sleep timing and structure are controlled by two oscillatory processes: an intrinsic 24-hour rhythm determined by the circadian ('about a day') pacemaker in the

hypothalamus (Process C), and a homeostatic process which monitors the duration of time spent awake and the duration of time spent asleep (Process S).

◆ NREM sleep comprises three stages (N1, N2, and N3), which represent increasingly 'deep' sleep states. Stage N3, or slow-wave sleep, usually occurs primarily in the first half of the night; it is highly correlated with prior time awake and is a measure of sleep deprivation. REM sleep is under strong circadian control and tends to be greatest in the second half of the night.

◆ The relationship between Process C and Process S determines sleep quantity, timing, and quality, as well as daytime function such as the time course of alertness, mood, and performance, and diurnal preference (morningness or eveningness). This relationship also underpins changes in sleep that occur in adolescence and ageing.

◆ Sleep and circadian rhythms directly affect a number of biomarkers of interest to epidemiologists; these effects should be taken into account when developing protocols and interpreting findings.

◆ Care should be taken when selecting the method used to assess sleep or circadian phase, the level of validation, and the method limitations, especially if consumer-level products are to be used.

◆ Single time-point assessment of biomarkers that have a rhythmic component may be misleading if not interpreted with respect to circadian phase or time of day. Knowledge of prior sleep may also be important for other biomarkers. New methods are in development to facilitate assessments more accurately and in as the most efficient way possible.

References

Åkerstedt, T., Ingre, M., Kecklund, G., Folkard, S. & Axelsson, J. 2008. Accounting for partial sleep deprivation and cumulative sleepiness in the Three-Process Model of alertness regulation. *Chronobiology International*, **25**, pp. 309–19.

Cajochen, C. 2007. Alerting effects of light. *Sleep Medicine Reviews*, **11**(6), pp. 453–64.

Czeisler, C. A. & Gooley, J. J. 2007. Sleep and circadian rhythms in humans. *Cold Spring Harbor Symposia on Quantitative Biology*, **72**, pp. 579–97.

Czeisler, C. A. & Klerman, E. B. 1999. Circadian and sleep-dependent regulation of hormone release in humans. *Recent Progress in Hormone Research*, **54**, pp. 97–132.

Dijk, D. J. & Czeisler, C. A. 1995. Contribution of the circadian pacemaker and the sleep homeostat to sleep propensity, sleep structure, electroencephalographic slow waves, and sleep spindle activity in humans. *The Journal of Neuroscience*, **15**, pp. 3526–38.

Dijk, D. J. & Lockley, S. W. 2002. Integration of human sleep-wake regulation and circadian rhythmicity. *Journal of Applied Physiology*, **92**, pp. 852–62.

Figueiro, M. G., Brainard, G. C., Lockley, S. W., Revell, V. L. & White, R. 2008. Light and Human Health: An overview of the impact of optical radiation on visual, circadian, neuroendocrine, and neurobehavioral responses. New York, NY: Illuminating Engineering Society of North America.

Lockley, S. W., Arendt, J. & Skene, D. J. 2007. Visual impairment and circadian rhythm disorders. *Dialogues in Clinical Neuroscience*, **9**, pp. 301–14.

Lucas, R. J., Peirson, S. N., Berson, D. M., Brown, T. M., Cooper, H. M., Czeisler, C. A., Figueiro, M. G., Gamlin, P. D., Lockley, S. W., O'Hagan, J. B., Price, L. L., Provencio, I., Skene, D. J. & Brainard, G. C. 2014. Measuring and using light in the melanopsin age. *Trends in Neurosciences*, **37**(1), pp. 1–9.

Morris, C. J., Yang, J. N. & Scheer, F. A. 2012. The impact of the circadian timing system on cardiovascular and metabolic function. *Progress in Brain Research*, **199**, pp. 337–58.

Stevens, R. G., Brainard, G. C., Blask, D. E., Lockley, S. W. & Motta, M. E. 2014. Breast cancer and circadian disruption from electric lighting in the modern world. *CA: A Cancer Journal for Clinicians*, **64**(3), pp. 207–18.

Van Cauter, E., Spiegel, K., Tasali, E. & Leproult, R. 2008. Metabolic consequences of sleep and sleep loss. *Sleep Medicine* **9** Suppl 1, pp. S23–S28.

Wright Jr., K. P., Gronfier, C., Duffy, J. F. & Czeisler, C. A. 2005. Intrinsic period and light intensity determine the phase relationship between melatonin and sleep in humans. *Journal of Biological Rhythms*, **20**, pp. 168–77.

Chapter 3

The function of sleep

Andrew J. K. Phillips

Introduction

Why do we spend so many hours sleeping? What are the physiological costs of not sleeping enough, and why did evolutionary pressures so ubiquitously select this solution over a state of constant activity? The functional basis for sleep remains one of the most important and elusive questions in neuroscience. Until recently, sleep functions were largely inferred from the deficits that insufficient sleep can cause, or guessed at based on the different patterns of sleep exhibited by other species, and how these may relate to their individual needs. In the past decade, however, great progress has been made in understanding the function of sleep, and we now recognize multiple key biological mechanisms that are enabled by sleep. This chapter reviews theories on the function of sleep, our current understanding, and remaining questions.

The null hypothesis of sleep function

New research has advanced us beyond the position of uncertainty set by Dement, whereby the only reason we sleep is because we get sleepy (Max, 2010). Nevertheless, it is instructive to consider a potential *null function* of sleep that was proposed before many mechanistic pathways were identified. Even if sleep had no other physiological functions, it would remain a practical mechanism for timing when animals interact with their environments. Ecological factors such as temperature, light, predation, food availability, and mate availability naturally vary with time of day. The relative cost vs benefit for an organism interacting with its environment is therefore a function of time of day. Humans, for instance, are ill-suited to performing tasks during the night, owing to specialized daytime vision and much poorer vision at night.

From this perspective, sleep can be viewed as a physiological state that gates the times of day at which we actively engage with our environment. Inactivity at certain times of day would therefore be an adaptive behaviour, although it must be balanced against potential dangers to the organism due to lack of conscious monitoring of the environment. Siegel (2009) has previously taken the devil's advocate position that the null function could be the *sole* function of sleep. This, however, is difficult to reconcile with current experimental facts demonstrating functions of sleep for both the body and brain, as well as profound adverse effects of sleep loss on physiological systems, which are reviewed later. Moreover, the discovery of *local sleep* demonstrates beyond doubt that sleep has use-dependent function. The depth of slow-wave sleep in a patch of cortex depends on the amount of prior use of that brain region, and sleep can even be locally induced in a region of an otherwise awake brain by repeatedly taxing that region, leading to temporary loss of function (Vyazovskiy et al., 2011).

Unihemispheric sleep is a special case of local sleep, in which animals sleep using only one brain hemisphere at a time. This phenomenon allows animals to obtain sleep while still actively monitoring their environment and moving about. It is commonly observed in birds and marine mammals, such as dolphins. Fur seals are observed to rapidly transition between bihemispheric (whole-brain) sleep when they are on land, like other terrestrial mammals, and unihemispheric sleep when they are in the water. If sleep's only function were the null function of gating when we are active, it would be difficult to satisfactorily explain the existence of local or unihemispheric sleep over a uniformly active—and therefore more functional—state of awareness.

The search for universal functions of sleep

Sleep has traditionally been connected with broad-scale changes in the activity of neurons in the central nervous system in mammals. This was first discovered in the late nineteenth century and early twentieth century by researchers developing electroencephalography to study the electrical activity of the brain. Studies of the sleeping brain led to identification of particular modes of brain activity corresponding to rapid eye movement (REM) and non-REM (NREM) sleep, which became the basis for sleep classification. More recently, a broader view of sleep has developed, including homologous states in other non-mammalian species. States similar to REM and NREM sleep have been observed in birds. Going further afield, periods of inactivity and reduced responsiveness to environmental stimuli that occur at consistent times of day have been observed in a range of simpler organisms, including *Drosophila* spp. and *Caenorhabditis elegans*.

Distinguishing these periods of inactivity from purely the output of a daily rhythmic oscillator (e.g. the circadian clock) is the fact that they are *homeostatically regulated*. When animals are forced to remain in the active state, they respond by increasing the length of the inactive state when this constraint is removed. In humans, this response manifests as sleeping longer after a period of insufficient sleep. Homeostatic regulation is an indirect but clear indication that the inactive state serves important functions, and when these are not performed they must be compensated for later. The inactive state shares common physiological functions between species as distantly related as primates and nematodes, which has led the inactive, homeostatically regulated state to be viewed as 'sleep', even in animals that lack a central nervous system or traditional measures of REM and NREM sleep.

The ubiquity of sleep among distantly related organisms has led to the scientific pursuit for functions of sleep that are universal between organisms. In certain cases noted later, functions do indeed appear to be conserved between species. It is worth remarking, however, that sleep does not appear to have any single universal function. Instead, it is best viewed as a collection of physiological processes that occur in parallel during the inactive state, which in combination improve the organism's performance during the active state, and thus the evolutionary fitness of the organism. For this reason, there is possibly no single answer to the question, "When did sleep first evolve?", since different processes and functions associated with sleep likely became coupled at different times in the evolutionary record, possibly at first driven simply by circadian fluctuations in cellular processes, including metabolism. In different organisms the demands of the active state differ, and so the composition, timing, and structure of sleep also differ. Within mammals alone, daily total sleep time varies between approximately 3 hours and 21 hours between species, and the amount of REM sleep varies between an almost negligible amount and over half of total sleep time.

Theories based on comparative analysis

One of the principal approaches to understanding the function of sleep has been to analyze correlations between sleep patterns and an animal's characteristics across species. Some studies of mammalian sleep have found weak but significant correlations between brain or body size or developmental variables and sleep variables such as total sleep time or time spent in REM sleep. One example is a negative correlation between body size and sleep duration (i.e. larger mammals sleep fewer hours on average). This approach, however, is limited by the fact that detailed observations of sleep have only been conducted in ~200–300 mammalian species out of a total of ~6,000 identified species, and by the fact that species have not all been studied under uniform conditions. The available data sample is also strongly biased towards certain phylogenetic classifications, such as rodents, which are common laboratory animals. When analyses are adjusted for the relative representation of different phylogenies, many of the previously reported correlations become statistically insignificant or even reverse in direction (Capellini et al., 2008).

Among the only trends that remain significant after correction for phylogeny and study conditions are (i) a negative correlation between metabolic rate and sleep duration, and (ii) a positive correlation between body size and the length of NREM/REM sleep cycles. Most mammals sleep polyphasically, meaning they alternate between wake and sleep cycles multiple times per day, with each sleep episode typically containing at least one NREM/REM sleep cycle. As shown in Figure 3.1, smaller species tend to have more of these cycles per day, and this trend can be explained by energetic constraints. Since metabolic rate scales with body size via Kleiber's law, smaller species are under greater demand than larger species to regularly awaken and seek out food sources. Agent-based simulations of evolution support the idea that shorter sleep cycles are positively selected when metabolic rate is higher, and models of sleep physiology suggest that the time constants of the sleep homeostatic system scale in accordance with Kleiber's law (Phillips et al., 2010). These findings indicate that sleep is intimately linked to metabolic function.

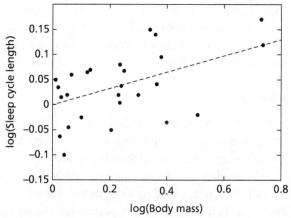

Fig. 3.1 Phylogeny-independent contrasts between sleep cycle length and body mass, with log transforms of both variables. The dashed line indicates a linear regression.

Reproduced with permission from Capellini I et al., 'Energetic constraints, not predation, influence the evolution of sleep patterning in mammals,' *Functional Ecology*, Volume 22, Issue 5, pp. 847–853, Copyright © 2008 British Ecological Society.

Sleep and metabolism

One of the earliest theories of sleep function was that it conserved energy, resulting in more efficient functioning of the organism, and therefore increased evolutionary fitness. For the brain, sleep is indeed critical to maintaining energy balance. Brain metabolism is significantly reduced in NREM sleep compared to wakefulness, and sleep generates an increase in the brain's main unit of energy currency, adenosine triphosphate (ATP). Other evidence also links sleep to brain metabolism. Adenosine is a key promoter of sleep, and its release in the brain is triggered by cellular energy demands. During wakefulness, the concentration of adenosine progressively increases in certain regions of the brain (e.g. the basal forebrain), reaching very high levels after sleep deprivation. When brain glycogen mobilization is blockaded using 1,4-dideoxy-1,4-imino-D-arabinitol, sleep duration is significantly increased. In addition, brain circuits that regulate sleep need are involved in regulating metabolism (Holst & Landolt, 2015).

Total energetic savings associated with sleep are, however, modest in mammals. In humans, whole-body metabolism is only about 10–20% lower in sleep than in inactive wakefulness, suggesting that sleep is not primarily for energy saving, unlike states such as torpor and hibernation, where metabolic activity is deeply reduced. Instead, during sleep, energy is devoted to numerous important maintenance tasks to improve functioning of physiological systems in both brain and body during wakefulness. These tasks are reviewed across the sections of this chapter that follow.

When individuals are restricted of sleep for multiple consecutive days, a syndrome of significant metabolic dysregulation is observed. This syndrome includes impaired insulin sensitivity, reduced glucose tolerance, and abnormal levels of the satiety and hunger hormones, leptin and ghrelin. The pathways involved in this complex, multi-system response are still being elucidated, but it is at least clear that sleep is important to maintaining normal metabolic function. For this reason, individuals who chronically sleep too little (< 6 hours) are at increased risk of diabetes, weight gain, and obesity (Spiegel et al., 2009).

Sleep and the body

While the brain has been the focal point for studies of sleep function, it is important to note that many of the processes conducted during sleep are beneficial to other systems in the body. It is now little exaggeration to say that sleep is beneficial for *every* system in the body. Epidemiological studies indicate that sufficient daily sleep duration is associated with improved health outcomes, including lower rate of mortality, and lessened risks of cardiovascular disease, diabetes, and obesity. Experimental studies have established a causal role for sleep in maintaining normal metabolic function, cardiovascular function, bone growth and repair, and immune function.

Recently, an intimate interaction between sleep and immune function has been uncovered. When individuals are sleep restricted, immune function is depressed, leading to greater risk of infection. When individuals are infected, sleepiness and sleep duration are increased, and these increases are beneficial to the immune response. Part of this interplay is achieved by immune-signalling molecules called cytokines. Some cytokines, such as interleukin (IL)-1, IL-6, and tumour necrosis factor-α (TNFα), have been shown to directly promote sleep (Imeri & Opp, 2009). Studies of prolonged sleep deprivation, which can be fatal in rats using the disc-over-water method, implicate impaired immune function in mortality.

Sleep and brain maintenance

Sleep has long been thought to play a key role in improving brain function, through either reconfiguration of neural networks or housekeeping tasks such as clearance of waste products from the brain. Indirect support for this idea came from the observation that individuals show grossly impaired cognitive performance when restricted of sleep, and the subjective feeling that a good night of sleep helps to clear and sharpen the mind. Detailed physiological mechanisms underlying this function have now been identified.

During wakefulness, when brain metabolism is elevated, various metabolites accumulate in the brain, including potential neurotoxins such as β-amyloid. It was recently demonstrated that a system exists for clearing these waste products from the brain during sleep, which has been called the *glymphatic system*. Specifically, interstitial spaces are significantly increased in volume during sleep, aiding convective exchange of interstitial fluid and cerebrospinal fluid. This results in much more rapid clearance of waste products during sleep than during wakefulness (Xie et al., 2013).

Sleep and synaptic plasticity

Evidence that sleep is involved in modifying brain plasticity and reconfiguring neural networks is now abundant. The general nature of these changes is still debated, however. Previously, Tononi and Cirelli postulated that a key function of sleep is *synaptic downscaling*, via mechanisms such as long-term depression (LTD). Specifically, they proposed that this downscaling is driven by slow waves during NREM sleep. They argued that synaptic downscaling is necessary owing to net strengthening of synapses during wakefulness by mechanisms such as long-term potentiation (LTP). If synaptic density increased continually without periods of downscaling, the increased synaptic density would greatly increase brain metabolic demands. Moreover, the ability of the neural network to encode new information would become saturated.

Convincing evidence of synaptic upscaling during wake, and synaptic downscaling during sleep, has been demonstrated in multiple brain circuits in *Drosophila* spp. Different, indirect measures of synaptic upscaling and downscaling with wake and sleep, respectively, have also been presented in rats (Tononi & Cirelli, 2014). The generalizability of this theory is currently contested, however, owing to clear examples of LTD occurring during wakefulness and LTP occurring during sleep with slow-wave activity. Indeed, some studies show that sleep primarily increases synaptic strength in some brain regions (Frank, 2014). Moreover, the theory does not provide any clear functional role for REM sleep, which comprises the majority of sleep during early stages of life in humans, when brain development is rapid. The precise effects of sleep on brain plasticity are therefore still being investigated.

Sleep and memory

Although we still lack an overarching understanding of sleep and synaptic plasticity, the fact that there are systematic changes in plasticity with sleep in certain brain regions, including the hippocampus, lends support to the theory that sleep is important to encoding and consolidating memories. Empirical data now confirm beyond doubt that a period of sleep shortly after exposure to new information (declarative memory) or training on a new task (procedural memory) improves later recall or performance. These effects of sleep in the immediate 24 hours after training persist for a long time, even up to years later (Diekelmann & Born, 2010). Moreover, the beneficial effects of sleep on memory have been demonstrated across multiple species, including humans, rats, and *Drosophila* spp.

One plausible mechanism by which sleep could improve memory is protection from interference. When awake, we are constantly bombarded by new information, which could interfere with the process of encoding information that was received earlier. When asleep, there is partial protection from environmental stimuli due to decreased interactions with the environment and changes to sensory processing. This purely passive process could therefore hypothetically account for some of the beneficial effects of sleep on memory.

Another plausible mechanism by which sleep could improve memory comprises active neurobiological processes that promote memory consolidation, such as changes in synaptic plasticity. Experiments that independently manipulate the timing of training, sleep, and recall suggest that sleep's role in improving memory is not purely passive, because sleep improves recall independent of how long individuals have been awake. Moreover, beneficial effects of sleep on memory have been shown to be resistant to subsequent inter-ference tasks (Ellenbogen et al., 2006).

A question that naturally arises when considering sleep function is, 'Why should it be necessary for many animals, including humans, to lose consciousness during sleep?' The null hypothesis of sleep function would explain this trait as one designed simply to prevent us interacting with our environments. When it comes to active functions of sleep, such as waste clearance and energy balance, the answer is not so obvious. Why can these processes not be completed 'in the background' of an otherwise conscious brain? Arguably, this would be less efficient for the organism. Periods of net energy gain and net waste clearance permit periods of net energy deficit and net production of wastes, which may correspond to higher cognitive function. A persistent conscious state would there-fore come at the cost of decreased cognitive function. Synaptic plasticity and learning pro-vide a complementary answer. Many functional networks change their activity between wake and stages of sleep. What may be optimal for manipulating, selecting, and storing memories may not be optimal for interacting with the environment. One of the potential advantages of sleep is the ability to conduct off-line simulations of wakefulness. It has been speculated that this may be the underlying basis for dreams, and could explain why dreams often involve unusual combinations of events, individuals, and circumstances. While this connection remains hypothetical, there is now clear evidence for memory re-play during sleep of events that were experienced during wakefulness.

Specific roles for REM and NREM sleep in the process of memory consolidation and learning remain unclear. The existence of a cycle between these stages is suggestive of an iterative process, in which each NREM sleep episode benefits from the insertion of a prior episode of REM sleep, and vice versa. Indeed, this is supported by evidence that informa-tion flow between the neocortex and hippocampus is reversed between REM and NREM sleep, suggesting an ongoing dialogue throughout the night. Empirical studies of sleep and memory have found associations between amounts or depth of specific sleep stages and performance on specific types of memory tasks. These findings, however, must be in-terpreted with considerable caution, as they are purely associations. It is unfortunately not possible to independently manipulate REM sleep or NREM sleep, as experimental disrup-tion of either stage affects the structure and progression of all subsequent stages of sleep. If the NREM/REM sleep cycle is actually the functional unit, due to interactions between NREM and REM sleep, it ultimately may not be very meaningful to attempt to tease apart functions for individual stages of sleep.

Summary

- Insufficient sleep has been associated with numerous adverse health outcomes at the population level, including obesity, diabetes, and cardiovascular disease.
- Insufficient sleep also impairs cognitive performance and increases risk of occupa-tional accidents.
- Experimental studies confirm that these are not only correlational, but also causal, associations.

- Sleep loss per se is potently harmful.
- The underlying biological mechanisms that generate sleep's protective effects remain an area of intense scientific investigation.
- Enormous strides have been made in the past decade towards identifying these mechanisms, with several mechanistic pathways now identified for sleep's effects on both the body and the brain.
- Understanding the nature of these pathways is important for managing or mitigating the effects of sleep loss on health, as well as providing accurate guidance to the general population on healthy sleep patterns.

References

Capellini, I., Nunn, C. L., McNamara, P., Preston, B. T. & Barton, R. A. 2008. Energetic constraints, not predation, influence the evolution of sleep patterning in mammals. *Functional Ecology*, **22**(5), pp. 847–53.

Diekelmann, S. & Born, J. 2010. The memory function of sleep. *Nature Reviews Neuroscience*, **11**(2), pp. 114–26.

Ellenbogen, J. M., Payne, J. D. & Stickgold, R. 2006. The role of sleep in declarative memory consolidation: passive, permissive, active or none? *Current Opinion in Neurobiology*, **16**(6), pp. 716–22.

Frank, M. G. 2014. Sleep and synaptic plasticity in the developing and adult brain. In: Meerlo, P., Benca, R. M. & Abel, T. ed(s). *Sleep, Neuronal Plasticity and Brain Function*. Berlin, Heidelberg: Springer, pp. 123–49.

Holst, S. C. & Landolt, H. P. 2015. Sleep homeostasis, metabolism, and adenosine. *Current Sleep Medicine Reports*, **1**(1), pp. 27–37.

Imeri, L. & Opp, M. R. 2009. How (and why) the immune system makes us sleep. *Nature Reviews Neuroscience*, **10**(3), pp. 199–210.

Max, D. T. 2010. The secrets of sleep. *National Geographic*, May 2010.

Phillips, A. J. K., Robinson, P. A., Kedziora, D. J. & Abeysuriya, R. G. 2010. Mammalian sleep dynamics: how diverse features arise from a common physiological framework. *PLoS Computational Biology*, **6**(6), e1000826.

Siegel, J. M. 2009. Sleep viewed as a state of adaptive inactivity. *Nature Reviews Neuroscience*, **10**(10), pp. 747–53.

Spiegel, K., Tasali, E., Leproult, R. & Van Cauter, E. 2009. Effects of poor and short sleep on glucose metabolism and obesity risk. *Nature Reviews Endocrinology*, **5**(5), pp. 253–61.

Tononi, G. & Cirelli, C. 2014. Sleep and the price of plasticity: from synaptic and cellular homeostasis to memory consolidation and integration. *Neuron*, **81**(1), pp. 12–34.

Vyazovskiy, V. V., Olcese, U., Hanlon, E. C., Nir, Y., Cirelli, C. & Tononi, G. 2011. Local sleep in awake rats. *Nature*, **472**(7344), pp. 443–447.

Xie, L., Kang, H., Xu, Q., Chen, M. J., Liao, Y., Thiyagarajan, M., O'Donnell, J., Christensen, D. J., Nicholson, C., Iliff, J. J., Takano, T., Deane, R. & Nedergaard, M. 2013. Sleep drives metabolite clearance from the adult brain. *Science*, **42**(6156), pp. 373–7.

Chapter 4

Sleep and cognition

Donald L. Bliwise and Michael K. Scullin

Introduction

This chapter will provide a selective review and commentary on the topic of sleep and cognition. Although this is perhaps somewhat deceptively a straightforward topic, a more detailed examination of the issues involved suggested a highly variegated and rich mixture of studies bearing potential relevance to it (Scullin & Bliwise, 2015). Even the most cursory examination of potential overlap yields a literature that is extensive in its diversity in methods and perspectives. Of relevance to epidemiologists is the fact that many of the studies are experimental and/or laboratory-based rather than population- based. As of 1 January 2016, a PubMed search of the terms 'sleep and cognition' yielded over 11,000 references, and 'sleep and memory' yielded nearly 6,000. Our approach to this massive body of work will make liberal use of other key reviews and commentaries that have encapsulated different components of the literature, and the reader is directed to these for a detailed rendering of primary source material. Alternatively, our approach here will be to create a more overarching commentary on these domains of literature, rather than to focus on a review of their specific content. To that end, we will rely upon the well-established causal criteria in epidemiology, now often simply referred to as 'Hill criteria' (Hill, 1965), with which to create a structure to attempt to reduce the diverse themes to workable categories of evidence. We will also make it clear whether we are discussing sleep as a normative occurrence, or sleep as it may have bearing in disease. The most relevant and conspicuous examples of the relevant diseases in a discussion of sleep and cognition relationships are: a) sleep apnoea and b) neurodegenerative disease.

Consistency of association

Over 50 studies report on the association between self-reported sleep complaints and measures of cognitive functioning in community-dwelling adults (Scullin & Bliwise, 2015). These studies overwhelmingly report significant associations between sleep variables and cognitive variables and only rarely report null findings. Formal meta-analyses have yet to appear on this topic, the one noteworthy exception being the recent paper on sleep durations (Lo et al., 2016), which reported no publication bias within the limitations of the kinds of studies reviewed by those authors (see the description of Lo et al.'s meta-analysis in the paragraph below, and also 'Strength of association'). Many of the studies cited were population-based and were based on very large samples, and some observed statistically significant associations even after controlling for demographics and selected confounders (e.g. hypertension). Some of the better studies have controlled for as many as 15 confounders (Song et al., 2015). However, apart from such considerations, a broad overview of this literature suggests that effect modification may indeed occur, quite possibly by gender, but more definitively by chronological age (Scullin & Bliwise, 2015). A good example of this is the study by Miller et al. (2014), which observed that short sleep was associated with poorer cognition in middle-aged adults, but not in older adults. Furthermore, older participants with greater levels of sleep disturbances showed higher cognitive functioning than those who slept well.

Lo et al.'s meta-analysis, which focused exclusively on self-reported habitual duration as its considered measure of sleep, reported that both short and long sleep—in both cross-sectional and prospective studies—showed associations with impaired cognition. In some sense, this is not surprising, since extremes of sleep duration have been associated with a variety of morbidities in such a U-shaped fashion (see Chapter 8). However, at another level, knowing that impaired cognition is associated with both short and long sleep begs the question of consistency. Self-reported sleep duration remains only one of the myriad of ways of characterizing sleep in human populations. Many epidemiological studies have shown associations between impaired cognition and variables such as sleep onset latency, night-time awakenings, awakening too early, napping, and daytime sleepiness, to name but a few. Often, a particular study reports an association with impaired cognition with one variable but not another, whereas another study does not. In this sense the consistency of findings may not be as great as is apparent from reading individual paper titles and abstracts. Additionally, in the case of total sleep time, some researchers define normality as 7–9 hours per night, inclusive as a basis for comparing short and long sleep, but this approach is not uniform. Six hours per night is sometimes considered normal and 9 hours is sometimes considered long. Some large studies use only the most extreme values to define abnormal sleep duration (3–4 hours/night). The lack of consistency with use of self-reports is not ameliorated by using actigraphy or polysomnography, where the number of options for defining permutations of sleep–wake state, quantification of the electroencephalogram (EEG), and counting disordered breathing events can expand exponentially. As perhaps best epitomized by the findings involving both short and long sleep duration, the inconsistency of associations across studies examining different metrics for sleep suggests that some of the reported positive findings may well represent Type I error (i.e. the likelihood that a result is significant by chance only).

Specificity of association

Although inconsistency of findings involving the sundry ways of characterizing human sleep remains one dilemma in this literature, the lack of specificity across various measures of cognition represents a different issue. The range of measures defining cognition in this literature is vast and includes tasks involving procedural memory, working memory, overnight memory consolidation, vocabulary, creativity, attention, visuo-spatial discrimination, and psychomotor speed, to name just a few. Some studies rely instead on brief, global assessments of mental status, such as the Mini-Mental State Exam (MMSE). By rough count, about a third of all cross-sectional studies and half of prospective studies examining sleep and cognition rely exclusively on such a measure, which contains one or two items from a number of different domains of cognitive function but does not assess any particular domain in depth. Contemporary neuroscience teaches that different mental functions can reflect widely varying neural networks. Knowledge that a general measure of cognition may be related to sleep is informative, but hardly conclusive, as some domains might be more related than others.

Laboratory-based studies in particular often hone in on specific aspects of cognition and sleep. In young adults, poorer performance in memory encoding and consolidation was associated with lower levels of slow-wave sleep, rapid eye movement sleep, and sleep spindle density. Using a simple test of task switching and psychomotor speed (Trail Making Test Part B), higher levels of REM sleep appeared protective for decline over intervals of 3–4 years (Song et al, 2015). Using a complex verbal task (the N-back task), verbal fluency related to slow-wave sleep, whereas verbal memory was more closely associated with REM sleep. A test involving visuo-spatial memory consolidation (mirror tracing) was positively related to the density of eye movements in REM. In studies such as these, it remains unclear whether other untested cognitive functions would demonstrate comparable associations to sleep, since by their very nature, the studies are limited by time and resources in their assessments of cognition. One could easily argue that the very fact that so many different functions relate to (different aspects of) sleep suggests that an association must be real, and that may well be the case. But to the extent that Hill's criteria demand some elements of specificity, the breadth of findings with such diverse measures might be portrayed as a potential weakness rather than a strength.

Strength of association

Lo et al. (2016) reported odds ratio (OR) confidence intervals (CI) for the association with poor cognitive function, which ranged from 1.27 to 1.56 for short sleep duration and 1.43 to 1.74 for long sleep duration. These moderate effects were based upon models that included the maximum number of covariates. Meta-analyses have not yet appeared for other metrics of self-reported sleep quality such as night-time awakenings, daytime sleepiness, or difficulty falling asleep.

There are fewer polysomnographic studies with which to estimate the strength of sleep/cognition associations. Some of the earliest reported very large effect sizes (e.g. $r^2 = 0.71$ between REM sleep and Wechsler Adult Intelligence Scale performance). Analyses from the MrOS Sleep Study cohort may provide a better true estimate of the strength of the association between cognitive function and various polysomnography variables (e.g. REM) with sufficient power to avoid Type II error (i.e. the likelihood that a true effect can be missed by chance). Song et al. (2015) reported that the duration of Stage N1 sleep (often viewed as a transitional stage of sleep) was strongly associated with clinically significant decline in the Trail Making Test Part B (OR = 2.17, 95% CI 1.34–3.52). Complementing these results was the finding that relatively low amounts of REM sleep were only marginally associated with clinically significant decline on the modified MMSE (OR = 1.29, CI 0.95–1.75). Other stages of sleep (e.g. N2, N3) showed no associations whatsoever. The MrOS study used only one night of polysomnography, a limited number of sleep variables, and only a few cognitive tests. These limitations preclude conclusive population-based estimates of the strength of association, albeit the findings remain provocative.

Temporality

Prospective data—many derived from population-based studies—also suggest that sleep complaints prospectively predict more rapid cognitive decline. In the Whitehall II study middle-aged adults were followed over 5 years. In those whose self-reported sleep duration decreased, there was a greater decline in reasoning, vocabulary, phonemic fluency, semantic fluency, and MMSE scores. Similar findings were obtained in the Nurses' Health Study, in which more than 15,000 nurses were followed over 6 years, and in the Finnish Longitudinal Study of Municipal Employees, which included a 28-year follow-up. Sleep complaints also tend to precede the diagnosis of Alzheimer's disease. In both the Women's Health Initiative Memory Study and the Uppsala Longitudinal Study of Adult Men, sleep complaints at baseline increased risk for Alzheimer's disease or dementia diagnosis by 33% and 51% approximately 7 years and 40 years later, respectively.

Longitudinal data often raise the possibility of bi-directional relationships, and the area of sleep and cognition is no exception. At least three longitudinal studies have reported that poor cognitive function at baseline predicted sleep disturbances (low REM and sleep fragmentation) up to 15 years later (Scullin & Bliwise, 2015). The mechanisms by which poor cognitive function would lead to later sleep disturbances remain unclear, but may include poor cognitive control over emotions and stressors (leading to difficulty sleeping), compromised cholinergic activity (explaining both poor memory function and diminished REM sleep), and atrophy in the prefrontal brain networks that regulate both cognitive functions and sleep state.

Biological plausibility

Data bearing upon whether sleep and cognition have a biologically plausible relationship represent a critical lynchpin in examining associations between the two phenomena. After all, if there is not a coherent and at least plausible mechanistic basis for such associations, then clinical studies from human populations, no matter how compelling and convincing, may be unfounded.

Basic science studies remain the ultimate source of our mechanistic understanding of how sleep and cognition may be related. Although a detailed description of the fundamental neuroscience in this area is far beyond the scope of this review, reference to a few key proven concepts provides some context for the types of data that speak to these issues. One key concept is sleep deprivation. Experimentally induced and often quite extensive (e.g. weeks) sleep deprivation in rats has provided invaluable insights into the multiple physiological functions of sleep. Insofar as brain function is concerned, sleep deprivation produces some of the same protein aggregates (e.g. β-amyloid) that characterizes the brains of patients with Alzheimer's disease (AD), perhaps the proto-typical human disease characterized by impaired cognition. Such depositions can be produced by partial chronic (4 hours per day for 21 days) sleep loss and are even detect-able within interstitial brain fluid within as little as 6 hours of acute sleep deprivation in mice especially inbred to carry genetic susceptibility to AD-type brain changes. This abnormal protein deposition may also represent what has more generally been referred to as the 'unfolded protein response' (UPR) in the mouse brain reported by other re-search. Whether such abnormal mechanisms linking sleep loss and degraded proteins are conserved in humans remains uncertain, but several studies have now reported that characteristically low sleep efficiency (assessed with actigraphy) is associated with higher levels of β-amyloid burden, as defined by cerebrospinal fluid markers and by neuroimaging. Neuropathological data from humans has also suggested that neuronal loss in a particular brain region thought to be crucial for maintaining sleep (the inter-mediate nucleus of the anterior hypothalamus) was linearly associated with ante-mortem actigraphic measurements of sleep fragmentation, recorded about 15 months before death. Those continuous associations were present in patients both with and without neuropathologically confirmed AD, though neuronal loss was significantly higher in the former, relative to the latter. Yet another degraded protein characterizing AD (tau) was also associated in regression models with poorer sleep among individuals with a geno-type strongly predisposing for AD (apolipoprotein E4).

Apart from measurements related to sleep disruption per se, a complementary, but dis-tinct, line of evidence emerges from studies that have specifically attempted to model the intermittent hypoxia that accompanies sleep apnoea in order to determine its effects on neuronal integrity. For example, there is compelling evidence that intermittent hyp-oxia hastens cell death in the CA1 layer of the hippocampus in rats, with the effect being particularly pronounced in older animals. Precisely how such apoptosis is accelerated remains uncertain, though likely candidate mechanisms include oxidative stress effects on neurons, inflammation, and activation of molecular hypoxic sensors that alter the per-meability of the blood–brain barrier. Ample evidence exists in humans of sleep apnoea as causal both for activation of reactive oxygen species (molecules that mark oxidative stress) and for a pro-inflammatory state.

Taken together, the evidence, much of which is based on animal studies, suggests potential neurobiological substrates whereby higher order brain function (in humans, cognition) could be impacted adversely by interruption of sleep per se or by specific sleep disorders characterized by abnormalities of gas exchange, i.e. sleep apnoea. The associations represent continuously scaled responses and, as such, they also meet this particular Hill criterion by thus representing a biological gradient in the association (Hill, 1965).

Experiment

Experimental studies, broadly defined as including clinical trials as well as experimental laboratory protocols, have substantial relevance to the topic of sleep and cognition. In this section, we will provide an overview of three distinct areas of evidence. As has been the case for other bodies of empirical literature to which we have alluded in this chapter, we again direct the reader to a number of previous reviews by both ourselves and others for reference to specific primary source material. The three areas covered here are: 1) sedative/hypnotic medication trials; 2) clinical trials for treatment of a specific sleep disorder, sleep apnoea, many of which have included measurements of cognition subsequent to nasal continuous positive airway pressure (CPAP) treatment; and 3) experimental studies of sleep deprivation and cognition that have considered age as an effect modifier. To the extent that all three areas involve manipulations of sleep as an independent variable, we consider them all to be experimentally derived data.

Sedative/hypnotic trials for insomnia have customarily assessed cognition as an outcome; however, the typical perspective used in those studies may not bear immediate relevance to the reader interested in the topic of this chapter. That is to say, improvements in sleep are not customarily viewed as conferring potential benefits for cognition in such trials, but rather, impaired cognition is viewed as a potential adverse effect of the medications being tested. We should first emphasize that whether patients with insomnia (those most likely to be taking sedative/hypnotics) show impaired cognition has been questioned repeatedly in the literature (Scullin & Bliwise, 2015). Nevertheless, in what have been literally hundreds of published pharmacological trials, tasks such as those involving psychomotor speed and immediate, explicit memory are typically administered over the course of the trial to patients administered a placebo or active drug during both baseline and after-drug treatment. Task administration is typically in the morning, after pill ingestion the prior night, to determine carryover effects. Absence of differences between placebo and active drug conditions before and after drug administration is considered a desired (null) outcome. Such safety considerations stand in stark contrast to a vastly smaller number of recent studies (less than ten) that have suggested that certain aspects of memory (e.g. consolidation) might be improved by hypnotic-induced sleep, particularly if specific EEG waveforms (e.g. spindles) are shown to increase by the medication studied.

Sleep apnoea represents another medical condition that often warrants treatment, and studies suggest a cross-sectional association between cognitive impairments and this disorder, though the magnitude of the associations may vary somewhat by age and/or by the presence of age-dependent comorbidities (Bliwise & Greenaway, 2011). Additionally, at least some longitudinal data have suggested that incident dementia or mild cognitive impairment may be associated with untreated sleep apnoea at baseline, though not all data concur. More relevant for this section of our chapter are dozens of treatment studies for sleep apnoea, which have frequently used CPAP and have examined cognitive/neuropsychological outcomes. One of the largest and best controlled studies, APPLES (Apnoea Positive Pressure Long-term Efficacy Study), indeed met a few of its primary endpoints in the neurobehavioural domain. However, an unappreciated aspect of this otherwise extensive multi-site trial was that the effect sizes among the measures of interest were small (Bliwise & Greenaway, 2011) because of what are frequently referred to as ceiling effects. In APPLES, only small effects may have been present because the patients treated were one standard deviation or higher above age-expected norms for baseline cognitive performance on these outcomes. With such strong cognitive functioning to begin with, there was simply little room for improvement. Other major recent CPAP trials involving sleep apnoea patients aged 65 years and above, the PREDICT (Positive Airway Pressure in Older People: a randomised controlled trial) trial, and the Spanish Sleep Network Trial showed significant improvements in sleepiness (Epworth Sleepiness Scale) and quality-of-life measures, but only equivocal results for measures of cognition per se (psychomotor function, reaction time, declarative memory) (Bliwise, 2015).

Perhaps the ultimate test of an intervention for sleep apnoea on cognition would be studies of sleep apnoea treatment among patients with frank dementia (e.g. Alzheimer's disease). These studies are extremely arduous to conduct, and may have the challenge of floor effects (i.e. cognition too poor to begin with, owing to reasons other than sleep loss, to expect to see large improvements), but a few small-scale trials have been completed (Ancoli-Israel et al., 2008; Troussière et al., 2014). Their results show modest effects on cognition, in some cases not withstanding statistical adjustments for multiple comparison testing, though sleepiness, mood, and quality-of-life measures demonstrated improvement. The recent trial by Troussière et al. is noteworthy to the extent that a self-selected subgroup of dementia patients who used CPAP for a median period of 3 years showed minimal change in general mental status over that interval, whereas those untreated showed the expected decline in cognition. The study results are provocative, but the number of cases was very small and the design was not randomized.

Experimental studies of sleep deprivation offer a third vantage point on experimental evidence relevant to sleep and cognition. Here, there is relative uniformity of the findings to the extent that the impact of sleep loss is diminished in older, relative to younger, persons (Scullin & Bliwise, 2015). These results raise the possibility that the function of sleep may differ as a function of age, a notion often given tacit lip service among the lay press (the belief that older people 'need' less sleep than younger people) (Bliwise & Scullin, 2016), but whether this holds true outside the sphere of cognition remains very much in doubt. Furthermore, basic science research implies that the need for sleep could even be greater in older, relative to younger, animals, since apoptosis (neuronal death) and protein aggregation (a hallmark for neurodegeneration) may be potentiated by sleep loss to a greater extent in older, relative to younger, animals (see 'Biological plausibility').

Summary

- Possible associations between sleep and cognition are provocative across different domains and hold the promise of prevention or reversibility. However, evidence is suggestive but hardly definitive.

- Hill's criteria can be used to assess the evidence in support of a causal effect.

- Consistency of association: studies on the association between self-reported sleep complaints and measures of cognitive functioning in adults overwhelmingly report significant associations between sleep variables and cognitive variables. However, inconsistency of associations is seen across studies examining different metrics for sleep.

- Specificity of association: there is a lack of specificity across various measures of cognition and various measures of sleep. The heterogeneity possibly reflects different associations between different domains of cognitive function and measures of sleep.

- Strength of association: important limitations preclude conclusive population-based estimates of the strength of association. However, moderate effects are seen when accounting for multiple confounding for some stages of sleep (e.g. N1) but not others (e.g. N2, N3).

- Temporality: prospective data from population-based studies suggest that sleep complaints predict more rapid cognitive decline.

- Biological plausibility: in animal experiments, sleep deprivation causes the formation of β-amyloid and tau proteins, seen in patients with Alzheimer's disease; hypoxia, through pro-inflammatory actions, may cause neuronal apoptosis.

- Experiment: three areas of evidence provide some insight into the possible causative link between sleep complaints and cognitive functions. They are: sedative/hypnotic medication trials, clinical trials of treatment of sleep apnoea, and experimental studies of sleep deprivation.

References

Ancoli-Israel, S., Palmer, B. W., Cooke, J. R., Corey-Bloom, J., Fiorentino, L., Natarajan, L., Liu, L., Ayalon, L., He, F. & Loredo, J. S. 2008. Cognitive effects of treating obstructive sleep apnea in Alzheimer's disease: a randomized controlled study. *Journal of the American Geriatrics Society*, **56**, pp. 2076–81.

Bliwise, D. L. & Greenaway, M. C. 2011. Will APPLES hit a ceiling? *Sleep*, **34**, pp. 249–50.

Bliwise, D. L. 2015. Never too old: beneficial neurobehavioral effects of continuous positive airway pressure in the elderly (Editorial). *The European Respiratory Journal*, **46**, pp. 13–15.

Bliwise, D. L. & Scullin, M. K. 2016. Normal aging. In: Kryger, M. H., Roth, T. & Dement, W. C. eds. *Principles and Practice of Sleep Medicine*. 6th ed. Philadelphia: Elsevier/Saunders, pp. 25–38.

Hill, A. B. 1965. The environment and disease: association or causation? *Proceedings of the Royal Society of Medicine*, **58**, pp. 295–300.

Lo, J. C., Groeger, J. A., Cheng, G. H., Dijk, D. J. & Chee, M. W. 2016. Self-reported sleep duration and cognitive performance in older adults: a systematic review and meta-analysis. *Sleep Medicine*, **17**, pp. 87–98.

Miller, M. A., Wright, H., Ji, C. & Cappuccio, F. P. 2014. Cross-sectional study of sleep quantity and quality and amnestic and non-amnestic cognitive function in an ageing population: the English longitudinal study of ageing (ELSA). *PLOS One*, **9**(6), e100991.

Scullin, M. K. & Bliwise, D. L. 2015. Sleep, cognition and normal aging: integrating a half-century of multidisciplinary research. *Perspectives on Psychological Science*, **10**, pp. 97–137.

Song, Y., Blackwell, T., Yaffe, K., Ancoli-Israel, S., Redline, S., Stone, K. L. & Osteoporotic Fractures in Men (MrOS) Study Group. 2015. Relationships between sleep stages and changes in cognitive function in older men: the MrOS Sleep Study. *Sleep*, **38**, pp. 411–21.

Troussière, A.-C., Charley, C. M., Salleron, J., Richard, F., Delbeuck, X., Derambure, P., Pasquier, F. & Bombois, S. 2014. Treatment of sleep apnoea syndrome decreases cognitive decline in patients with Alzheimer's disease. *Journal of Neurology, Neurosurgery, and Psychiatry*, **85**, pp. 1405–8.

A more detailed listing of references cited in this chapter can be obtained by contacting Professor Bliwise directly at dbliwis@emory.edu.

Chapter 5

An overview of sleep–wake circuitry: Circuit nodes, pathways, and transmitters

Anne Venner and Patrick M. Fuller

Introduction

Over the course of a typical 24-hour day, the brain cycles through three behavioural states, each of which is operationally defined by the level of behavioural arousal and electrocortical activity. Electrocortical activity refers to the net electrical activity across the brain cortex during a particular behavioural state, and is recorded using an electrophysiological measuring method called electroencephalography (EEG). Wakefulness, is characterised by high-frequency, low-amplitude waves (which are thought to represent differences in the timing of processing of motor, perceptual, and cognitive functions) and by a high level of alertness or vigilance, often occurring concurrently with motor behaviours. Sleep, on the other hand, comprises at least two distinct states: rapid eye movement (REM) sleep and non-rapid eye movement (NREM) sleep. REM sleep (also called paradoxical sleep or active sleep) is characterised by saccadic eye movements, cortical activity that mimics the high-frequency, low-amplitude EEG waves of waking, and muscle paralysis. It is of interest that dreaming is very commonly reported when people are woken during REM sleep. NREM sleep, by contrast, and in particular deep NREM sleep, is characterised by low-frequency, high-amplitude waves (often termed 'slow wave activity') on the cortical EEG, low responsivity to external stimuli, and limited eye movements and dreams.

To the extent that both good quality, as well as a good quantity of, sleep is the *sine qua non* for optimal wake, our behaviour during wake can similarly influence both the quality and quantity of our subsequent sleep. This functional interrelationship between sleep and wake reflects, perhaps not surprisingly, an interdependent circuit organisation used by the brain to organise, initiate, and maintain wake and sleep. Experimental work seeking to define and understand the neural circuitry that the brain uses to regulate sleep and wake dates back to the early twentieth century, with the vast majority of this experimental work performed in rodents. Over the last decade in particular however, the advent of genetically engineered mouse models has allowed scientists to selectively manipulate neurochemically and anatomically defined cell types within the brain, thereby enabling a considerably more detailed understanding of sleep–wake circuitry. Scientists have, for example, been able to locate and characterise different populations of neurons (or nodes) within the brain that are predominantly associated with specific states of sleep and arousal. Using genetically driven anatomical mapping techniques, they have then been able to establish functional linkages between these discrete circuit nodes, in turn illuminating complex and orchestrated networks that form the structural basis for wake and sleep regulation. Scientists, such as ourselves, continue to ask the following questions:

1. What brain circuit nodes, transmitters, and pathways are sufficient and/or necessary to produce and maintain behavioural and EEG *wake*?

2. What brain circuit nodes, transmitters and pathways are sufficient and/or necessary to produce and maintain behavioural and EEG *sleep*?

In this chapter, we will provide an overview of several parallel, yet interrelated, neural circuits through which the brain can control sleep and wake. We will then discuss some of the factors that can influence the activity of these sleep–wake circuits and thereby influence which behavioural state predominates in the brain.

Circuit # 1. The wake-promoting parabrachial-basal forebrain (PB-BF)-cortical axis and its regulation by the parafacial zone

Given that the major source of excitatory inputs to the brain's cortex emanates from the *thalamus,* this subcortical structure has long been considered necessary for generating the EEG correlates of cortical arousal and a wakeful state. Yet, curiously, destruction of thalamic cells has little impact on arousal level or total waking time and does not eliminate sleep–wake cycles (Fuller et al., 2011). Without doubt, complete lesions of the thalamus lead to severe cognitive impairments, but do not result in profound sleepiness. Hence, the structural integrity of the thalamus is not, in fact, a fundamental requirement for the initiation and maintenance of wakefulness (Figure 5.1A).

The cortex also receives projections from other subcortical brain regions, however, including the basal forebrain (BF), which, like the thalamus, has long been linked with arousal control. The BF is a large brain region that receives considerable input from the brainstem, and contains a wide variety of neurons, including cholinergic, glutamatergic, and GABAergic neurons (neurons that produce GABA, γ-aminobutyric acid). Of great interest, lesions of the BF produce coma, whilst selective activation of the various BF cell populations bias, to a large degree, the waking state. For example, specific activation of BF GABAergic neurons potently drives (likely through a process called 'dis-inhibition') wakefulness, whereas inhibition of these cells increases sleep (Anaclet et al., 2015). Interestingly, activation of parvalbumin-containing BF cells (a subpopulation of GABAergic cells) increases high-frequency waves on the cortical EEG without increasing behavioural wakefulness, whilst their inhibition reduces high-frequency cortical power EEG waves.

As indicated, the BF receives considerable inputs from the brainstem, most notably from excitatory glutamatergic neurons in the parabrachial (PB) nucleus. Lesions of the

PB nuclear complex produce behavioural unresponsiveness and a continuous prominent slow-wave EEG pattern, which is strikingly similar to the coma-like state following lesions of the BF. Given these findings, it has been proposed that projections from the parabrachial nucleus, relayed by the BF to the cerebral cortex (i.e. a PB-BF-cortical pathway), form the backbone of a powerful wake-promoting circuit that is indispensable for wakeful consciousness (Fuller et al., 2011) (Figure 5.1A).

It was recently shown that the PB complex receives dense innervation from sleep-active GABAergic neurons in the parafacial zone (PZ, so-called because these neurons are located lateral and dorsal to the facial nerve). This finding was of great interest given that disruption of GABAergic neurotransmission in PZ neurons produces insomnia, and acute activation of PZ neurons unambiguously drives NREM sleep and cortical slow waves. In other words, GABAergic PZ neurons may produce normal sleep by 'switching off' the PB-BF-cortical pathway, which, as described earlier, appears to be a primary brain circuit regulating the level of behavioural and EEG arousal. A functional synaptic PZ-PB-BF-cortical circuit was recently confirmed using a new technique called optogenetics (Anaclet et al., 2014) (Figure 5.1A).

Circuit # 2. The sleep-promoting ventrolateral preoptic area inhibits arousal nodes: the 'flip-flop switch'

It has been known for over 50 years that the preoptic area (POA) of the brain contains sleep-active neurons. More recent work has shown that a particularly important collection of sleep-active neurons resides in the ventrolateral region of the POA—the VLPO (Sherin et al., 1996). VLPO neurons contain the inhibitory transmitters GABA and galanin, and importantly, cell-body specific lesions of VLPO neurons produce chronic insomnia and sleep fragmentation in rats (Lu et al., 2000). Hence, neurons of the VLPO are thought to play a major role in helping our brain go to sleep. From an anatomical standpoint, VLPO neurons are reciprocally connected with several arousal-promoting brainstem and hypothalamic nuclei, including:

1) *Noradrenergic neurons of the locus coeruleus* (LC). Acute inhibition of LC neurons increases the number of transitions into NREM sleep, whilst their activation produces arousal in mice.

2) Wake-active *dopaminergic neurons of the ventral periaqueductal grey* (vPAG) region. Lesions of vPAG neurons produce a major reduction in wakefulness.

3) *Histaminergic neurons of the tuberomamillary nucleus* (TMN). TMN neurons fire selectively during wakefulness, and drugs that antagonise histamine produce sedation.

4) *Serotonergic neurons in the dorsal raphe* (DR). DR neurons are predominantly wake-active (Figure 5.1B).

The interaction between the VLPO and the foregoing components of the brainstem and hypothalamic arousal systems has been demonstrated to be mutually inhibitory and, as such, these pathways have been conceptualized, functionally, as a 'flip-flop' switch, analogous to that of an electronic circuit (Saper et al., 2010). In this circuit arrangement, the

(a) PB-BF-cortical axis

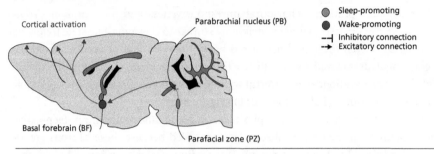

Cortical activation

Parabrachial nucleus (PB)

● Sleep-promoting
● Wake-promoting
⊣ Inhibitory connection
→ Excitatory connection

Basal forebrain (BF)

Parafacial zone (PZ)

(b) Flip-flop switch

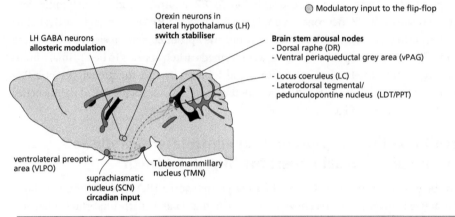

Orexin neurons in lateral hypothalamus (LH) **switch stabiliser**

○ Modulatory input to the flip-flop

LH GABA neurons **allosteric modulation**

Brain stem arousal nodes
- Dorsal raphe (DR)
- Ventral periaqueductal grey area (vPAG)

- Locus coeruleus (LC)
- Laterodorsal tegmental/
  pedunculopontine nucleus (LDT/PPT)

ventrolateral preoptic area (VLPO)

Tuberomammillary nucleus (TMN)

suprachiasmatic nucleus (SCN) **circadian input**

(c) Basal ganglia control of arousal

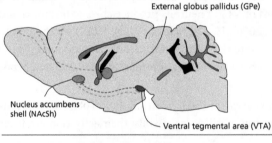

External globus pallidus (GPe)

Nucleus accumbens shell (NAcSh)

Ventral tegmental area (VTA)

(d) Circuitry controlling REM sleep

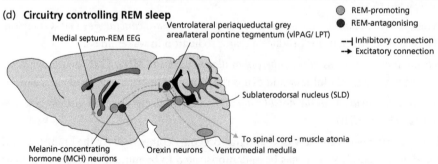

Ventrolateral periaqueductal grey area/lateral pontine tegmentum (vlPAG/ LPT)

Medial septum-REM EEG

● REM-promoting
● REM-antagonising
⊣ Inhibitory connection
→ Excitatory connection

Sublaterodorsal nucleus (SLD)

To spinal cord - muscle atonia

Melanin-concentrating hormone (MCH) neurons

Orexin neurons

Ventromedial medulla

Fig. 5.1 Circuitries mediating state change switching.

A. The inhibitory PZ switches off wake-promoting neurons in the PB to induce NREM sleep. The PB elicits wake through excitatory projections through the BF to the cortex. B. The sleep-promoting VLPO inhibits wake-promoting brainstem and hypothalamic arousal nodes to induce

VLPO represents the 'sleep side' whereas the brainstem and hypothalamic nodes represent the 'wake side'. The flip-flop model further predicts that an additional group of neurons, the *orexin neurons of the lateral hypothalamus (LH)*, act as a switch stabiliser, thereby preventing unwanted transitions into sleep, and stabilising wake. Indeed, loss of orexin, as occurs in the sleep disorder narcolepsy, results in 'sleep attacks', excessive daytime sleepiness, and state transitions from wake directly into REM sleep. Other influences, such as the internal circadian clock (see 'Timing of wake and sleep by the hypothalamic circadian clock'), and so-called 'allostatic' inputs to the switch (for example, GABAergic neurons of the lateral hypothalamus (Venner et al., 2016), which send an inhibitory projection to the VLPO and bias the switch towards the waking state), also play an important role in determining which way the switch should be flipped. The flip-flop switch is, by its nature, self-reinforcing: the side that is firing reduces its own inhibitory feedback, improving stability of the arousal state (wake or sleep) and avoiding 'intermediary' states. Thus, the flip-flop switch ensures relatively rapid switching between states as well as stability of state. At the same time, flip-flop switches can possess the undesirable property of abruptly undergoing unwanted state transitions, the frequency of which may increase. However, if one side of the switch becomes weakened, this can bias the switch towards a midpoint where smaller perturbations may trigger undersirable and abrupt state transitions.

Circuit # 3. Basal ganglia control of arousal

The basal ganglia (BG) consist of four major nuclei, including the striatum (caudate, putamen, and nucleus accumbens), globus pallidus, subthalamic nucleus, and substantia nigra. Sleep–wake disturbances are common in BG disorders (e.g. Parkinson's disease and Huntington's disease), suggesting a possible fundamental role for BG structures in sleep–wake regulation. It is also of interest that *GABAergic neurons of the shell of the nucleus accumbens (NAcSh)*, located in the ventral striatum, are the primary arousal target of caffeine. Caffeine is one of the most widely available and popular psychoactive 'wake-promoting' drugs and is a common ingredient in beverages such as coffee and fizzy

---

NREM sleep. The VLPO is itself inhibited by these same arousal nodes, resulting in a bistable flip-flop switch. Modulatory influences outside the core flip-flop circuitry, such as the orexin neurons and newly revealed wake-promoting GABA neurons in the LH (Venner et al., 2016) and circadian input act upon the flip-flop circuitry to bias it in a particular direction. C. Dopaminergic neurons in the VTA are profoundly wake-promoting. They inhibit the sleep-promoting NAcSh, likely through activation of D2 receptors. In parallel, the external globus pallidus increases sleep, most likely through inhibitory projections to the cortex. D. The SLD causes REM-sleep through its projections to the medial septum and to the spinal cord. It is under the inhibitory control of the 'REM-off' vlPAG/ LPT which is itself under inhibitory control from the SLD as well as several other REM-promoting nodes, such as the MCH neurons and GABAergic neurons of the ventromedial medulla. The vlPAG/LPT is excited by orexin neurons. In the absence of orexin neurons, the strength of the 'REM-off' region is impaired and this facilitates transitions into the REM sleep, for example in narcolepsy.

Reproduced courtesy of Dr Patrick M. Fuller and Dr Anne Venner.

drinks. Knockdown of the adenosine 2A receptor ($A_{2A}R$) in the NAcSh completely blocks the wake-promoting actions of caffeine (Lazarus et al., 2011). Moreover, lesions of NAcSh neurons result in a ~ 25% increase in wakefulness, indicating that their functional role is to promote sleep. NAcSh neurons project to several arousal-promoting nuclei including the LH and the PB, and—with particular density—to the midbrain ventral tegmental area (VTA). It has been recently demonstrated that *dopaminergic VTA* neurons are required for maintaining normal levels of arousal since their inhibition results in increased sleep amounts and preparatory sleep behaviours such as nest-building in mice. In addition, acute activation of dopaminergic VTA terminals in the sleep-promoting nucleus accumbens (NAc) significantly decreases the latency to wake, likely through inhibition of the NAc via dopamine type 2 receptors (Eban-Rothschild et al., 2016). Lesions of the *external globus pallidus (GPe)*, another major structure of the basal ganglia, produce a 50 per cent increase in wake; hence, neurons of the GPe may also be sleep-promoting. Neurons in the GPe release GABA and project widely to the cortex and are therefore anatomically and functionally well-situated to inhibit cortical activation and bias the sleep state (Figure 5.1C).

REM sleep circuitry

In healthy humans and animals, NREM sleep precedes REM sleep and REM sleep occupies a much smaller percentage of our nightly sleep time than NREM sleep. Circuitry within the pontine brainstem has long been implicated as having 'executive' control over REM sleep. To this end, neurons of the *sublaterodorsal nucleus (SLD)* of the pontine brainstem are known to be important for REM sleep, as lesions of these neurons result in a 40 per cent decrease in REM sleep over a 24-hour period (Lu et al., 2006). From an anatomical perspective, SLD neurons send ascending projections to the *medial septum*, a brain region responsible for driving hippocampal activity that is characteristic of the REM sleep state, as well as descending projections to the ventral 'motor' horn of the *spinal cord*, where they promote muscle atonia during REM sleep. This latter connection is particularly critical for preventing humans and animals from 'acting out' their dreams. When muscle atonia fails during REM sleep, as it does in the human sleep disorder 'REM behavioural disorder', it is common for the afflicted individual and/or their bed partner to become severely injured. SLD neurons themselves are excited by inputs from cholinergic neurons (which favour the REM state) and inhibited by inputs from the *ventrolateral periaqueductal grey area (vlPAG) and the lateral pontine tegmentum (LPT)*. Predictably, lesions of the LPT/vlPAG result in a doubling of the amount of REM sleep and more frequent wake-REM transitions. Interestingly, the LPT/vlPAG is itself under reciprocal inhibitory control from SLD neurons, as well as from neurons of the *ventromedial medulla*, and possibly from *melanin-concentrating hormone (MCH)* neurons of the lateral hypothalamus. The LPT/vlPAG also receives inputs from *LH orexin* neurons, which themselves are critical for maintaining sleep–wake states. It is therefore possible that orexinergic activation of the vlPAG prevents REM sleep, and when these neurons are not active, REM is 'permitted' to occur (Figure 5.1D).

Timing of wake and sleep by the hypothalamic circadian clock

The *suprachiasmatic nuclei (SCN) of the hypothalamus* are fundamental for the mainten-ance of daily or circadian (from the Latin, *circa* (about) *dies* (days)) rhythms, including the daily sleep–wake rhythm. Studies have shown that the SCN play an important role in determining the duration, intensity, and propensity of sleep. For example, experimentally placed lesions of the SCN in monkeys and rodents result in the loss of 24-hour sleep–wake rhythms and a reduction in the amount of deep NREM sleep (Edgar et al., 1993). How the SCN clock regulates sleep timing, duration, and intensity is not fully understood, but has been conceptualised in a two-process model as an interaction between a homeostatic drive for sleep (i.e. a sleep 'pressure' or 'need' for sleep that builds during the waking day and declines exponentially during the night as we sleep) and a circadian process that is inde-pendent of sleep and waking. This model has been used to explain how humans maintain consolidated bouts of waking (~ 16 hours) and sleep (~ 8 hours) each day and night. From a circuitry standpoint, remarkably little is known about how the SCN govern timing and consolidation of sleep. One popular theory is that the SCN control, via a multi-synaptic pathway, the regulation and release of melatonin in the brain's pineal gland. Circulating levels of melatonin are about ten-fold higher during the night (in both diurnal and noc-turnal animals) and so may serve as a biological 'signal' for night. Indeed, exogenously ad-ministered melatonin in humans can promote early sleep onset and longer sleep duration.

Not sleeping enough?

The inability to sleep (generally referred to as 'insomnia') is a widespread clinical com-plaint, but the aetiology of this condition is complex and varies from patient to patient. For example, it has been suggested that neural cell loss from sleep-promoting nodes, such as the VLPO (a common pathology in the ageing population), or due to viral-induced injury (e.g. victims of the Spanish flu in the 1920s), can result in insomnia secondary to an imbalance in the arousal network—that is, the arousal influence is stronger than the sleep influence, thereby biasing the waking state. Alternatively, in many cases, insomnia may be the result of hyperactivity of wake-promoting circuitry, triggered by anxiety, de-pression, and/or stress. For example, rats exposed to a stressful stimulus show increased cellular activity in many of the arousal nodes described earlier, including the LC, TMN, and non-orexinergic (putatively GABAergic) neurons of the LH (Cano et al., 2008). This hyper-activation in turn drives the brain towards a waking state and is strong enough to overwhelm the sleep and circadian processes that would otherwise be pushing the brain towards a sleep state.

Sleeping too much?

Sleeping too much is a less frequently recorded complaint; however, it is a common occur-rence during bacterial and viral infections. For example, immune responses to pathogenic microbes produce several factors that cause an increase in NREM sleep (and decrease in REM sleep) following an infection. One such factor is the cytokine prostaglandin D2, which, through activation of receptors on the meninges of the ventral aspect of the brain, increasing extracellular adenosine, that then activates A_{2A}Rs located on neurons of the shell of the nucleus accumbens to promote sleep (Urade & Hayaishi, 2011). Understanding how immune mediators (e.g. cytokines) produce infection-induced sleep is an important and ongoing area of sleep research. Another common complaint is excessive daytime sleepiness (EDS). While EDS most commonly reflects a homeostatic response to not getting sufficient sleep during the night (i.e. staying up late to watch TV, play video games, etc.), there are a host of neuropsychiatric and neurodegenerative disorders in which EDS is a co-morbidity, such as narcolepsy with cataplexy, some forms of depression, and Parkinson's disease.

Conclusion

In the span of this brief chapter we have attempted to summarise a vast amount of experimental data with the hope of presenting a coherent description of how various neural circuits contribute to the control of sleep and arousal. One thing that remains abundantly clear is that our understanding of the neural circuitry subserving arousal states remains incomplete. For example, in almost all of the circuitries described here, very little is known about which particular inputs are important for initiating or generating state-change control. We also fully expect that other nodes and networks important for arousal-state control have yet to be elucidated. It is also remarkable to consider that it is almost impossible, by means of ablation or lesion of a single node or nucleus (with the exception of extremely large lesions of the PB or BF), to permanently and completely eliminate either wake or sleep. Two implications of this fascinating observation are that the circuitry subserving arousal-state control is highly redundant, and that the final behavioural and EEG 'outcome' is likely determined by integration of these distinct circuits by higher order brain regions. Where and how this integration occurs are key questions for future investigations.

Summary

- How and when we wake and sleep are under the control of complex neural circuitry, consisting of neuronal populations (or nodes), neurotransmitters, and pathways that form orchestrated wake- or sleep-promoting networks.
- Loss of orexin signalling—as occurs in narcolepsy and narcolepsy with cataplexy—leads to excessive daytime sleepiness, sleep attacks, and wake–REM transitions.
- Stress induces hyper-activity in arousal-promoting nodes, which may, in turn, be responsible for triggering insomnia.
- Caffeine promotes wake through antagonism of adenosine 2A receptors located on neurons within the shell of the nucleus accumbens.
- Cell damage in neurons responsible for REM atonia is a common pathology in many neurodegenerative diseases, such as Parkinson's disease, and causes REM behavioural disorder.

- ◆ Viral- or age- induced cell loss in the VLPO can lead to insomnia and/ or disrupted sleep.
- ◆ During sickness, the immune system produces prostaglandins that can increase time spent in NREM sleep and inhibit time spent in REM sleep.

References

Anaclet, C., Ferrari, L., Arrigoni, E., Bass, C. E., Saper, C. B., Lu, J. & Fuller, P. M. 2014. The GABAergic parafacial zone is a medullary slow wave sleep-promoting center. *Nature Neuroscience*, **17**(9), pp. 1217–24.

Anaclet, C., Pedersen, N. P., Ferrari, L. L., Venner, A., Bass, C. E., Arrigoni, E. & Fuller, P. M. 2015. Basal forebrain control of wakefulness and cortical rhythms. *Nature Communications*, **6**, p. 8744.

Cano, G., Mochizuki, T. & Saper, C. B. 2008. Neural circuitry of stress-induced insomnia in rats. *The Journal of Neuroscience*, **28**(40), pp. 10167–84.

Eban-Rothschild, A., Rothschild, G., Giardino, W. J., Jones, J. R. & de Lecea, L. 2016. VTA dopaminergic neurons regulate ethologically relevant sleep-wake behaviors. *Nature Neuroscience*, **19**(10), pp. 1356–66.

Edgar, D. M., Dement, W. C. & Fuller, C. A. 1993. Effect of SCN lesions on sleep in squirrel monkeys: evidence for opponent processes in sleep-wake regulation. *The Journal of Neuroscience*, **13**(3), pp. 1065–79.

Fuller, P. M., Sherman, D., Pedersen, N. P., Saper, C. B. & Lu, J. 2011. Reassessment of the structural basis of the ascending arousal system. *The Journal of Comparative Neurology*, **519**(5), pp. 933–56.

Lazarus, M., Shen, H. Y., Cherasse, Y., Qu, W. M., Huang, Z. L., Bass, C. E., Winsky-Sommerer, R., Semba, K., Fredholm, B. B., Boison, D., Hayaishi, O., Urade, Y. & Chen, J. F. 2011. Arousal effect of caffeine depends on adenosine A2A receptors in the shell of the nucleus accumbens. *The Journal of Neuroscience*, 6, **31**(27), pp. 10067–75.

Lu, J., Greco, M. A., Shiromani, P. & Saper, C. B. 2000. Effect of lesions of the ventrolateral preoptic nucleus on NREM and REM sleep. *The Journal of Neuroscience*, **20**(10), 3830–42.

Lu, J., Jhou, T. C. & Saper, C. B. 2006. Identification of wake-active dopaminergic neurons in the ventral periaqueductal gray matter. *The Journal of Neuroscience*, **26**(1), pp. 193–202.

Saper, C. B., Fuller, P. M., Pedersen, N. P., Lu, J. & Scammell, T. E. 2010. Sleep state switching. *Neuron*, **68**(6), pp. 1023–42.

Sherin, J. E., Shiromani, P. J., McCarley, R. W. & Saper, C. B. 1996. Activation of ventrolateral preoptic neurons during sleep. *Science*, **271**(5246), pp. 216–19.

Urade, Y. & Hayaishi, O. 2011. Prostaglandin D2 and sleep/wake regulation. *Sleep Medicine Reviews*, **15**(6), pp. 411–18.

Venner, A., Anaclet, C., Broadhurst, R. Y., Saper, C. B. & Fuller, P. M. 2016. A novel population of wake-promoting GABAergic neurons in the ventral lateral hypothalamus. *Current Biology*, **26**(16), pp. 2137–43.

Chapter 6

The genetics of sleep

Michelle A. Miller

Introduction

Sleep in an individual is the result of a complex interaction between his/her genes and numerous environmental characteristics. Animal studies have demonstrated that the amount, distribution, and rebound of sleep are genetically linked. From twin studies in humans it has been estimated that heritability for sleep patterns is around 44% (Partinen et al., 1983). To date, however, an underlying genetic basis for only a few sleep disorders has been established. This, in part, may be due to the complex interactions between environmental conditions and an individual's underlying genetic composition. Nevertheless, new genetic techniques may aid this search and should lead to a greater understanding of the disease pathogenesis and progression which will aid the development of new drug therapies and a more personalized medicine approach to treatment.

Genes, normal sleep regulation, and circadian rhythm

Many biological processes exhibit a circadian rhythm, which is, roughly, a 24-hour cycle in the biochemical, physiological, or behavioural processes. In mammals, the sleep–wake cycle is regulated by the sleep homeostat (a measure of an individual's time awake versus time asleep) and by the central circadian clock/oscillator which is located in the hypothalamic suprachiasmatic nucleus (SCN). The circadian clock is composed of many genes and proteins that interact together and have both positive and negative feedback loops (Leloup & Goldbeter, 2004).

Whilst circadian rhythms are endogenously generated, they can also be entrained by external cues such as daylight or feeding. Amongst healthy living people there are individuals who prefer to sleep and wake early—sometimes referred to as 'morning people', or 'larks'—and there are individuals who prefer to go to sleep later and wake up at later times during the day and are referred to as 'evening people', or 'owls'. Research in this area is ongoing, but a number of genes, including the period genes, have been identified as being important in sleep–wake regulation. Among others, the CLOCK and BMAL1 elements promote the expression of the period (PER 1, 2, and 3) and cryptochrome (CRY 1 & 2) genes, some of which have demonstrated polymorphic variation. For example, a variable-tandem–repeat polymorphism in PER3 affects human sleep structure (Parish et al., 2013). Further investigation has demonstrated that individuals with the PER3[5/5] genotype are more likely to show morning preference ('larks'), than PER3$^{4/4}$ individuals, who are evening types ('owls') (Dijk & Archer, 2010).

The importance of genetic variations in the development of sleep disorders will be discussed in the following sections. It is expected that the utilization of new genetic techniques, including genome-wide association studies (GWASs), will bring about further breakthroughs in this area or research.

Genes and sleep disorders

Much of the earlier research regarding sleep and genes was to understand the genetic basis of circadian rhythms and was mainly examined using *Drosophila* and rodent models. Studies are now being conducted in large human populations. For example, the CoLaus Study is aiming to phenotype a large adult population and study genes involved in both normal sleep regulation as well as those that may be of importance in the development of sleep disorders (Firmann et al., 2008). Most sleep disorders arise from the result of complex interactions between an individual's genetic composition and environmental factors. It would be interesting to identify and study possible genes and gene products which may contribute to sleep disorders in children as they are less likely to be influenced by the age-associated co-morbidities present in adult populations. However, there are some sleep disorders that affect certain children, and ideally, these would need to be excluded from such studies.

Sleep phase disorders

Some individuals have disorders of their circadian rhythm. In certain circumstances this may result from extrinsic factors—for example, shift-work sleep disorder, which affects people who work nights or rotating shifts. However, in other individuals there appears to be an intrinsic disorder. These individuals appear to have a much later timing of their sleep onset and have a peak period of alertness in the middle of the night. This is known as delayed sleep phase syndrome (DSPS). Other individuals have advanced sleep phase syndrome (ASPS), which causes difficulty staying awake in the evening and staying asleep in the morning. One study has shown that mutations in the human period 2 gene are responsible for an autosomal dominant form of familial ASPS (Parish et al., 2013).

Obstructive sleep apnoea

Obstructive sleep apnoea (OSA) is the most common sleep disorder and affects both adults and children. Complete or partial obstruction of the upper airway results in a number of symptoms, including snoring, sleep fragmentation, transient hypoxia, and excessive daytime sleepiness. It has been shown to have multiple effects on the body, including effects on the cardiovascular system. Many of the risk factors for OSA have a large heritable component. The apnoea–hypopnoea index (AHI) is one of the key diagnostic factors for OSA, and one study suggested that 40% of its variance could be explained by familial factor (Parish et al., 2013). Patients with OSA syndrome have elevated tumour necrosis factor-α (TNF-α) levels. The -308A TNF-α gene polymorphism, which is responsible for increased TNF-α production, is more likely to be found in individuals with OSA syndrome and their siblings than in population controls (Parish et al., 2013). Positive associations between OSA and polymorphic variants in other candidate genes, including the apolipoprotein E4 (ApoE4) gene and leptin receptor gene polymorphism (GLN223 ARG), have also been reported (Dauvilliers & Tafti, 2008; Parish et al., 2013).

Narcolepsy

A number of sleep disorders, including narcolepsy, have been associated with the human leukocyte antigen (HLA) on chromosome 6. Narcolepsy is a disabling sleep condition, and whilst believed to be genetically complex, environmental factors may also be important. Evidence from different populations has highlighted the importance of various HLA loci and combinations of different HLA alleles in determining narcolepsy susceptibility. The neuropeptide orexin (hypocretin) also appears to be important (Parish et al., 2013).

Kleine–Levin syndrome

Kleine–Levin Syndrome (KLS) is a rare disorder mainly occurring in adult males. It is characterized by recurrent hypersomnia and various behavioural abnormalities, including compulsive hyperphagia. However, the individuals normally present as entirely normal between episodes. Whilst the underlying aetiology of this disorder is not known, some familial clustering has been observed (Dauvilliers & Tafti, 2008). One study, which investigated a particular family using extensive HLA typing to characterize each family member, reported that six of the affected family members were homozygous for DQB1*02. However, two out of six of the unaffected family members were also homozygous for the same variant (BaHammam et al., 2008).

Insomnia

Four sleep disorders have been shown to arise from a single gene mutation. These include familial ASPS and a severe form of narcolepsy. The other two single-gene mutation disorders that have been characterized are forms of insomnia. Fatal familial insomnia (FFI), which is thought to arise from a mutation in a proton prion gene (Goldfarb et al., 1992), is characterized by an inability to sleep and rapidly leads to death. While a number of factors may lead to chronic primary insomnia, evidence from a family study suggests that it may also arise as a result of a single gene mutation which occurs in the GABRB3 gene (Buhr et al., 2002). Further longitudinal family studies are required to determine whether other genetic and environmental factors may be important for this condition in the general population (Dauvilliers & Tafti, 2008).

Parasomnias

Sleep disorders that involve abnormal movements, emotions, and behaviours that occur when an individual is either entering into sleep, sleeping, between sleep stages, or awaking from sleep, are generally characterized as parasomnias.

Sleepwalking

Sleepwalking often has a strong family history, which suggests that there may be an underlying genetic susceptibility possibly triggered by precipitating factors, including conditions that increase slow-wave sleep. One recent study suggested that there may be an association between a particular HLA subtype DQB1*05 and sleepwalking (Lecendreux et al., 2003).

Primary nocturnal enuresis

Primary nocturnal enuresis (PNE) is defined in a child aged 7 years or over who has never been dry at night. There is often a strong family history in PNE, and genetic linkage studies have identified a number of different chromosomal loci, which may be of importance in this condition. These suggest the presence of genetic heterogeneity and polygenetic inheritance patterns within PNE families (Dauvilliers & Tafti, 2008).

Restless legs syndrome and periodic limb movements in sleep

Restless legs syndrome (RLS) is a common sleep disorder, which is characterized by the urge to move the legs. It is often accompanied by an unpleasant sensation in the legs as well. Periodic limb movements in sleep (PLMS) is a sleep disorder where the patient moves limbs involuntarily during sleep. A number of genetic studies of these conditions have been conducted (Dauvilliers & Tafti, 2008; Parish et al., 2013). It has been concluded that whilst there is substantial evidence to support a genetic component for RLS, it is equally apparent that there is a large degree of heterogeneity within this condition. It is likely to be a polygenic disorder and may involve different sets of genes in different families or populations. Familial forms of PLMS have also been identified, and persons with a positive family history seem to have an earlier onset of symptoms as compared to those without a family history (Parish et al., 2013).

Sleep, genes, inflammation, and cardiovascular risk

Evidence for a link between short sleep and cardiovascular risk, and potential underlying biochemical and inflammatory mechanisms, is increasing (Ferrie et al., 2007; Miller et al., 2009). Diurnal rhythms have a large influence on normal cardiovascular physiology. Normal blood pressure across the diurnal cycle exhibits a 10% dip at night, followed by an increase at around the awakening time. Cardiovascular incidents, such as myocardial infarcts, are approximately three times more likely to occur in the early morning than late at night (Martino & Sole, 2009). Plasminogen activator inhibitor (PAI)-1 is a primary regulator in the fibrinolytic cascade. The level of this activator displays circadian variation, with the level peaking in the morning. This variation is believed to be under the control of the PER2 gene and its regulatory elements, CLOCK and BMAL (Martino & Sole, 2009).

A number of sleep conditions, including OSA, are associated with an increase in inflammatory markers (Parish et al., 2013), which are important in the development of cardiovascular disease (CVD). Further work is required to investigate the possibility that genetic determinants of sleep acting, for example, on the oxidative and immune pathways may be an important determinant of an individual's cardiovascular risk. The effect of potential diurnal variation on gene expression and the level of possible biomarkers for disease (e.g. CVD) needs to be fully appreciated, understood, and adjusted for, where possible (Miller et al., 2009). This is of particular importance in studies focused on the search for new disease biomarkers.

Summary

- The genetic regulation of normal sleep and sleep disorders is complex and often shows strong environmental interactions.

- There has been an increased awareness of the contribution of genetic components to the pathology of sleep disorders.

- Research in this field is expanding rapidly, and the number of sleep conditions with known underlying genetic components is growing.

- Techniques may include the use of genome-wide scanning, utilization of sleep manipulation, and the use of well-characterized families and twin studies to investigate the underlying familial components.

- The focus of genetic studies on sleep needs to be directed not only towards understanding the intrinsic biology of sleep regulation, but also towards characterizing and observing other possible phenotypic associations which may be associated with sleep.

- Proper family investigation into the rare, but heritable, fatal sleep conditions, such as fatal familial insomnia, is of paramount importance.

- Sleep conditions are observed in children as well as adults.

References

BaHammam, A. S., Gadelrab, M. O., Owais, S. M., Alswat, K. & Hamam, K. D. 2008. Clinical characteristics and HLA typing of a family with Kleine-Levin syndrome. *Sleep Medicine*, **9**(5), pp. 575–8.

Buhr, A., Bianchi, M. T., Baur, R., Courtet, P., Pignay, V., Boulenger, J. P., Gallati, S., Hinkle, D. J., Macdonald, R. L. & Sigel, E. 2002. Functional characterization of the new human GABA(A) receptor mutation beta3(R192H). *Human Genetics*, **111**(2), pp. 154–60.

Dauvilliers, Y. & Tafti, M. 2008. The genetic basis of sleep disorders. *Current Pharmaceutical Design*, **14**(32), pp. 3386–95.

Dijk, D. J. & Archer, S. N. 2010. PERIOD3, circadian phenotypes, and sleep homeostasis. *Sleep Medicine Reviews*, **14**(3), pp. 151–60.

Ferrie, J. E., Shipley, M. J., Cappuccio, F. P., Brunner, E., Miller, M. A., Kumari, M. & Marmot, M. G. 2007. A prospective study of change in sleep duration: associations with mortality in the Whitehall II cohort. *Sleep*, **30**(12), pp. 1659–66.

Firmann, M., Mayor, V., Vidal, P., Bochud, M., Pécoud, A., Hayoz, D., Paccaud, F., Preisig, M., Song, K. S., Yuan, X., Danoff, T. M., Stirnadel, H. A., Waterworth, D., Mooser, V., Waeber, G. & Vollenweider, P. 2008. The CoLaus study: a population-based study to investigate the epidemiology and genetic determinants of cardiovascular risk factors and metabolic syndrome. *BMC Cardiovascular Disorders*, **8**, p. 6.

Goldfarb, L. G., Petersen, R. B., Tabaton, M., Brown, P., LeBlanc, A. C., Montagna, P., Cortelli, P., Julien, J., Vital, C., Pendelbury, W. W., et al. 1992. Fatal familial insomnia and familial Creutzfeldt-Jakob disease: disease phenotype determined by a DNA polymorphism. *Science*, **258**, pp. 806–8.

Lecendreux, M., Bassetti, C., Dauvilliers, Y., Mayer, G., Neidhart, E. & Tafti, M. 2003. HLA and genetic susceptibility to sleepwalking. *Molecular Psychiatry*, **8**(1), pp. 114–17.

Leloup, J. C. & Goldbeter, A. 2004. Modeling the mammalian circadian clock: sensitivity analysis and multiplicity of oscillatory mechanisms. *Journal of Theoretical Biology*, **230**(4), pp. 541–62.

Martino, T. A. & Sole, M. J. 2009. Molecular time: an often overlooked dimension to cardiovascular disease. *Circulation Research*, **105**(11), pp. 1047–61.

Miller, M. A., Kandala, N. B., Kivimaki, M., Kumari, M., Brunner, E. J., Lowe, G. D., Marmot, M. G. & Cappuccio, F. P. 2009. Gender differences in the cross-sectional relationships between sleep duration and markers of inflammation: Whitehall II study. *Sleep*, **32**(7), pp. 857–64.

Parish, J. M. 2013. Genetic and immunologic aspects of sleep and sleep disorders. *Chest*, **143**(5), pp. 1489–99.

Partinen, M., Kaprio, J., Koskenvuo, M., Putkonen, P. & Langinvainio, H. 1983. Genetic and environmental determination of human sleep. *Sleep*, **6**(3), pp. 179–85.

Chapter 7

Sleep disorders: Types and approach to evaluation

Lawrence J. Epstein

Introduction

Our understanding and recognition of sleep disorders have grown tremendously since the opening of the first clinical centre dedicated to the treatment of patients with sleep disorders, the Stanford Sleep Disorders Clinic, in 1970. Once limited to passively observing people while sleeping, technology now allows us to study the functioning of the brain and other organs during sleep, improving our understanding of the problems that lead to dysfunction and illness.

The third edition of the *International Classification of Sleep Disorders* (ICSD-3) (AASM, 2014) describes over 70 sleep disorders, and 50–70 million Americans have a chronic sleep disorder (Colton, 2006). The disorders are grouped into the following general categories: *insomnia, sleep-related breathing disorders, central disorders of hypersomnolence, circadian rhythm sleep–wake disorders, parasomnias,* and *sleep-related movement disorders.* It is beyond the scope of this discussion to cover all the sleep disorders. Instead, each category will be described and the most common disorder within the category reviewed.

Insomnia

Insomnia is the most commonly reported sleep problem and the most prevalent sleep disorder. The term insomnia describes a number of disrupted sleep patterns, including difficulty getting to sleep, difficulty maintaining sleep, earlier than desired awakening, and difficulty going to bed on an appropriate schedule. For the pattern to be considered a clinical disorder, it must also result in daytime impairment.

Insomnia is categorized as either short-term or chronic insomnia depending on whether the disturbance has been present for more or less than 3 months. A precipitating cause, a particular stressor, can often be identified. Short-term insomnia may resolve itself with no intervention, but clinical intervention may be required to prevent development of chronic insomnia.

Chronic insomnia occurs in about 10% of the population. Daytime impairment includes fatigue, sleepiness, concentration or memory impairment, or impaired social, family, or academic performance. Insomnia is associated with increased work-related accidents, increased absenteeism and presenteeism, impaired work performance, and increased risk of developing depression and anxiety (Sarsour, 2011). Difficulty with sleep is one of the biggest factors in poor academic performance in college students.

Insomnia develops from a series of predisposing, precipitating, and perpetuating factors (Spielman, 1987). Predisposing factors include biological factors such as the elevated metabolic and stress hormone levels found in insomnia patients, psychological factors such as tendency to worry or ruminate excessively, and social factors such as a disruptive bed partner. A precipitating factor, such as a high stress situation, can trigger one of the insomnia patterns. Once the disrupted pattern is established, perpetuating factors prevent the person from re-establishing a good sleep pattern. For example, use of caffeine to combat fatigue from sleep loss can further interfere with sleep.

There are several subtypes of insomnia, and patients often demonstrate multiple types. Patients with *psychophysiological insomnia* demonstrate heightened arousal responses and learned, or conditioned, associations to the sleep situation that interfere with their ability to get to sleep. Such associations often manifest as excessive worrying about being able to sleep and annoyance and frustration while in bed unable to sleep. In *paradoxical insomnia*, the person markedly overestimates the time spent awake during the night. Insomnia related to *inadequate sleep hygiene* occurs when the person engages in behaviours that disrupt or interfere with sleep, such as having an irregular sleep–wake schedule or performing mentally or physically arousing activities (exercising, stimulating games, emotional conflict) in close proximity to bedtime or while in bed.

Insomnia can present at any time, including childhood. *Behavioural insomnia of childhood* results from poor sleep training or poor limit setting by parents. *Idiopathic insomnia* describes an almost lifelong problem with sleep, often going back to infancy or early childhood.

Insomnia due to a mental disorder, medical condition, drug, or substance describes sleep disturbance related to other conditions. There is a bi-directional relationship between mental disorders and insomnia. Patients with depression and anxiety frequently develop insomnia, and having insomnia increases the risk of later developing depression or anxiety.

Identifying predisposing, precipitating, and perpetuating factors and characterizing involved subtypes are the first steps in addressing the problem. There are three primary approaches to the treatment of chronic insomnia: correction of secondary causes, behavioural therapy, and pharmacotherapy. Combination therapy using two, or all three, approaches is often required.

Cognitive-behavioural therapy for insomnia (CBTi) applies an array of behavioural techniques to correct predisposing and perpetuating factors. *Sleep restriction* reduces the time spent in bed to consolidate the sleep period and improve sleep efficiency. *Stimulus control therapy* replaces sleep routines that become cues for anxiety about sleep and lead to arousal. A variety of *relaxation therapies* (e.g. progressive muscle relaxation, biofeedback, meditation, imagery training) may be helpful when anxiety and stress are contributors to the insomnia. *Cognitive restructuring therapy* alters excessive preoccupation with sleep, disruptive attitudes and beliefs, and misattributions that hinder sleep. *Sleep hygiene education* teaches how to identify and change the lifestyle and environmental factors that interfere with sleep. Comparison studies show that sleep restriction and stimulus control therapy are the most effective as monotherapies, but that CBTi, which combines multiple techniques, results in the greatest improvement (Schutte-Rodin, 2008).

Pharmacotherapy for insomnia should be considered when the patient is significantly distressed or impaired by their insomnia, and preferably after a trial with CBTi and resolution of secondary causes. When used, medications should be given in the lowest effective dosage for the shortest period of time. Whenever possible, patients should receive CBTi during pharmacotherapy.

The first-line drugs are the benzodiazepine receptor agonists (BzRAs). They are effective for short-term and chronic insomnia and safe when used appropriately. The medications in this class are differentiated by their time to onset of action, length of half-life and selectivity for the subtypes of the alpha receptor of the γ-aminobutyric acid (GABA) A receptor complex. Less selective agents are more likely to have muscle relaxant effects, anxiolytic actions, and side-effects. Medication selection should be individualized to the patient's insomnia pattern and subtype. For instance, a quick-acting, short half-life agent is better suited for sleep-onset insomnia, while a medium half-life agent would be better for sleep maintenance problems.

Sedating antidepressants are the most commonly prescribed sleeping medications, though not specifically approved for insomnia. Comparative trials with the BzRAs have not been conducted. Melatonin receptor agonists are approved for the treatment of sleep-onset insomnia. They effectively shift the circadian sleep phase, but are weak sedating agents. Over-the-counter sleep medications contain sedating antihistamines. Short-term improvement in sleep has been demonstrated with such medications, but long-term efficacy is unknown.

The newest sleeping medication is an orexin receptor antagonist. Orexin, also called hypocretin, is a central nervous system neuropeptide that promotes wakefulness. By blocking the binding of orexin peptides, the medication blocks the wakefulness signal, allowing sleep. It improves both sleep onset and sleep maintenance, but comparative data with other medications is not available.

Comparative trials of CBTi vs BzRAs show similar short-term effectiveness for both sleep-onset and sleep-maintenance problems, with CBTi producing longer lasting improvement. Combined therapy with pharmacotherapy and CBTi may be beneficial for some patients, but no consistent advantage or disadvantage over CBTi alone has been shown.

Sleep-related breathing disorders

These disorders do not share a common mechanism, but rather, are all the result of the physiological changes that occur when changing from the waking to the sleeping state. The abnormalities in respiration result in metabolic derangements such as hypoxaemia and hypercapnia, and lead to fragmented, non-restful sleep. This category includes: the *obstructive sleep apnoea* (OSA) disorder, in which the airway is blocked; the *central sleep apnoea* syndromes, characterized by an open airway but reduced or no effort to breathe; and the *sleep-related hypoventilation* disorders, in which anatomical, congenital, or central nervous system problems result in insufficient ventilation (AASM, 2014). This section will focus on OSA, the most common disorder.

OSA is prevalent, presenting with awake symptoms in 2%–7% of the general population, with higher rates in males, older individuals, and the obese population. Patients present with complaints of snoring, daytime sleepiness, and witnessed breathing pauses during sleep. Other symptoms include sensations of choking, morning headaches, nocturia, and memory and concentration problems. OSA patients have a 2- to 7-fold increase in motor vehicle crashes.

The symptoms and associated health problems are the consequence of the pathophysiological events that occur during obstruction. OSA patients have a smaller upper airway than those with no OSA. Airway patency is maintained during wakefulness by a wake-state driven compensatory increase in the neurological stimulation of the upper airway dilator muscles. This increased muscle tone is lost when the person falls asleep; the muscles relax and the airway collapses, blocking air flow. During blockage, oxygen levels drop and carbon dioxide levels increase, both prompting greater and greater efforts to breathe. The airway remains blocked until the struggle to breathe triggers an arousal from sleep, which reinstates the wake stimulation of the muscles, opening the airway. The arousal increases sympathetic activity throughout the body, with increases in heart rate and blood pressure. When the airway is open, breathing resumes and the blood–gas abnormalities correct. With equilibrium restored, the person falls back to sleep, muscle tone drops, and the airway collapses. This cycle can be repeated hundreds of times each night.

The repetitive awakenings lead to daytime sleepiness. The arousal-triggered increase in sympathetic activity and apnoea-related hypoxaemia cause vasoconstriction and elevated blood pressure. Over time, systemic hypertension develops. As a result, OSA is a risk factor for the development of hypertension, stroke, coronary artery disease, congestive heart failure, atrial fibrillation, and increased mortality. OSA also increases the risk of development of type 2 diabetes, independent of the association of OSA with obesity.

OSA is diagnosed by demonstrating an abnormal number of obstructive events during an overnight sleep study in the presence of symptoms and risk factors. Two types of sleep studies are used to diagnose OSA. Overnight polysomnography (PSG) is performed in a sleep laboratory and records sleep stages, respiratory effort, air flow, heart rate, limb movement, snoring, and oxyhaemoglobin saturation. Home sleep apnoea tests are limited channel studies that measure respiratory effort, air flow, and oxyhaemoglobin saturation, but are quite sensitive for patients with moderate-to-severe OSA. The presence of > 15 obstructive events/hours of sleep is diagnostic of moderate-to-severe OSA, while 5–15 obstructive events/hour in the face of clinical symptoms is diagnostic of mild OSA.

There are several modalities of treatment for OSA: medical, surgical, and behavioural. The first-line therapy for mild, moderate, and severe OSA is positive airway pressure (PAP) therapy, which utilizes an air blower to splint open the airway and prevent collapse.

There are several types of PAP devices. The most common is a continuous positive airway pressure (CPAP) device, which delivers a constant pressure throughout inspiration and expiration. A bi-level (BPAP) device varies the pressure during the different phases of the respiratory cycle, with higher pressures required during inspiration. Autotitrating (APAP) devices adjust the PAP delivered to keep the airway open. The device detects changes in upper airway resistance and patency and responds by increasing or decreasing pressure. Though highly effective, the major limitation to PAP therapy is patient acceptance and tolerance.

Oral appliances that move the lower jaw or base of the tongue forward, preventing airway collapse, are an alternative OSA treatment. The devices are successful at eliminating OSA in 50%–70% of cases of mild to moderate OSA. Behavioural therapies include weight loss in obese individuals, positional therapy to prevent supine sleep in those with supine-only OSA, and avoidance of alcohol and medications with muscle relaxant properties.

Multiple surgical procedures have been developed to increase the size of the upper airway at the site of collapse. These include nasal turbinectomy and septoplasty, removal of the uvula and part of the soft palate, and tongue reduction. Such procedures are successful at eliminating OSA in 40%–55% of cases. Jaw reconstruction surgery, which advances the mandible and maxilla, has a success rate of up to 90% and tracheostomy is 100% effective, though both are not typically first-line surgeries. Bariatric surgery, through weight loss, typically improves OSA as well. The newest procedure is genioglossal nerve stimulation surgery, in which an electrode placed around the genioglossal nerve stimulates airway dilator muscles during inspiration, preventing airway collapse. Overall success rate, long-term effectiveness, and proper patient selection are still under evaluation.

OSA should be approached as a chronic disease requiring long-term management. Patients need to be educated on the patho-physiology, risk factors, natural history, and clinical consequences of OSA, and the treatment selected for a particular patient will depend on OSA severity, contributing risk factors, and patient preference (Epstein, 2009).

Central disorders of hypersomnolence

Disorders of hypersomnolence, or excessive sleepiness, impair the person's ability to be alert and function at peak performance during the major waking episodes of the day. As a result, cognitive abilities, work performance, and learning are impaired, and excessively sleepy people are at risk for both workplace and motor vehicle accidents. This grouping comprises disorders that cause excessive sleepiness but are not caused by fragmented sleep or misaligned circadian rhythms (AASM, 2014).

The most common disorder in this group is *insufficient sleep syndrome*, caused by volitional failure to obtain the amount of sleep required to maintain alertness and wakefulness. There is great individual variability in sleep need, but a recent consensus statement recommended that adults should regularly get at least 7 hours of sleep per night to promote optimal health. Sleeping < 7 hours has been associated with adverse health outcomes, including obesity, diabetes, hypertension, heart disease, stroke, depression, and increased risk of death (Watson, 2015). The other disorders in this group include: *Kleine–Levin syndrome; idiopathic hypersomnia; hypersomnia due to a medical disorder, medication, substance, or psychiatric disorder;* and *narcolepsy* (discussed below).

Narcolepsy is characterized by excessive daytime sleepiness and features of rapid eye movement (REM) sleep dissociation. The person experiences episodic attacks of profound sleepiness on top of a background of chronic sleepiness. The sleep attacks can occur multiple times a day; are difficult to resist; cause concentration, learning, and memory impairment; and increase the risk of motor vehicle accidents.

REM sleep is characterized by the rapid eye movements that give the stage its name, dreaming, muscle atonia to prevent dream-associated movement, and a high-frequency, low-voltage EEG (electroencephalogram) pattern. REM sleep dissociation is defined as the occurrence of these features during wakefulness or other stages of sleep. *Cataplexy* is the occurrence of muscle atonia during wakefulness, resulting in uncontrollable muscle weakness, which can range from knee buckling, to head drooping, to full-body weakness and a drop attack.

When the atonia occurs just as the person is falling asleep or waking up it is called *sleep paralysis*, which the patient can experience as a terrifying inability to move or speak. Visual and auditory hallucinations, called *hypnagogic hallucinations*, can occur at the onset of, or wakening from, sleep and represent dreaming imagery occurring during the transition between wake and sleep.

The primary diagnostic tool is the multiple sleep latency test (MSLT), a series of four to five naps every 2 hours during day. The MSLT quantifies sleepiness by measuring the time to fall asleep and records evidence of REM dissociation. Hypersomnolence is defined as an average time to fall asleep (mean sleep latency) of < 8 minutes on all naps. REM sleep typically occurs in the latter portions of the night and not during short naps, so the appearance of REM periods on the MSLT is atypical.

The diagnosis of narcolepsy requires symptoms of sleepiness and REM dissociation and a demonstration of hypersomnolence by objective testing. A mean sleep latency of < 8 minutes plus two or more REM periods during the MSLT are diagnostic of narcolepsy, with most narcoleptics averaging under 3 minutes. When cataplexy is present, the disorder is labelled narcolepsy type 1, while narcolepsy type 2 is characterized by the sleepiness and MSLT findings without cataplexy.

Narcolepsy type 1 is caused by the loss of hypocretin-producing cells in the hypothalamus, resulting in low levels of hypocretin (also called orexin) in the cerebral spinal fluid (CSF). Hypocretin is a component of wake-promoting cortical neuronal systems. Hypocretin deficiency results in loss of sleep–wake stability with subsequent unstable transitions between wakefulness, non-rapid eye movement (NREM) sleep, and REM sleep (Chow, 2016). This manifests clinically as abnormal daytime sleepiness with sleep attacks and cataplexy. A strong association with HLA DQB1*0602 suggests a possible autoimmune mechanism for the cell loss. A CSF hypocretin level of < 110 pg/ml along with sleepiness is also diagnostic of narcolepsy type 1 and is found in 90%–95% of narcoleptics with cataplexy.

Patients with narcolepsy type 2 are excessively sleepy and have similar MSLT findings, but do not have cataplexy, and their hypocretin levels are > 110 pg/ml. Sleep paralysis and hypnogogic hallucinations may be present. The aetiology of narcolepsy type 2 is unclear.

Treatment for both types of narcolepsy is directed at managing symptoms—predominantly excessive sleepiness. Stimulant medications are the mainstay of treatment. Options include amphetamine-derivative drugs, central nervous system wake-promoting agents, and caffeine. Sodium oxybate was originally used to treat cataplexy, but has also been shown to reduce sleepiness and may be used as monotherapy for both. Other anti-cataplexy medications include the tricyclic antidepressants, selective serotonin re-uptake inhibitors, and venlafaxine.

Narcolepsy is another chronic disorder requiring lifelong management. Patient support and education are important in helping individuals deal with the impact of the disorder.

Circadian rhythm sleep–wake disorders

Circadian rhythms are endogenous biological rhythms controlled by the master pacemaker in the suprachiasmatic nucleus of the anterior hypothalamus, and include the timing of the sleep–wake cycle. The rhythms are near 24 hours in duration to synchronize with the earth's light–dark cycle. The circadian phase is synchronized, or entrained, with the local time by timing of light exposure. For most people, the circadian sleep phase occurs during the night and early morning hours, but there is individual variability to the start of the sleep phase, ranging from early evening to early morning. For optimal sleep length and quality, the sleep period should match the timing of the sleep phase of the circadian rhythm.

Circadian disorders occur from mistiming of the internal rhythm with the sleep–wake cycle followed by the individual. This can occur when the person's desired work, school, or social schedule doesn't align with their internal sleep phase, as in *shift-work disorder, advanced sleep–wake phase disorder,* and *delayed sleep–wake phase disorder* (DSWPD). Inability to entrain to the ambient light–dark cycle can occur owing to an inability to sense light, as in *non-24-hour sleep–wake rhythm disorder,* seen commonly in blind individuals, or functional abnormalities in the clock, as seen in *irregular sleep–wake rhythm disorder.* Difficulty tolerating the mismatch of the circadian cycle and ambient schedule after multi-time-zone travel is the basis for *jet lag disorder* (AASM, 2014). DSWPD is described below.

Patients with DSWPD have a delay in the timing of their major sleep period, usually 2 hours or more, compared to their desired sleep time or to the time required by their work or school schedule. They typically present with complaints of difficulty getting to sleep or difficulty getting up at their desired time. Their sleep is normal if they follow the schedule dictated by their internal rhythm. They will often report being late to school or work because of inability to get up on time, and are sleepy during the day from not getting sufficient sleep. This can lead to poor work performance, low school grades, job termination, or disciplinary measures for missing school classes.

The delayed sleep pattern typically begins in adolescence and is a chronic pattern lasting until late in life, when the circadian clock naturally advances as part of the ageing process. The delay in the sleep phase can be exacerbated behaviourally through volitional sleep delay for the social activities that accompany adolescence and early adulthood, or by exposure to light in the evening, which further delays the internal clock.

The diagnosis of DSWPD is made when symptoms have lasted for more than 3 months and there is evidence of a delayed cycle either by sleep log or actigraphy or by measurement of a delayed dim light melatonin onset. A sleep study is not necessary except to demonstrate the absence of another sleep disorder.

Treatment falls into two categories: adjusting the work/school/social schedule to the circadian phase, or advancing the circadian sleep phase. The sleep phase can be advanced by applying light at the appropriate time, following the nadir of the core body temperature, or taking exogenous melatonin in the evening a few hours before the onset of secretion of endogenous melatonin, which typically occurs 2–3 hours before habitual bedtime. Once the cycle is shifted, the person must maintain the new schedule to avoid reverting to the natural schedule.

Parasomnias

Parasomnias are undesirable behaviours during sleep that can cause sleep fragmentation, injuries, and social distress to the patient and their bed partner. The disorders are categorized according to the stage of sleep during which they occur—either REM-related or NREM-related (AASM, 2014).

The NREM parasomnias are partial arousal disorders. The person arouses from the deeper stages of NREM sleep, and engages in strange behaviours, but does not achieve full alertness. Almost any conceivable behaviour has been described, including walking, talking, eating, cooking, driving, and sexual behaviour. The person is often difficult to awaken, but if awakened, has little recall of the event. The NREM parasomnias occur commonly in childhood, and typically resolve on their own, but may recur later, sometimes triggered by stress, illness, or medications. The primary clinical consequence is sleep disruption and potential for injury when ambulating while not fully alert.

The REM parasomnias involve disruption of the typical REM features. Repeated *nightmares* (disturbing and well-remembered dreams) can disrupt sleep and make it difficult to return to sleep, causing psychological distress. *Sleep paralysis* is the continuation of REM sleep atonia into wakefulness. One of the most intriguing parasomnias is *REM sleep behaviour disorder* (RBD), in which the REM muscle atonia is not complete and the person exhibits abnormal behaviours that represent acting out their dreams.

Whereas the NREM parasomnias do not represent significant neuropathology, RBD may represent signs of neurodegenerative disease and has been associated with Parkinson's disease and Lewy body dementia. Some antidepressant medications can also trigger RBD (Howell, 2015).

Treatment suppresses behaviours in patients at risk for injury to themselves or others. The first step is making the sleep environment safe in the event of the patient getting out of bed. Pharmacotherapy with BzRAs is effective in both REM and NREM parasomnias.

Tricyclic antidepressants may also be used, and melatonin has been effective in some RBD cases.

Sleep-related movement disorders

These disorders are characterized by stereotyped movements that disturb sleep or its onset, including *sleep-related bruxism, leg cramps, myoclonus,* and *rhythmic movement disorder* (AASM, 2014). Most common is periodic limb movement disorder (PLMD), which occurs in about 8% of adults. PLMD patients demonstrate recurrent episodes of repetitive limb movements that occur in a stereotypical fashion, cause sleep fragmentation, and lead to daytime sleepiness or cognitive or behavioural impairment. The limb movements (mostly legs but can occur in the arms) are recorded on PSG.

PLMD is often associated with another movement disorder, the *restless legs syndrome* (RLS), which is a sensorimotor disorder that causes awake symptoms but interferes with getting to sleep or staying asleep. Patients report an irresistible urge to move their legs, typically worse during inactivity, occurring predominantly in the evening or night and relieved by movement. RLS occurs in 5%–10% of adults, and most also demonstrate periodic limb movements of sleep. Risk factors for RLS include medications (antihistamine, antidepressants), pregnancy, renal failure, and iron deficiency.

Treatment for RLS and PLMD is indicated when sleep is disrupted and daytime symptoms occur. Iron replacement for serum ferritin < 50–70 ug/L may diminish symptoms. First-line therapy is typically dopamine agonists. Other effective agents include alpha-2-delta agonists, BzRAs, and opioids (Mackie, 2015).

An approach to sleep disorders

Patients don't present with a complaint of, 'I have REM sleep behaviour disorder'; rather, they have symptoms of disturbed sleep. Typically, they have one of three complaints: ' I can't sleep', 'I can't stay awake', or 'Something strange happens at night'. These symptoms guide the clinical evaluation and suggest particular disorders (Table 7.1).

Table 7.1 Guide to identifying sleep disorders by presenting complaint

Presenting complaint	Suspected sleep disorders
'I can't sleep'	Insomnia, circadian rhythm disturbances (shift work, jet lag, delayed sleep–wake phase disorder), restless legs syndrome
'I can't stay awake'	Insufficient sleep/sleep deprivation, sleep-related breathing disorders (obstructive sleep apnoea, central sleep apnoea), periodic limb movement disorder, central disorders of hypersomnolence, circadian rhythm disturbances (advanced sleep–wake phase disorder, delayed sleep–wake phase disorder, shift work, jet lag)
'Strange things happen at night'	Parasomnias (REM-related, NREM-related), restless legs syndrome

Reproduced courtesy of the author.

Summary

◆ Sleep disorders are common, with over 70 described sleep disorders that disrupt the sleep of an estimated 50–70 million Americans.

◆ Sleep disorders disrupt the health, cognitive, and restorative benefits of sleep.

◆ The different disorders fit in the broad categories of: insomnia, sleep-related breathing disorders, central disorders of hypersomnolence, circadian rhythm sleep–wake disorders, parasomnias, and sleep-related movement disorders.

◆ Insomnia is the most common sleep disorder, with chronic insomnia affecting about 10% of the population, and includes difficulty getting to sleep, difficulty maintaining sleep, earlier than desired awakening, and difficulty going to bed on an appropriate schedule.

◆ Sleep-related breathing disorders can be due to obstruction of the airway, irregular breathing patterns with an open airway, or hypoventilation.

◆ Narcolepsy is characterized by excessive daytime sleepiness and features of rapid eye movement (REM) sleep dissociation, including muscle weakness (cataplexy), sleep paralysis, and hypnagogic hallucinations.

◆ Circadian rhythm disorders occur from mistiming of the internal rhythm with the sleep–wake cycle followed by the individual, and can be due to advanced or delayed shifting of the sleep phase or from external causes such as shift work or multi-time-zone travel.

◆ Movement disorders may be specific types of movements, such as in periodic limb disorder of sleep or rhythmic movement disorder, or may be more generalized movements as seen with the parasomnias, which can be REM sleep-related or non-rapid eye movement (NREM) sleep-related.

◆ The suspected sleep disorder and subsequent sleep evaluation are determined by the type of initial complaint.

References

American Academy of Sleep Medicine (AASM). 2014. *International Classification of Sleep Disorders.* 3rd ed. Darien, IL: American Academy of Sleep Medicine.

Chow, M. & Cao, M. 2016. The hypocretin/orexin system in sleep disorders: preclinical insights and clinical progress. *Nature and Science of Sleep*, **8**(3), pp. 81–6.

Colton, H. R. & Altevogt, B. M. eds. 2006. Sleep disorders and sleep deprivation: An unmet public health problem. Washington DC: Institute of Medicine, National Academies Press.

Epstein, L. J., Kristo, D., Strollo, P. J., Friedman, N., Malhotra, A., Patil, S. P., Ramar, K., Rogers, R., Schwab, R. J., Weaver, E. M., Weinstein, M. D; Adult Obstructive Sleep Apnea Task Force of the American Academy of Sleep Medicine. 2009. Clinical guideline for the evaluation, management and long-term care of obstructive sleep apnea in adults. *Journal of Clinical Sleep Medicine*, **5**(3), pp. 263–76.

Howell, M. J. & Schenck, C. H. 2015. Rapid eye movement sleep behavior disorder and neurodegenerative disease. *JAMA Neurology*, **72**(6), pp. 707–12.

Mackie, S. & Winkelman, J. W. 2015. Long-term treatment of restless legs syndrome (RLS): an approach to management of worsening symptoms, loss of efficacy, and augmentation. *CNS Drugs*, **29**(5), pp. 351–7.

Sarsour, K., Kalsekar, A., Swindle, R., Foley, K. & Walsh, J. K. 2011. The association between insomnia severity and healthcare and productivity costs in a health plan sample. *Sleep*, **34**(4), pp. 443–50.

Schutte-Rodin, S., Broch, L., Buysse, D., Dorsey, C. & Sateia, M. 2008. Clinical guideline for the evaluation and management of chronic insomnia in adults. *Journal of Clinical Sleep Medicine*, **4**(5), pp. 487–504.

Spielman, A. J., Caruso, L. & Glovinsky, P. 1987. A behavioral perspective on insomnia. *The Psychiatric Clinics of North America*, **10**, pp. 541–53.

Watson, N. F., Badr, M. S., Belenky, G., Bliwise, D. L., Buxton, O. M., Buysse, D., Dinges, D. F., Gangwisch, J., Grandner, M. A., Kushida, C., Malhotra, R. K., Martin, J. L., Patel, S. R., Quan, S. F. & Tasali, E. 2015. Recommended amount of sleep for a healthy adult: a joint consensus statement of the American Academy of Sleep Medicine and Sleep Research Society. *Sleep*, **38**(6), pp. 843–4.

Part 2

Health

Chapter 8

Sleep and cardio-metabolic disease

Francesco P. Cappuccio and Michelle A. Miller

Introduction

We spend about a third of our life asleep. We spend more time asleep as babies and children and then generally settle into a pattern of 7–8 hours per night. Sufficient sleep is necessary for optimal daytime functioning, performance, and wellbeing, yet the amount of sleep that people get varies greatly.

The quantity and quality of sleep show secular trends alongside changes in modern society that require longer hours of work, more shift work, and '24/7' availability and use of commodities. These changes have reduced the average duration of sleep and modified the patterns of sleep across westernized populations, with increased reporting of fatigue, tiredness, and excessive daytime sleepiness. Data published from the National Sleep Foundation in 2005 reported a significant decline in the average duration of sleep of Americans over the last 100 years, with a loss of more than 2 hours per night, from the average 9.0 hours per night in 1910 to the average 6.8 hours per night reported in 2005. This sleep curtailment has been attributed by many to mainly lifestyle changes.

Sleep and self-reported ill-health

Epidemiological studies of self-reported sleep and health status began to appear about 50 years ago. However, in the last 20 years there has been an explosion of population science on the relationship between sleep quantity and quality as well as a variety of health outcomes, and the implications for public health have become apparent (Cappuccio et al., 2010a). An exploratory study using an anonymous questionnaire probing self-reported sleep and ill-health in over 17,000 college students, aged 17–30 years, from 27 non-health-related universities from 24 countries, showed that short sleep durations (< 7 hours per night) were associated with poorer self-rated health in men and women, while longer sleep durations were not related to poorer self-rated health (Steptoe et al., 2006). Countries with the shortest sleep duration had the worst self-rated health (all in Far East Asia), with 30–40 per cent of ill-health reported in Japan and South Korea, and 20–30 per cent in Thailand and Taiwan. These results clearly do not imply a causal relationship but point to a new interest in the health and social implications of sleep deprivation and the potential importance for public health.

Short sleep and obesity

In the last few decades there has been a significant increase in the prevalence of obesity worldwide; the World Health Organization has declared it a global epidemic. The rise in obesity has been paralleled by a steady constant reduction in the average sleep time, as indicated by the results of national surveys in the USA over the last century. The 'inverse' parallel trends have sparked a new interest in exploring the possible connection between these two distinct, and apparently independent, patterns.

Children and adolescents

Obesity in childhood has reached epidemic proportions in recent years and is a cause of physical and psychological problems, including low self-esteem. It often continues into adulthood, where it causes major morbidity, disability, and premature death, including type 2 diabetes and cardiovascular disease. Several studies have reported associations between short sleep duration and the risk of obesity in children and adolescents, with increased estimated risk as high as 90 per cent (Cappuccio et al., 2008). The early studies have been predominantly cross-sectional—that is, they measured duration of sleep and presence of obesity at the same time point—and therefore, whilst suggestive of possible relationships, were unable to support a cause–effect association. In other words, their results could have been consistent with two hypotheses: that a reduced duration of sleep could be the cause of obesity, or, on the contrary, that obesity was the main cause of reduced sleep (Figure 8.1). Both explanations are plausible. It is important, therefore, to ascertain whether the reduced duration of sleep (the exposure of interest) preceded

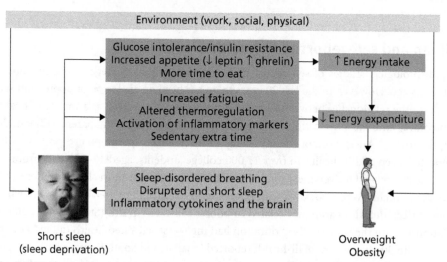

Fig. 8.1 Bi-directional model possibly explaining the associations between short sleep duration and obesity.

Reproduced from Cappuccio FP and Miller MA. Editorials: Is prolonged lack of sleep associated with obesity? *British Medical Journal*, Volume 342: d3306, copyright © 2011, with permission from BMJ Publishing Group Ltd.

the development of obesity (the outcome of interest). To address the temporal sequence whereby the 'exposure' of interest should precede the 'outcome' to support a link of 'causality', prospective longitudinal studies in children have shown that short duration of sleep may indeed precede the development of overweight or obesity, in support of a plausible causal link between short duration of sleep and the development of obesity. The potential public health implications of a causal association would be far reaching. However, whilst highly encouraging, these studies had limitations in that sleep assessment had often been based on parental reports or self-reports rather than on direct measurements, and body mass index had been the main outcome measure of obesity. More recently, however, more objective measures of sleep—using actigraphy—and more specific measures of adiposity (fat mass vs lean body mass) seem to confirm the association originally described.

Adults

Short sleep is also associated with the risk of obesity in cross-sectional studies of adults (approx. 55 per cent increased risk). However, prospective studies are less clear in establishing the temporal sequence, and further studies are still ongoing. One reason offered to explain why the prospective association is less clear is that, with time, additional more powerful factors (physical inactivity, overfeeding) intervene, masking the effect of sleep deprivation in the determination of weight gain.

How would short duration of sleep cause obesity?

There are several lines of evidence to suggest plausible mechanisms. In short-term, severe sleep curtailment experiments in healthy volunteers, sleep curtailment causes an increase in energy intake and a reduction in energy expenditure through activation of hormonal responses that regulate appetite and energy balance. During sleep deprivation there are reciprocal changes in leptin, a hormone produced by fat cells (adipocytes) which regulates energy stores and satiety, and ghrelin, a hormone produced by the stomach which enhances appetite. These two hormones regulate hunger and satiety. In normal circumstances, when energy stores are low and the stomach is empty, leptin falls and ghrelin increases to stimulate energy intake and appetite. Conversely, when the body has accumulated sufficient energy through food, leptin increases and ghrelin falls. During sleep deprivation this system is activated so that leptin is suppressed and ghrelin is stimulated, determining hunger, increased appetite, and greater energy intake and storage in adipocytes with concomitant reduction in energy expenditure (Spiegel et al., 2004; Taheri et al., 2004). These responses to sleep deprivation, if sustained over a longer period of time, would facilitate weight gain. Sleeping less would also give people more time to eat and to engage in other sedentary activities, as exemplified by children and adolescents who like to stay up late to play on their computer or watch TV or to interact with social networks whilst snacking.

In principle, the associations seen between sleep deprivation and overweight or obesity are open to the possibility of a 'reverse causality' pathway, whereby obesity causes short or disrupted sleep (or both) because of breathing problems at night and the effect of inflammatory markers on the brain's regulation of the circadian rhythm (Figure 8.1). The results of controlled intervention studies in healthy volunteers, the results of prospective associations between short sleep duration and weight gain, and the compelling evidence on other metabolic effects lend support to the first 'causal hypothesis'.

Short sleep, glucose metabolism, and diabetes

Type 2 diabetes (the commonest form of diabetes in the world) is a chronic condition characterized by the inability of the body to utilize glucose from the circulation (glucose intolerance), with the result of high circulating levels of glucose in the bloodstream (hyperglycaemia). This is caused either by a resistance of the peripheral tissues (especially muscle) to the action of the hormone insulin to take up glucose into the cell (insulin resistance), or by the lack of appropriate production of insulin from the pancreas in response to a glucose load. One of the most important risk factors for the development of type 2 diabetes is overweight or obesity. The latter is characterized by an increasing degree of glucose intolerance due to insulin resistance, eventually leading to overt type 2 diabetes. Diabetes is one of the most powerful, though preventable, causes of cardiovascular diseases (i.e. coronary heart disease, stroke, and kidney disease).

Short sleep and glucose metabolism

Short-term, acute, laboratory, and cross-sectional observational studies indicate that disturbed or reduced sleep is associated with glucose intolerance, insulin resistance, reduced acute insulin response to glucose, and a reduction in the disposition index, thus predisposing individuals to type 2 diabetes (Spiegel et al., 2009). Moreover, the same metabolic dysregulations can be observed in association with disruptions in sleep quality (Spiegel et al., 2009). These acute observations are fully reversible when sleep quantity and quality are reversed. Therefore, the effects of acute, short-term sleep deprivation or disruption are reversible. Yet, many individuals believe they adapt to chronic sleep loss easily, or that recovery requires only a single extended sleep episode. This is not the case. The cumulative detrimental effects of sustained and prolonged chronic sleep loss (deprivation) are not reversed, so that prolonged lifestyle habits of sleep curtailment may lead to long-term adverse health and safety consequences (Cohen et al., 2010). Finally, prolonged sleep restriction with concurrent circadian disruption decreases resting metabolic rate and increases post-prandial plasma glucose (from inadequate insulin secretion) (Buxton et al., 2012). So, sleeping less and at the wrong time of the circadian cycle has compounding negative effects on glucose and insulin metabolism.

This area of research has produced so far the most compelling and convincing evidence of the direct influence of sleep on metabolic, as well as genetic, pathways. In the first clinical study linking sleep restriction to an alteration of a molecular metabolic pathway, the authors studied seven healthy volunteers in a randomized crossover trial of 4 days of sleep deprivation (4.5 hours per night) and 4 days of normal sleep (8.5 hours per night). They monitored the stages of sleep with polysomnography, and adherence to bedtime with actigraphy. Caloric intake and meals were kept constant throughout the study. At the end of each period the participants underwent an intravenous glucose tolerance test (IVGTT)—to measure total body insulin sensitivity—and a subcutaneous abdominal fat biopsy to isolate adipocytes. The researchers then exposed the adipocytes 'in vitro' to incremental insulin concentrations to measure the ability of insulin to increase the phosphorylation of Akt, an important step in the insulin-signalling pathway (Broussard et al., 2012). The results show that sleep deprivation is associated with a 30% reduction in the phosphorylation of Akt, indicating reduced peripheral insulin response. This was paralleled by an expected reduction in total body insulin sensitivity. These results substantially challenge the traditional views that the primary purpose of sleep is confined to restorative effects on the central nervous system, pointing to a much wider influence of sleep on bodily functions, including metabolism, adipose tissue, cardiovascular function, and possibly more.

To further this concept there is evidence, using gene transcriptome analysis, that sleep restriction can up- and down-regulate the expression of genes mainly associated with not only circadian rhythms and sleep homeostasis (rather expected), but also with those involved in oxidative stress and metabolism (Möller-Levet et al., 2013).

Short sleep and diabetes

From the experimental data discussed, we can summarize as follows: in *short-term, acute*, laboratory, and cross-sectional studies, disturbed or reduced sleep is associated with glucose intolerance, insulin resistance, reduced acute insulin response to glucose and a reduction in the disposition index, reduced peripheral insulin response, and up- and down-regulation of the expression of genes involved in metabolic pathways, all predisposing factors to the development of type 2 diabetes.

It is, therefore, obvious to ask the question: does sleep deprivation predict the risk of developing type 2 diabetes? The causality of the association, and the generalizability of the results and their extrapolation to *longer-term* effects of *sustained* sleep disturbances, however, will require the verification that short sleepers have a greater risk of developing type 2 diabetes in prospective population studies to establish a temporal sequence between exposure and outcome (excluding 'reverse causality').

The aggregate analysis of prospective longitudinal studies carried out in populations around the world supports the concept that individuals who sleep less than 6 hours per night have, on average, a 28 per cent greater risk of developing type 2 diabetes than those sleeping 6–8 hours per night (Cappuccio et al., 2010b). The risk is even greater when disrupted quality of sleep is considered (as difficulty in initiating or maintaining sleep), with risks estimated to rise to 57 per cent and 84 per cent, respectively.

Short sleep and hypertension

What is hypertension?

High blood pressure (or hypertension) is the third biggest risk factor for disease in England after smoking and poor diet. It is the largest known risk factor for cardiovascular disease and related disability. Often described as a 'silent killer' because it rarely causes symptoms, high blood pressure was responsible for about 75,000 deaths in England in 2015. The diseases caused by high blood pressure are coronary heart disease, stroke, kidney disease, and vascular dementia. They cost the NHS over £2.1 billion every year.

High blood pressure affects over 12.5 million people in England alone—31 per cent of men and 25 per cent of women in 2015. About half of the adult population do not know what their blood pressure is and about 70% of adults with high blood pressure (approx. 5.5 million people in England) have undiagnosed hypertension.

Up to 80 per cent of premature death from cardiovascular disease can be prevented through better public health. Whilst some risk factors (age, ethnicity, gender, genetics) cannot be modified, addressing modifiable risk factors will yield significant health and economic gains. Reducing excessive dietary salt, improving poor diet and reducing obesity, avoiding excessive alcohol consumption, increasing levels of physical activity, and improving socio-economic conditions and mental health are all cost-effective public health interventions.

When these actions are not sufficient, drug therapy is used to reduce blood pressure and the burden of cardiovascular complications.

Role of sleep

In physiological conditions, our blood pressure follows a diurnal pattern with a fall at night whilst we rest and sleep (referred as 'nocturnal dip'). This fall is due to a variety of mechanisms, including supine position, muscle relaxation, and reduced sympathetic tone. However, in recent years, it has become apparent that many individuals may not present the expected nocturnal dip in blood pressure ('non-dippers'). This phenomenon may present both in those with normal 'day-time' blood pressure as well as in those with high 'day-time' blood pressure. Non-dippers have a higher risk of developing cardiovascular disease than dippers.

Early findings from UK and US studies suggest associations between sleep duration and hypertension risk. Specifically, cross-sectional analyses showed a significant, consistent association between short sleep duration (< 5 hours per night) and risk of hypertension. In some studies, the association was stronger among women, which was attenuated in prospective analyses after multivariate adjustment (Cappuccio et al., 2007). A recent review of the available studies estimates the risk of developing hypertension in short sleepers at 21 per cent (Meng et al., 2013). The effect of sleep disturbances, of quantity as well as quality, on the incidence of hypertension is detected also independently of the severity of sleep-breathing problems (as measured by the apnoea–hypopnoea index, or AHI). The effect is detectable early in childhood and adolescence, affecting both daytime and night-time blood pressure, suggesting that sleep disturbances not only raise night blood pressure by disrupting sleep, but exert prolonged carry-over effects on daytime blood pressure, leading to hypertension. Finally, in a group of elderly men studied with polysomnography and followed up for many years, it has been established that short sleep is an independent predictor of the development of hypertension, predominantly because of a significant reduction in slow-wave sleep, the restorative stage of sleep (Fung et al., 2011).

An important step in epidemiological research to imply causality is the evidence of 're-versibility'—that is, the evidence that if one is able to modify the risk factor, the outcome should be modified in the direction of the observed relationship. One of the main limitations in this field of research is the absence of a standard validated tool for extending sleep (without the use of hypnotics or other pharmacological agents) in a sustained matter. Sleep extension can be achieved in a variety of ways, but it invariably will involve multiple behavioural modifications aided by structural changes in environmental factors that exert pressure on our time (e.g. extended commuting time to go to work, light and noise pollution, unsocial working hours) and, therefore, the opportunities we have to engage in 'sleep'. One encouraging experiment was carried out with success in 22 participants with stage 1 hypertension who were randomized to either a 6-week period aimed at increasing bedtime by 1 hour daily (sleep extension group) or to a 6-week period (sleep maintenance group) aimed at maintaining habitual bedtime (Haack et al., 2013). During the trial, the sleep extension group increased the sleep duration (directly measured by actigraphy) by an average of 35 minutes per night compared to the sleep maintenance group. At the same time, their blood pressure—measured throughout the 24 hours—was reduced by an additional 7/4 mmHg by the end of the interventions, suggesting a direct beneficial effect of sleep extension on blood pressure.

Short sleep and other conditions

Lipids

Blood lipid profiles characterized by high levels of total cholesterol and low-density lipo-protein (LDL)-cholesterol, high triglycerides, and/or low levels of high-density lipoprotein (HDL)-cholesterol are well-established risk factors for cardiovascular disease. They are also more commonly associated with other metabolic abnormalities such as obesity, insulin resistance, and diabetes. Some longitudinal evidence suggests an association between short duration of sleep and an unfavourable pattern of blood lipid profile, particularly detectable in adolescents (Gangwisch et al., 2010). However, a recent review of all the available evidence pooled together, whilst suggesting a trend for a 10 per cent greater risk of developing hypercholesterolaemia in those sleeping 5 hours or less, does not provide unequivocal evidence for an independent effect of sleep deprivation on lipid metabolism (Kruisbrink et al., 2017).

Vascular calcifications

The concept of a possible causal link between sleep deprivation and cardio-metabolic risk is strengthened by the evidence obtained from the Coronary Artery Risk Development in Young Adults (CARDIA) cohort in Chicago. In this study, black and white men and women aged 18–30 years were studied and followed up for 5 years. At baseline, sleep metrics (duration and fragmentation measured by wrist actigraphy, daytime sleepiness, overall quality, self-reported duration) were examined and a CT (computed tomography) scan of their heart was obtained to measure calcifications of their coronary arteries. A similar CT scan was repeated 5 years later. After excluding the confounding effect of a variety of be-havioural, lifestyle, and metabolic factors, participants who slept 5 hours or less exhibited a sharp increase in the risk of developing coronary calcifications—risk factors for myocar-dial infarction (i.e. heart attacks). The rate of development of calcification was 33 per cent greater for every hour of sleep curtailment (King et al., 2008). The effect was twice as strong in women as in men, although the reason for this gender difference is not known.

Short sleep and health outcomes

From what we have described so far, it is apparent that sleep deprivation—whether short- or long-term—is strongly and consistently associated with a variety of biological mech-anisms (hormonal changes in regulation of energy balance and appetite; activation of inflammatory markers; glucose intolerance and insulin resistance; molecular effects in adipocytes; up- and down-regulation of gene expression; vascular calcifications) and risk factors (overweight and obesity; type-2 diabetes; hypertension) that, collectively, are strong predictors of the likelihood of developing cardiovascular disease. If these associ-ations were to reflect a cause–effect relationship, we would expect to find that those with long-term sleep deprivation (i.e. those who regularly sleep less than the average for the population) would be more likely to develop cardiovascular disease (e.g. coronary heart disease and stroke) and die more often from it (Figure 8.2).

Coronary heart disease

In large population studies, people have been asked about their sleeping habits and have been followed up for many years, often decades, and their health outcomes have been re-corded carefully over the years. When these studies have been collated and analyzed, it has

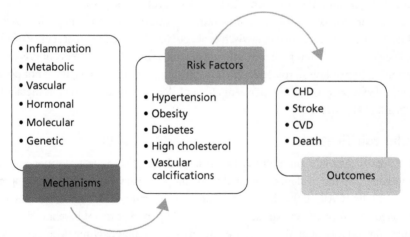

Fig. 8.2 Sleep deprivation and cardio-metabolic disease: from mechanisms, to risk, to outcomes.
Adapted with permission from Cappuccio FP and Miller MA. Are short bad sleep nights a hindrance to a healthy heart? *Sleep*, Volume 34, Issue 11, pp. 1457–1458, Copyright © 2011 Associated Professional Sleep Societies, LLC.

become apparent that, despite the variability between studies due to different populations, various methods of assessments, and so on, those who were reporting shorter duration of sleep (usually < 5 or 6 hours per night) were more likely to experience an episode of coronary heart disease and to die from it than those usually sleeping, on average, 6–8 hours per night. The early studies indicate an average increase in risk of 48 per cent (Cappuccio et al., 2011). The risk of developing coronary heart disease is further enhanced if the short sleep is also associated to poor-quality sleep (Chandola et al., 2010), suggesting an independent role of quantity, as well as quality, of sleep on cardiovascular risk.

Stroke

Similar to what we have seen for coronary heart disease, short sleepers display a greater risk of developing fatal and non-fatal strokes over a long term (Cappuccio et al., 2011), equivalent to an approximately 15 per cent higher risk (Leng et al., 2015).

Mortality

One of the most surprising results of the epidemiological studies exploring the relationships between short duration of sleep and health outcomes is the description of a 12 per cent increased risk of all-cause mortality in short sleepers (Cappuccio et al., 2010c). This finding has been consistently confirmed in independent analyses from different researchers and in different countries. These results, if attributable to a direct cause–effect, would reinforce the general concept that sleep is such a fundamental function in human biology that a sustained habit of insufficient sleep (currently estimated as < 5–6 hours per day on a regular basis) would be a likely contributor of premature death. It is of interest to highlight that a careful study in a representative British population has established that the higher risk of mortality that is seen in people who tend to curtail their average sleeping time is due mainly to an increase in cardiovascular mortality rather than non-cardiovascular mortality (Ferrie et al., 2007).

In summary, Figure 8.3 describes the current state of knowledge that links sleep disturbances of quantity and quality with health outcomes. It is immediately apparent that the traditional belief that sleep pertains exclusively to the brain is being challenged by recent evidence suggesting that sleep exerts a much wider control than previously thought on several organs and systems, from the heart to the kidney, and the metabolic pathways to adipose tissue to the vasculature. The concept that sleep is an idle state of a suspended mind, closer to a state of death, must be abandoned. Sleep is an active physiological process greatly needed by our body to sustain vital functions, in the short as well as in the longer term. Its trading for extra wakefulness is not without consequences.

Napping and risk

A long-established practice in Mediterranean areas, daytime napping—commonly known as 'siesta'—is often associated with good health through a postulated stress relief mechanism. However, daytime sleepiness, often characterized by daytime napping, has been

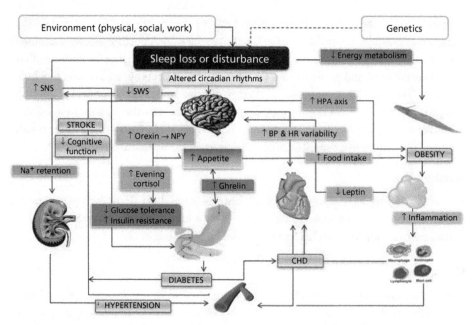

Fig. 8.3 Possible mechanistic pathways linking short duration of sleep and adverse cardiovascular health.

BP, blood pressure; HbA1c, haemoglobin A1c; HDL, high-density lipoprotein cholesterol; HR, heart rate; LDL, low-density lipoprotein cholesterol; PAI-1, plasminogen activator inhibitor-1; SNS, sympathetic nervous system; SWS, slow-wave sleep; Trigs, triglycerides.

Reproduced with permission from Miller MA and Cappuccio FP. Biomarkers of cardiovascular risk in sleep deprived people. *Journal of Human Hypertension*, Volume 27, pp. 583–588, Copyright © 2013 Macmillan Publishers Limited.

regarded as an early sign or risk indicator of a range of health problems, such as depression, cognitive impairment, Parkinson's disease, and other chronic debilitating illnesses. Whilst early evidence in Mediterranean countries suggested that 'siesta' would be associated with favourable cardiovascular outcomes, the contemporary association between daytime napping and mortality risk is uncertain. Most previous studies have originated from Mediterranean countries in which the incidence of, and the rate of, death from cardiovascular disease tends to be low. Several prospective studies from Israel show an increased mortality rate associated with 'siesta' among older people, whereas one study from Greece suggested that 'siesta' is protective against heart-related deaths, especially in working men. In addition, conflicting US-based research has found an increased risk of death associated with daytime napping in both men and women. Only naps of long durations were found to be significant. In Japan, another study suggested that daytime napping was associated with increased risk of all-cause and cardiovascular death, but this association was largely explained by concomitant comorbidity. Clearly, the population evidence so far is inconsistent and it may largely depend on differences in cultural, environmental, and demographic factors. It therefore remains unclear whether daytime napping is beneficial or a risk factor for, or marker of, ill-health.

A recent programme of research on the effects of daytime napping on health outcomes was completed in a representative sample of British men and women. This programme was carried out in the EPIC-Norfolk (Norfolk cohort of the European Prospective Investigation into Cancer and Nutrition) prospective study, in which over 16,000 participants provided information on their sleeping patterns, including sleep duration, time in bed, and daytime napping. They were then followed up for up to 13 years (Leng et al., 2014). After allowing for potential known confounders, daytime napping was significantly associated with an increased risk of dying. For naps of < 1 hour, the risk was increased by an average 14%, whereas for naps > 1 hour the risk increased further to an average 32%. The risk was also more pronounced for deaths from respiratory diseases and in individuals aged > 65 years. In the same study, daytime napping has been associated with an increased risk of developing type 2 diabetes (2.5-fold higher), especially when associated with short duration of sleep (< 6 hours per night) (Leng et al., 2016a). Finally, a similar increased risk of chronic respiratory disease was detected amongst shorter (< 1 hour) and longer (≥ 1 hour) naps, with a dose-dependent effect of 52% and 72% increased risk, respectively (Leng et al., 2016b).

Long sleep duration and ill-health

It is important to mention that the associations between duration of sleep and health outcomes, whether morbid or fatal, show clear-cut and consistent U-shaped curves, with the lowest risk usually seen between 6h and 8h per night and increased risks also detectable for 'long' duration of sleep (>8h per night)(Cappuccio et al., 2010b, c; 2011). However, the evidence does not fulfil all the necessary criteria for implying causality (in particular absence of plausible biological mechanisms); the current interpretation is that 'long' duration of sleep is, rather, a marker or a symptom of pre-clinical ill-health. However, further research is needed.

Summary

- There is a strong and consistent association between short duration of sleep and cardio-metabolic risk factors and outcomes.
- The associations may reflect causality as:
  - the effects are *strong*: large relative risks
  - they are *consistent*: confirmed in different populations for several end-points
  - they show a *temporal sequence*: short sleep preceding end-points
  - there is a *dose–response effect*: consistent threshold effects
  - there is *biological plausibility*: several potential mechanisms are involved (genetic, molecular, cellular, physiological, and so on)
  - there is *reversibility*: confirmed when tested under controlled trial conditions (at least short-term ones).

- Daytime napping and long duration of sleep are also associated with ill-health and worse health outcomes.

- These associations are more likely to reflect the fact that napping and long sleep may be markers of compensation for sleep deprivation (forced daytime napping) or of sub-clinical chronic and/or debilitating ill-health.

References

Broussard, J. L., Ehrmann, D. A., Van Cauter, E., Tasali, E. & Brady, M. J. 2012. Impaired insulin signalling in human adipocytes after experimental sleep restriction. *Annals of Internal Medicine*, **157**, pp. 549–57.

Buxton, O. M., Cain, S. W., O'Connor, S. P., Porter, J. H., Duffy, J. F., Wang, W., Czeisler, C. A. & Shea, S. A. 2012. Adverse metabolic consequences in humans of prolonged sleep restriction combined with circadian disruption. *Science Translational Medicine*, **4**(129), p. 129ra43.

Cappuccio, F. P., Stranges, S., Kandala, N.-B., Miller, M. A., Taggart, F. M., Kumari, M., Ferrie, J. E., Shipley, M. J., Brunner, E. J. & Marmot, M. G. 2007. Gender-specific associations of short sleep duration with prevalent and incident hypertension: the Whitehall II Study. *Hypertension*, **50**, pp. 694–701.

Cappuccio, F. P., Taggart, F. M., Kandala, N.-B., Currie, A., Peile, E., Stranges, S. & Miller, M. A. 2008. Meta-analysis of short sleep duration and obesity in children and adults. *Sleep*, **31**, pp. 619–26.

Cappuccio, F. P., Miller, M. A. & Lockley, S. W. 2010a. *Sleep, Health & Society: from aetiology to public health*. Oxford: Oxford University Press, pp. 1–471 (ISBN 978-0-19-956659-4).

Cappuccio, F. P., D'Elia, L., Strazzullo, P. & Miller, M. A. 2010b. Quantity and quality of sleep and incidence of type-2 diabetes: a meta-analysis of prospective studies. *Diabetes Care*, **33**, pp. 414–20.

Cappuccio, F. P., D'Elia, L., Strazzullo, P. & Miller, M. A. 2010c. Sleep duration and all-cause mortality: a systematic review and meta-analysis of prospective studies. *Sleep*, **33**(5), pp. 585–92.

Cappuccio, F. P., Cooper, D., D'Elia, L., Strazzullo, P. & Miller, M. A. 2011. Sleep duration predicts cardiovascular outcomes: a systematic review and meta-analysis of prospective studies. *European Heart Journal*, **32**, pp. 1484–92.

Chandola, T., Ferrie, J. E., Perski, A., Akbaraly, T. & Marmot, M. G. 2010. The effect of short sleep duration on coronary heart disease risk is greatest among those with sleep disturbance: a prospective study from the Whitehall II cohort. *Sleep*, **33**, pp. 739–44.

Cohen, D. A., Wang, W., Wyatt, J. K., Kronauer, R. E., Dijk, D. J., Czeisler, C. A. & Klerman, E. B. 2010. Uncovering residual effects of chronic sleep loss on human performance. *Science Translational Medicine*, **2**(14), p. 14ra3.

Ferrie, J. E., Shipley, M. J., Cappuccio, F. P., Brunner, E., Miller, M. A., Kumari, M. & Marmot, M. G. 2007. A prospective study of change in sleep duration: associations with mortality in the Whitehall II cohort. *Sleep*, **30**, pp. 1659–66.

Fung, M. M., Peters, K., Redline, S., Ziegler, M. G., Ancoli-Israel, S., Barrett-Connor, E., Stone, K. L; Osteoporotic Fractures in Men Research Group. 2011. Decreased slow wave sleep increases risk of developing hypertension in elderly men. *Hypertension*, **58**, pp. 596–603.

Gangwisch, J. E., Malaspina, D., Babiss, L. A., Opler, M. G., Posner, K., Shen, S., Turner, J. B., Zammit, G. K. & Ginsberg, H. N. 2010. Short sleep duration as a risk factor for hypercholesterolemia: analyses of the National Longitudinal Study of Adolescent Health. *Sleep*, **33**(7), pp. 956–61.

Haack, M., Serrador, J., Cohen, D., Simpson, N., Meier-Ewert, H. & Mullington, J. M. 2013. Increasing sleep duration to lower beat-to-beat blood pressure: a pilot study. *Journal of Sleep Research*, **22**, pp. 295–304.

King, C. R., Knutson, K. L., Rathouz, P. J., Sidney, S., Liu, K. & Lauderdale, D. S. 2008. Short sleep duration and incident coronary artery calcificationet al. *JAMA*, **300**(24), pp. 2859–66.

Kruisbrink, M., Robertson, W., Ji, C., Miller, M. A., Geleijnse, J. M. & Cappuccio, F. P. 2017. Association of sleep duration and quality with blood lipids: a systematic review and meta-analysis of prospective studies. *BMJ Open*, **7**, e018585.

Leng, Y., Wainwright, N. W. J., Cappuccio, F. P., Surtees, P. G., Hayat, S., Luben, R., Brayne, C. & Khaw, K. T. 2014. Daytime napping and the risk of all-cause and cause-specific mortality: a 13-year follow-up of a British population. *American Journal of Epidemiology*, **179**(9), 1115–24.

Leng, Y., Cappuccio, F. P., Wainwright, N. W. J., Surtees, P. G., Luben, R., Brayne, C. & Khaw, K. T. 2015. Sleep duration and risk of fatal and non-fatal stroke: a prospective study and meta-analysis. *Neurology*, **84**, 1072–79.

Leng, Y., Cappuccio, F. P., Surtees, P. G., Luben, R., Brayne, C. & Khaw, K. T. 2016a. Daytime napping, sleep duration and increased 8-year risk of type 2 diabetes in a British population. *Nutrition, Metabolism, and Cardiovascular Diseases*, **26**, pp. 995–1003.

Leng, Y., Wainwright, N. W. J., Cappuccio, F. P., Surtees, P. G., Hayat, S., Luben, R., Brayne, C. & Khaw, K. T. 2016b. Daytime napping and increased risk of incident respiratory diseases: symptom, marker, or risk factor? *Sleep Medicine*, **23**, pp. 12–15.

Meng, L., Zheng, Y. & Hui, R. 2013. The relationship of sleep duration and insomnia to risk of hypertension incidence: a meta-analysis of prospective cohort studies. *Hypertension Research*, **36**, pp. 985–95.

Möller-Levet, C. S., Archer, S. N., Bucca, G., Laing, E. E., Slak, A., Kabiljo, R., Lo, J. C., Santhi, N., von Schantz, M., Smith, C. P. & Dijk, D. J. 2013. Effects of insufficient sleep on circadian rhythmicity and expression amplitude of the human blood transcriptome. *Proceedings of the National Academy of Sciences of the United States of America*, **110**(12), E1132–E1141.

Spiegel, K., Tasali, E., Penev, P. & Van Cauter, E. Sleep curtailment in healthy young men is associated with decreased leptin levels, elevated ghrelin levels, and increased hunger and appetite. *Annals of Internal Medicine*, **141**, pp. 846–50.

Spiegel, K., Tasali, E., Leproult, R. & Van Cauter, E. 2009. Effect of poor and short sleep on glucose metabolism and obesity risk. *Nature Reviews Endocrinology*, **5**, pp. 253–61.

Steptoe, A., Peacey, V. & Wardle, J. 2006. Sleep duration and health in young adults. *Archives of Internal Medicine*, **166**, pp. 1689–92.

Taheri, S., Lin, L., Austin, D., Young, T. & Mignot, E. 2004. Short sleep duration is associated with reduced leptin, elevated ghrelin, and increased body mass index. *PLoS Medicine*, **1**, e62.

Chapter 9

Sleep and respiratory disorders

Bradley A. Edwards and Garun S. Hamilton

Introduction

Sleep is something that we spend a third of our lives doing. This is such a significant amount of time to devote to a function that has been conserved through millions of years of evolution. So it may not be surprising that sleep loss/poor quality sleep is associated with a number of adverse health consequences. As discussed in this book, poor sleep in general increases the risk of developing various physical and mental health conditions. However, several sleep-related breathing and respiratory disorders impact our ability to achieve a good night's sleep. The aim of this chapter is to provide an overview of how some of these common disorders contribute to poor sleep, with a particular focus on the most common sleep-related breathing disorder, obstructive sleep apnoea (OSA), review how these disorders impact both the individual and society, and discuss some of the key challenges we face in terms of moving forward as a field.

Obstructive sleep apnoea

Obstructive sleep apnoea (OSA) is by far the most common and prevalent sleep-related breathing disorder and is characterized by repetitive collapse (apnoea) or partial collapse (hypopnoea) of the pharyngeal airway during sleep. These airway obstructions lead to increasingly powerful respiratory efforts until the airway re-opens and breathing is restored, often in association with an arousal from sleep. Such transient events also expose the sufferer to intermittent hypoxia and hypercapnia, large swings in intrathoracic pressure, and surges in sympathetic activation. Clinically, an individual is diagnosed with OSA when they experience these apnoeas/hypopnoeas at least five times an hour (apnoea–hypopnoea index (AHI) ≥ five events/hour). An AHI of between 15 events/hour and 30 events/hour is considered as moderate OSA, while an AHI of ≥ 30 events/hour is considered as severe OSA.

Prevalence

The current adult population prevalence estimates of moderate-to-severe OSA are in the approximate range of 6%–17% (Senaratna et al., 2016), depending on how OSA is defined. Prevalence increases significantly with age, with up to 49% of middle-aged and elderly individuals having moderate or severe OSA (AHI ≥ 15 events/hour). Unfortunately, as many as 80% of this population are currently undiagnosed and untreated. The reason for such high numbers is complex, but may be attributed to the fact that many individuals perceive OSA as unimportant and do not understand the significant impact that this disorder can have on their lives. Furthermore, some individuals who have been living with the condition for an extended period of time are either truly asymptomatic or have become acclimatized to their symptoms (see 'Diagnosing/screening for OSA and its challenges'), such that it has become their baseline level of function.

Obesity and OSA

A number of factors increase an individual's risk for developing OSA, but by far the greatest risk factor is the presence of obesity—specifically, central obesity. Obesity is a growing epidemic and is one of the western world's leading health care concerns. Not surprisingly, the incidence and prevalence of OSA are expected to rise with the increasing obesity rates. Large epidemiological studies have reported a striking dose–response association between the prevalence of OSA and increased body mass index (BMI) and neck/waist circumferences. The Wisconsin Sleep Cohort found that a 10% weight gain led to a 6-fold increase in the odds of developing moderate-to-severe OSA, independent of confounding factors such as age and baseline measures of body habitus. Conversely, a 10% weight loss predicted a modest improvement in OSA severity (26% decrease in AHI) (Peppard et al., 2000), a finding supported by the Sleep Heart Health Study. As such, obesity and OSA are exceptionally common health problems which frequently co-exist, with both being associated with adverse cardio-metabolic outcomes. Obesity is thought to play a role in the pathogenesis of OSA in a number of ways, including alterations in upper airway structure and function promoting greater collapsibility, a reduction in resting lung volumes, and a disturbance of the relationship between respiratory drive and load compensation. While obesity is the largest independent risk factor for developing OSA, there is also emerging evidence that OSA itself may predispose to the development of obesity (Ong et al., 2013), thereby creating a vicious positive feedback cycle.

Other risk factors

The risks of developing OSA are, however, not solely related to obesity. In both sexes the syndrome is more prevalent with increasing age, reaching very high rates in patients aged over 65 years. Males appear to have a higher rate of OSA than women, with a ratio of 2:1 to 10:1, depending on the study. Any condition resulting in an anatomical abnormality which narrows the posterior airspace can predispose to the development of OSA. This includes nasal obstruction, retro- or micrognathia, tonsillar hypertrophy, and macroglossia. Several studies have demonstrated a higher risk for developing OSA if there is a family history of the disorder, with increasing risk with increasing number of affected relatives suggestive of a genetic link. Lastly, use of alcohol or sedative medication can contribute to the development of OSA through their relaxant effect on the upper airway muscles.

Health consequences of OSA on individuals, and its impact on healthcare systems

Loud snoring, daytime sleepiness, tiredness, and non-restorative sleep are the most common symptoms of OSA, presumably caused by the associated sleep fragmentation due to frequent arousals. However, if left untreated, OSA is also associated with increased risk of a range of health problems, including cardiovascular disease, metabolic disturbances, neurocognitive impairment, mental health disorders (i.e. depression), cancer, and a 2- to 3-fold increased risk of all-cause mortality (Marin et al., 2005). In general, the adverse consequences of OSA increase with increased OSA severity. The evidence for all of these adverse effects of OSA is strong for severe OSA, but either weak or not present for mild OSA. However, OSA is a highly heterogeneous disorder with underlying causes and consequences that vary substantially between patients. For example, there are patients with severe OSA who are not subjectively or objectively sleepy. Conversely, there are patients with only mild OSA who experience severe sleepiness. Nonetheless, the sleepiness and impaired alertness associated with untreated OSA may also be safety hazards.

Driving-related risk

Almost 20% of all serious car crash injuries in the general population are associated with driver sleepiness. This makes driver sleepiness the largest identifiable and preventable cause of accidents in all modes of transport—surpassing alcohol and drugs. As highlighted above, one of the most commonly reported symptoms of OSA is excessive daytime sleepiness, and this may explain the increased risk of motor vehicle accidents seen in this population. However, it remains unclear which individuals with OSA are at particularly significant risk given that the relationship between crash risk and measures of OSA severity and subjective sleepiness is non-linear. Nevertheless, in the largest and most rigorous study to date of commercial drivers (Garbarino et al., 2016), OSA drivers who were never treatment-compliant had a 5-fold increase in the rate of serious preventable crashes, while drivers who were always treatment-adherent had a crash rate statistically similar to that of matched controls. A major challenge for the field of sleep medicine is to develop a simple test which accurately predicts risk of motor vehicle and workplace accidents. No such test currently exists and it is likely that the optimal test would be state dependent (involving some type of current 'fit for duty' score) as impaired vigilance from OSA and other sleep disorders is a dynamic rather than a static problem.

Safety in the workplace

Given the increasing societal obesity trends and prevalence of the disorder, it was inevitable that OSA would manifest as an important health and safety concern in the workplace. In the United States, the rates of obesity in emergency service personnel (i.e. police, firefighters, and ambulance workers) are either on par with, or higher than, those of the general public, despite the fitness screening required for the job. Importantly, as highlighted earlier, OSA remains largely undiagnosed in this population. Recent evidence suggests that the presence of OSA (regardless of whether it was diagnosed via PSG or by questionnaires) is associated with a 2-fold excess in the risk of occupational accidents. Recent evidence suggests that the presence of OSA (regardless of whether it was diagnosed via polysomnography or by questionnaires) is associated with a 2-fold excess in the risk of occupational accidents. Some industries, such as commercial trucking and aviation, have OSA screening policies in place; however, these vary widely according to country and state, and the most appropriate method to screen for OSA in occupational settings is uncertain. Given that individuals working in such settings are largely responsible for the health and safety of the population, we need evidence-based policies to be implemented to ensure that we can improve the safety of both the emergency services workers as well as the general public.

Effect on the economy

In addition to the burden of the disorder on the individual, OSA also has a profound impact on the healthcare infrastructure and economy. Estimates of the cost of diagnosing and treating OSA to the hospital system in Australia totalled A$70.3 million per year as of 2010. Additionally, other medical costs for services relating to OSA amounted to AUS$96.6 million, and the total cost of treatment devices such as continuous positive airway pressure (CPAP) machines was AUS$81.5 million (Deloitte Access Economics and The Sleep Health Foundation, 2012). Furthermore, motor vehicle accidents that were due to all sleep disorders cost the healthcare system, government, and insurance industry a combined AUS$472 million. OSA-related lost productivity also caused an AUS$1,092 million loss to the economy, primarily stemming from depression and related symptoms linked with the disorder. Perhaps more surprising is the reported cost of undiagnosed OSA to the economy. A recent report commissioned by the American Academy of Sleep Medicine (AASM, 2016) demonstrated that the cost of caring for undiagnosed OSA patients is almost four times the cost of diagnosing and treating OSA. Therefore, it is imperative that we improve our diagnosis of the disorder as well as provide efficacious and efficient treatment to patients with OSA, targeting both neurocognitive and cardiovascular sequelae.

Diagnosing/screening for OSA and its challenges

Currently, in-laboratory polysomnography (PSG) remains the gold standard diagnostic instrument for a diagnosis of OSA and other sleep disorders. However, laboratory PSG is costly and labour intensive, which has led to a rapid increase in home sleep testing as technology has matured over the past few years. There are different types and complexities of home sleep tests, ranging from full PSG carried out at home to various 'limited channel' devices, which only record one or more key breathing signals. The relative uptake of these different tests between countries has been largely driven by different costs and healthcare system reimbursement models. Although home sleep tests are generally good at 'ruling in' moderate to severe OSA in individuals with a high probability for the disorder, their relative simplicity has led not only to better access to diagnosis and treatment for patients, but also to an increase in testing performed in less symptomatic individuals. This has often been accompanied by calls to 'screen' high-risk groups for OSA. However, a major challenge for the field is that because OSA is so highly prevalent in the general community and has such a large proportion of asymptomatic or minimally symptomatic disease, widespread testing for OSA will almost certainly turn up a high proportion of positive cases, the clinical significance of which is uncertain. As yet, it is unknown whether there are any population health benefits from widespread screening for OSA, and furthermore the cost-effectiveness of this approach is unknown. Currently, the key group requiring sleep testing remains those who volunteer significant symptoms of the disorder to their healthcare practitioner.

Treating OSA and its challenges

The gold standard treatment for OSA is CPAP, which involves the delivery of pressurized air through a nasal or oral-nasal mask and acts by pneumatically splinting open the airway during sleep. It highly safe and effective at reducing OSA severity and overall can improve cardiovascular morbidity/mortality and daytime sleepiness, without any known serious or harmful side-effects. The main limitation of therapy, however, is treatment adherence. Only approximately 50% of patients prescribed CPAP continue to use it adequately in the long term, although this percentage can vary between 46% and 89% depending on definitions of adherence and length of follow-up. A good argument can be made that reported adherence values (46–89%) are an overestimate of the OSA population, since they typically include in the denominator patients with diagnosed OSA who have initially accepted CPAP as a treatment. The proportion of CPAP-adherent patients would certainly be low if calculations also accounted for: 1) the number of patients who have OSA but decline a diagnostic study specifically because they believe they will not use CPAP, 2) the number of patients who are diagnosed with OSA but then decline a CPAP titration, and 3) the number of patients who have a negative experience at their CPAP titration and decline to accept CPAP therapy, so never acquire a CPAP device.

Common alternative therapies recommended for patients that either cannot tolerate CPAP or simply would prefer a different option include upper airway surgery, mandibular advancement splints, weight loss, and lateral sleeping. However, a common limitation of these therapies is that they are often variably effective and/or tolerated, and currently there are no ideal tools which accurately predict treatment response—meaning that patients tend to work through these CPAP-alternative treatments in an ad-hoc fashion. Further measures to improve CPAP adherence, better methods of predicting success with non-CPAP therapies, and programmes to prevent the development of obesity in communities are urgently needed to improve the health consequences of OSA at a population level.

Other respiratory disorders/diseases and sleep

There are a number of other respiratory disorders (discussed below) which, by themselves, often produce abnormalities in sleep and breathing during sleep. Unfortunately,

OSA can often co-exist with many of these disorders, which not only compounds the sleep disturbances experienced by the patient, but may also increase morbidity.

Chronic obstructive pulmonary disease and OSA (overlap syndrome)

Chronic obstructive pulmonary disease (COPD) is a serious, progressive, and disabling condition that limits air flow in the lungs. It is estimated that approximately 10% of the population aged over 40 years have COPD, a prevalence which is expected to rise to epidemic proportions owing to historical smoking trends, the ageing of the population, and air pollution.

When both OSA and COPD occur together in the same individual it is known as 'overlap syndrome'. Overlap syndrome has a population prevalence of 1.0%–3.6% and mainly affects older individuals, given that COPD is rare under the age of 50 years (Shawon et al., 2016). Compared to subjects with either condition alone, those with overlap syndrome have higher rates of cardiovascular disease and hospital admissions and a worse quality of life. Furthermore, COPD itself (with or without the presence of OSA) can impact on sleep quality. Subjects with overlap syndrome have worse sleep quality than those with only OSA, and several studies have reported that those with moderate to severe COPD have increased sleep fragmentation, fatigue, and daytime sleepiness. In particular, sleep quality worsens at the time of a COPD exacerbation. Despite the effects of moderate to severe COPD on sleep quality, mild COPD has not been associated with significant sleep disturbance.

Asthma and OSA

Individuals with asthma generally report worsening of symptoms during the night. In support of this, emergency room visits for asthma-related issues are more common at night, and there is also evidence to demonstrate that the majority of asthma-related deaths occur between 6 p.m. and 3 a.m. Furthermore, after a night's sleep, asthma is worse in the morning than in the evening. It is well-known that airway function declines during the night, whether the patient sleeps or not, though the decline is exaggerated by sleep. Hence, sleep may be one of the important factors in night-time asthma exacerbation.

There is an association between asthma and OSA, and those with asthma have been shown to have a higher incidence of developing OSA than those without (Teodorescu et al., 2015). However, it is unknown whether there is a causative link between the two conditions as the mechanisms underlying this association have not been clearly delineated. OSA has been linked with increased symptoms of breathlessness in people with asthma (as well as the general population), but the co-morbid obesity is an important potential confounder in this regard. There are also conflicting data as to whether there is any increase in bronchial hyperresponsiveness in OSA subjects compared to BMI-matched controls. As with COPD, those with more severe (or poorly controlled) asthma may have sleep disturbance secondary to nocturnal asthma symptoms. Nocturnal and early-morning asthma symptoms are therefore a marker of the need to consider escalating asthma therapy.

Obesity hypoventilation syndrome

Obesity hypoventilation syndrome (OHS) is a very severe form of sleep-disordered breathing. It is a complication of obesity, but individuals with morbid obesity (BMI > 40 kg/m^2) are particularly at risk. OSA is co-morbidly present in up to 90% of individuals, but the key distinguishing feature is the presence of chronic alveolar hypoventilation, as defined by an elevation of daytime arterial CO_2 levels (PaCO$_2$ ≥ 45 mmHg). Other causes of the hypercapnia need to be excluded. In OHS there is sleep-related hypoventilation, which, over time, leads to chronic daytime respiratory failure, with elevated CO_2 levels and chronic hypoxia. Individuals with OHS have a high mortality rate from respiratory failure and cardiovascular disease, and furthermore have high levels of social disability. Because of the extreme obesity they are usually poorly mobile and have high rates of co-morbid metabolic disease. Some patients present to their doctors with symptoms of OSA because of the associated sleep fragmentation, but a significant proportion only come to medical attention when an inter-current illness (or physiological stress such as surgery) precipitates acute respiratory failure. A major challenge with OHS is recognition and institution of appropriate treatment. Although CPAP is effective in many subjects with OHS, other patients require chronic non-invasive ventilation delivered via a nasal or oral-nasal mask to adequately augment their breathing overnight. Weight loss is also far more critical than in OSA, given the risk of respiratory failure with the condition. Given that obesity prevalence continues to increase across the world, OHS is likely to become more of a problem in the future.

Summary and future directions

In summary, sleep-related breathing disorders are very common and can have a dramatic impact on an individual's sleep, which can be particularly worsened when they occur together with other respiratory diseases. The prevalence of these disorders, particularly OSA and OHS, will continue to rise synergistically with the rising rates of obesity in the population. For OSA, one of the largest problems we need to tackle as a field is the incredible proportion of individuals that are undiagnosed. This is largely driven by the public misconception that snoring or daytime sleepiness is a normal part of life, yet both of these are signs that something more serious (e.g. OSA) may be lurking in the shadows. Public awareness campaigns to better educate the general public (as well as general practitioners) are going to be critical. For those diagnosed with OSA, the development of new telemedicine tools, predictive analytics, and personalized medicine, which can determine the best treatment for an individual, will allow physicians to deliver better care than we are currently achieving. Furthermore, the development of more accurate, and simpler, home testing for OSA, a rapidly developing consumer sleep technology market, and wireless CPAP compliance monitoring and feedback via smart-phone apps will likely improve the successful diagnosis and treatment of OSA. Thus, there is plenty more work to be done.

Summary

- Sleep-related breathing disorders are very common and can have a dramatic impact on an individual's sleep.
- The prevalence of these disorders will continue to rise synergistically with the rising rates of obesity in the population.
- An incredible proportion of patients remain undiagnosed.
- There is public misconception that snoring or daytime sleepiness is a normal part of life.

References

AASM (American Academy of Sleep Medicine). 2016. *Hidden health crisis costing America billions: underdiagnosing and undertreating obstructive sleep apnea draining healthcare system.* [Frost & Sullivan]. [Online]. [Accessed 1 January 2018]. Available from: https://aasm.org/resources/pdf/sleep-apnea-economic-crisis.pdf

Deloitte Access Economics and the Sleep Health Foundation. 2012. *Re-awakening Australia—the economic cost of sleep disorders in Australia.* [Online]. [Accessed 1 January 2018]. Available from: https://www2.deloitte.com/au/en/pages/economics/articles/sleep-health.html

Garbarino, S., Guglielmi, O., Sanna, A., Mancardi, G. L. & Magnavita, N. 2016. Risk of occupational accidents in workers with obstructive sleep apnea: systematic review and meta-analysis. *Sleep*, **39**, pp. 1211–18.

Marin, J. M., Carrizo, S. J., Vicente, E. & Agusti, A. G. 2005. Long-term cardiovascular outcomes in men with obstructive sleep apnoea-hypopnoea with or without treatment with continuous positive airway pressure: an observational study. *Lancet*, **365**, pp. 1046–53.

Ong, C. W., O'Driscoll, D. M., Truby, H., Naughton, M. T. & Hamilton, G. S. 2013. The reciprocal interaction between obesity and obstructive sleep apnoea. *Sleep Medicine Reviews*, **17**(2), pp. 123–31.

Peppard, P. E., Young, T., Palta, M., Dempsey, J. & Skatrud, J. 2000. Longitudinal study of moderate weight change and sleep-disordered breathing. *JAMA*, **284**, 3015–21.

Senaratna, C. V., Perret, J. L., Lodge, C., Lowe, A. J., Campbell, B. E., Matheson, M. C., Hamilton, G. S. & Dharmage, S. C. 2017. Prevalence of obstructive sleep apnoea in the general population: a systematic review. *Sleep Medicine Reviews*, **34**, 70–81. doi: 10.1016/j.smrv.2016.07.002

Shawon, M. S., Perret, J., Senaratna, C. V., Lodge, C., Hamilton, G. S. & Dharmage, S. C. 2017. Current evidence on prevalence and clinical outcomes of co-morbid obstructive sleep apnea and chronic obstructive pulmonary disease: a systematic review. *Sleep Medicine Reviews*, **32**, 58–68. doi: 10.1016/j.smrv.2016.02.007

Teodorescu, M., Barnet, J.H., Hagen, E.W., Palta, M., Young, T. B. & Peppard, P. E. 2015. Association between asthma and risk of developing obstructive sleep apnea. *JAMA*, **313**, pp. 156–64.

Chapter 10

Sleep and neurological disorders

Daniel A. Cohen and Asim Roy

Introduction

Sleep states are associated with physiological changes that affect the functioning of multiple organ systems, but sleep is fundamentally a nervous system process. Mutually inhibitory sleep and arousal brain circuits interact so that sleep and wakefulness switch on and off in a coordinated fashion. Endogenous circadian rhythms that regulate the timing of sleep and wakefulness are controlled by pacemaker activity in the suprachiasmatic nucleus (SCN) of the hypothalamus. Respiratory patterns in sleep are driven by brainstem mechanisms that integrate information about carbon dioxide and oxygen exchange at the lungs; the mechanics of breathing itself is a product of reflex brainstem mechanisms that control upper airway dilator muscles and spinal cord outputs to power the respiratory muscles to promote ventilation. Diseases of the nervous system can disrupt these processes at multiple levels and cause sleep disorders. In turn, sleep disorders may negatively impact the structure and function of the nervous system through a variety of mechanisms (Figure 10.1).

Neurological diseases impacting sleep

Neurological diseases and sleep–wake regulation

The ability to sustain stable sleep and wakefulness is governed by a functional switch that arises from the mutually inhibitory connections between brainstem ascending arousal circuits and sleep-promoting neurons in the ventrolateral hypothalamus. The state of the switch predominantly depends on interactions between processes of sleep homeostasis, which is an accumulated drive for sleep from recent waking activity, and the phase of the endogenous circadian rhythm generated by pacemaker activity in the hypothalamic SCN. Structural brain injury can directly damage key components of the sleep–wake and circadian circuitry or disrupt the white matter connections between these regions and their outputs to other brain circuits, functionally disconnecting these systems and leading to conditions of excessive daytime sleepiness or fragmented sleep.

The most studied category of neurological diseases causing sleep–wake disorders are neurodegenerative diseases, which are a heterogeneous collection of conditions associated with progressive cognitive and motor disability. Abnormal folding and aggregation of several disease-related proteins preferentially target specific neuronal populations, leading to recognizable clinical phenotypes. The main focus of sleep studies in neurodegenerative

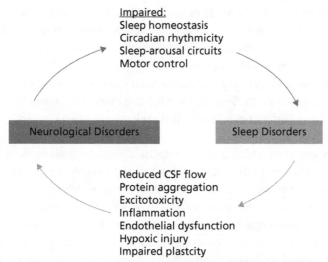

Fig. 10.1 Schema for understanding sleep disorders in neurological disease. Neurological disorders and sleep disorders show a bi-directional relationship. Pathology of the nervous system disrupts the sleep–wake circuitry and the circadian regulation of sleep and wakefulness. Sleep disorders mediate worsened nervous system structure and function through a variety of mechanisms, including inflammation, hypoxic injury, abnormal brain protein aggregation, and impaired synaptic plasticity.
Reproduced courtesy of Daniel A. Cohen and Asim Roy.

conditions has been in Alzheimer's disease and Parkinson's disease. Dysfunction of serotonergic, noradrenergic, dopaminergic, and cholinergic components of the arousal system have all been reported in neurodegenerative diseases. These changes may not only lead to hypersomnia but also change the underlying structure of sleep, including the reduction in slow-wave sleep and REM (rapid eye movement) sleep seen in neurodegenerative diseases compared to such sleep in healthy ageing. Degeneration of orexin neurons may contribute to a narcolepsy phenotype in which there is rapid and unpredictable switching between the states of sleep and wakefulness. Primary degeneration of the SCN has been reported (Wu & Swaab, 2005), which leads to lower amplitude and more variable circadian rhythms. In addition, patients with neurodegenerative diseases often lack typical exposure to environmental time cues to entrain the circadian system, most importantly daily bright light exposure. As a result, sleep may be scattered into multiple, short bouts spread over the 24-hour cycle, a condition known as the circadian disorder—irregular sleep–wake type. As neurodegeneration advances, there is typically progressive disorganization of sleep–wake patterns.

Neurological diseases causing sleep-related sensorimotor disorders

Parkinson's disease (PD), dementia with Lewy bodies (DLB), and multiple system atrophy are neurodegenerative conditions associated with abnormal accumulation of α-synuclein protein within neurons. These conditions account for the overwhelming majority of cases of REM sleep behavioural disorder (RBD), a condition in which there is a failure of the normal muscle atonia during REM sleep. RBD is characterized by excessive, potentially injurious behaviours occurring during REM sleep that often correspond to the contents of a dream; these dreams tend to be aggressive or violent in nature. RBD increases the risk of injury to both patients and their bed partners, for example secondary to punching and kicking movements that may correspond to a fighting theme of a dream. There is growing evidence that the majority of people with RBD will go on to develop Parkinson's disease or other Parkinson-like syndromes.

Restless legs syndrome (RLS) and the associated periodic limb movements of sleep (PLMS) are common in both central and peripheral nervous system disorders, with estimates of a 3–10 times higher prevalence than in age-matched controls. The pathophysiology of the sensorimotor abnormalities in RLS/PLMS is not fully understood, but a reduction in dopaminergic transmission is thought to play a key role. Reduction in central dopaminergic neurons, such as in PD, or damage to descending dopaminergic pathways to the spinal cord, as in demyelinating diseases such as multiple sclerosis, may account for the higher prevalence seen in these conditions. In addition, abnormal sensory input from peripheral nerve disorders such as diabetic neuropathy can also increase the likelihood of these disorders.

Abnormalities in the regulation of muscle tone can be seen in a wide array of central and peripheral nervous system disorders, and the resultant painful muscle spasms and cramps during sleep can be a significant source of sleep fragmentation and reduced sleep quality. Additionally, impaired mobility such as occurs in PD can impair sleep quality, potentially by causing pressure injury from maintaining a fixed sleep position for too long. In fact, long-acting dopaminergic medications used before bed can improve bed mobility and subjective sleep quality.

Neurological disease as a cause of sleep-disordered breathing

Focal central nervous system injury such as from stroke may cause sleep-disordered breathing. While associated conditions such as obesity may partially explain the association between sleep-disordered breathing and stroke, some evidence suggests that the nervous system injury can directly cause sleep-disordered breathing. For example, sleep-disordered breathing, particularly central sleep apnoea, improves from the acute phase to the subacute phase of a stroke. Stroke may increase the risk of central sleep disordered breathing by damaging brainstem structures involved with respiratory pattern generation and chemoreflex control of breathing; stroke may also cause obstructive sleep apnoea (OSA) from brainstem or hemispheric lesions that impair coordination of upper airway muscles.

Disorders of peripheral nerves, muscles, or the intervening neuromuscular junction are strongly associated with sleep-disordered breathing, with estimates as high as 70% in this population. Sleep-disordered breathing in this population may present in two primary forms: 1) OSA, and 2) hypercapnoeic hypoventilation. Depending on the disease, there may be an evolution in the type of sleep-disordered breathing, with upper airway obstruction developing early in the course of neuromuscular weakness, and later, the development of hypoventilation.

Coordinated neuromuscular recruitment of upper airway muscles is essential to maintain airway patency in the face of negative intraluminal upper airway pressures during inspiration. Neuromuscular disorders can affect the recruitment of pharyngeal dilator muscles or reduce the amount of force they generate, promoting upper airway collapsibility and OSA. Even if the muscle force generation is preserved, damage to autonomic fibres may interfere with upper airway reflex responses to mechanical forces. For example, in patients with diabetic autonomic neuropathy, obstructive events last longer and there is a greater degree of hypoxaemia than in those with spared autonomic function (Bottini et al., 2008). Autonomic dysfunction may also disrupt baroreceptor-mediated chemosensitivity to carbon dioxide, leading to central apnoeas. Treatment of neuromuscular disease may also contribute to sleep-disordered breathing; for example, steroid treatment in disorders such as myasthenia gravis, an autoimmune condition affecting the neuromuscular junction, may cause myopathy of the upper airway muscles and weight gain, which may be additional factors that may increase the risk of OSA.

Respiratory failure with hypercapnia and hypoxia is one of the leading causes of death and disability in patients with significant neuromuscular impairment, and respiratory insufficiency generally begins during sleep. Ventilation falls during normal sleep, particularly during REM sleep, in which tone to accessory respiratory muscles is reduced and the diaphragm drives ventilation in relative isolation. Nocturnal ventilation in neuromuscular disease falls in parallel to declining respiratory muscle strength; daytime pulmonary function tests may be useful for predicting nocturnal hypoventilation, but they are not always reliable. Therefore, a high index of suspicion is warranted with a low threshold for obtaining a nocturnal polysomnogram. Complications of hypoventilation include: hypoxia, hypercapnia, pulmonary hypertension, and right-sided heart failure. Treatment of nocturnal hypoventilation using non-invasive positive pressure ventilation can significantly improve survival and quality of life in patients with neuromuscular diseases such as those with amyotrophic lateral sclerosis.

Sleep disorders affecting nervous system structure

Sleep fragmentation as a cause of neuronal harm

Sleep serves a homeostatic function to promote recovery from waking activity. For example, with increasing hours awake, cortical neuronal excitability and firing rates progressively increase, which are both metabolically demanding and carry the potential for excitotoxicity and neuronal cell injury (Vyazovskiy et al., 2009); cortical firing rates are restored to a lower, more sustainable level following sleep. Insufficient sleep can harm the nervous system by the following additional mechanisms: chronic sleep restriction causes an increase in pro-inflammatory cytokines, which can lead to cell injury and exacerbate immune-mediated neurological conditions such as multiple sclerosis or myasthenia gravis; and cerebrospinal fluid (CSF) clearance is reduced in wakefulness compared to sleep, so reduced CSF flow from chronic sleep restriction may mediate the toxic accumulation of amyloid-β, a protein implicated in the pathogenesis of Alzheimer's disease (Kang et al., 2009). Impaired CSF flow and clearance of abnormal metabolic waste products from the brain may prove to be associated with many types of neurodegenerative diseases. In fact, since total sleep time is typically reduced in ageing, it is possible that this mechanism contributes to some of the normal cognitive decline expected with the ageing process.

Sleep-disordered breathing as a cause of stroke

Sleep-disordered breathing causes intermittent hypoxia, which can directly harm neurons by triggering neuronal apoptosis, glial scar formation, and altered morphology and connectivity of neurons. However, sleep-disordered breathing may cause nervous system injury by additional mechanisms as well, including alterations in glucose regulation, endothelial dysfunction, increased sympathetic nervous system tone, increased blood viscosity, and platelet activation, which all increase the risk of atherosclerosis and ischaemic stroke. In fact, sleep apnoea patients have increased intima-media thickness of the carotid artery (Silvestrini et al., 2002), a marker of atherosclerosis and stroke risk. Sleep apnoea may also increase the risk of cardioembolic stroke, mediated by atrial fibrillation or right-to-left intracardiac shunting through a patent foramen ovale and paradoxical embolization secondary to the intrathoracic pressure changes associated with apnoeas.

Sleep disorders affecting nervous system function

Sleep disorders exacerbating cognitive deficits

There is a wealth of data demonstrating cognitive deficits from sleep restriction in healthy volunteers, particularly poor sustained attention. Individuals with baseline cognitive impairment are particularly vulnerable to the impact of sleep disorders, as they have decreased cognitive reserve to compensate for this physiological stress. In fact, treatment of OSA by adenotonsillectomy in a paediatric population with attention deficit hyperactivity disorder (ADHD) improved the neurobehavioural symptoms to the same degree (or greater) as methylphenidate pharmacotherapy for attention (Huang et al., 2007). Circadian disruption in AD has been postulated to contribute to an evening increase in agitation, or 'sundowning'. Sleep disorders in dementia can also increase waking confusion. Excessive daytime sleepiness in neurodegenerative disease is associated with reduced functional status and the need for more assistance with activities of daily living. Nocturnal sleep disruption in the setting of dementia syndromes is taxing to caregivers and is one of the main factors leading to institutionalization in a long-term care facility.

Sleep and neuroplasticity

In recent years, there is a growing body of literature linking sleep to processes of neuroplasticity, the experience-dependent changes that occur at a synaptic level. Processes of neuroplasticity shape the functional connections between neural networks that become specialized for different types of information processing. Impaired plasticity during childhood development may increase the probability of cognitive or emotional disorders. For example, a prospective 5-year longitudinal study demonstrated a significantly higher chance of developing ADHD by 5.5 years of age for infants aged 6–12 months with severe sleep difficulties, particularly sleep initiation problems (Thunstrom, 2002). Conceivably, impaired plasticity can also reduce the functional recovery from nervous system injury such as stroke, traumatic brain injury, or other static insults such as anoxic brain injury following cardiac arrest. However, data on functional neurological outcomes by treating sleep disorders are lacking.

Sleep and paroxysmal neurological disorders

Epilepsy, defined as a propensity for unprovoked seizures, is one of the most common disorders in neurology. Individual seizures reflect abnormal, excessive, synchronized discharges in a population of neurons, and the clinical manifestations depend on the specific neural networks that are involved. The seizure threshold is influenced by sleep–wake state, and many seizures occur predominantly during sleep, particularly non-REM sleep. In fact, the probability of detecting abnormal electroencephalographic activity that is diagnostic of epilepsy increases 3-fold during sleep. It is well established that sleep disruption is one of the most common factors that lowers the seizure threshold and provokes seizure activity. Treatment of a primary sleep disorder improves seizure control. Positive airway pressure treatment for sleep-disordered breathing, for example, can improve seizure control in the majority of adult patients. Treatment of insomnia, either by pharmacological therapy or cognitive-behavioural therapy, would be predicted to improve seizure control. However, evidence for this in clinical populations with epilepsy is currently lacking.

Paroxysmal seizure phenomena during sleep can be difficult to distinguish from parasomnias. A brief frontal lobe seizure, for example, may appear similar to a confusional arousal. Episodic nocturnal wanderings are a manifestation of frontal lobe epilepsy that can be indistinguishable from sleepwalking. Adding to the difficulty in distinguishing seizures from parasomnias, electroencephalograms are often normal during frontal lobe seizures, and there is often normal awareness without confusion immediately following the event. Seizures are often abrupt in onset, with explosive activity, but the key distinguishing feature of seizures is the stereotyped nature of the spells. In fact, recurrent and stereotyped dreams are also a well-defined manifestation of seizures.

Headache is a common neurological disorder, occurring in up to one-third of adults. The relationship between headaches and sleep is clinically important in certain headache patients. Early observations noted that certain headaches would occur exclusively during sleep, particularly REM sleep (Dexter, 1979). Changes in sleep during the prior one to three nights may be a useful predictor of headache. Therefore, a brief sleep history should be incorporated into the evaluation of all headache patients, and sleep logs should be encouraged in order to determine headache triggers. Sleep disorders including OSA, circadian rhythm disorders, PLMS, and insomnia have been associated with an increase specifically in morning headaches.

Potential mechanisms for the relationship between sleep-disordered breathing and headache may relate to intermittent hypoxaemia, blood pressure surges, and increased intracranial pressure during obstructive apnoeas. These physiological changes may be particularly important in the autonomic cephalgias, with resultant activation of the trigeminal nucleus and the genesis of headache (Welch, 2003). Sleep deprivation can lower pain thresholds (Onen et al., 2001), and therefore sleep disruption or deprivation from a variety of causes can increase headache.

Conclusions

Scientific investigation of the relationships between sleep and neurological disorders is at a relatively early stage. More randomized, controlled treatment trials will ultimately help to determine the optimal timing and treatment modalities for the sleep disorders in these patients and the impact this will have on improving neurological health, enhancing neurological function, and reducing the care burden for this population.

Summary

- Damage to the nervous system or impaired neural development can cause a wide array of sleep disorders.

- In turn, sleep disruption may impair neuroplastic processes that are important for functional recovery after nervous system insults.

- Sleep disorders in patients with neurological disease can negatively affect quality of life for both the patients and the caregivers.

- Cardiovascular, metabolic, and immune process changes associated with sleep disorders may exacerbate the underlying neuropathological changes in neurological disease.

- Early intervention for sleep disorders in these patients may substantially improve neurological outcomes.

References

Bottini, P., Redolfi, S., Dottorini, M. L. & Tantucci, C. 2008. Autonomic neuropathy increases the risk of obstructive sleep apnea in obese diabetics. *Respiration*, **75**, pp. 265–71.

Dexter, J. D. 1979. The relationship between stage III + IV + REM sleep and arousals with migraine. *Headache*, **19**, pp. 364–9.

Huang, Y. S., Guilleminault, C., Li, H. Y., Yang, C. M., Wu, Y. Y. & Chen, N. H. 2007. Attention-deficit/hyperactivity disorder with obstructive sleep apnea: a treatment outcome study. *Sleep Medicine*, **8**, pp. 18–30.

Kang, J. E., Lim, M. M., Bateman, R. J., Lee, J. J., Smyth, L. P., Cirrito, J. R., Fujiki, N., Nishino, S. & Holtzman, D. M. 2009. Amyloid-beta dynamics are regulated by orexin and the sleep-wake cycle. *Science*, **326**(5955), pp. 1005–7.

Onen, S. H., Alloui, A., Gross, A., Eschallier, A. & Dubray, C. 2001. The effects of total sleep deprivation, selective sleep interruption and sleep recovery on pain tolerance thresholds in healthy subjects. *Journal of Sleep Research*, **10**, pp. 35–42.

Silvestrini, M., Rizzato, B., Placidi, F., Baruffaldi, R., Bianconi, A. & Diomedi, M. 2002. Carotid artery wall thickness in patients with obstructive sleep apnea syndrome. *Stroke*, **33**, pp. 1782–5.

Thunstrom, M. 2002. Severe sleep problems in infancy associated with subsequent development of attention-deficit/hyperactivity disorder at 5.5 years of age. *Acta Paediatrica*, **91**, pp. 584–92.

Vyazovskiy, V. V., Olcese, U., Lazimy, Y. M., Faraguna, U., Esser, S. K., Williams, J. C., Cirelli, C. & Tononi, G. 2009. Cortical firing and sleep homeostasis. *Neuron*, **63**, pp. 865–78.

Welch, K. M. 2003. Contemporary concepts of migraine pathogenesis. *Neurology*, **61**, S2–S8.

Wu, Y. H. & Swaab, D. F. 2005. The human pineal gland and melatonin in aging and Alzheimer's disease. *Journal of Pineal Research*, **38**, pp. 145–52.

Chapter 11

Sleep and epilepsy—chicken or egg?

Dora A. Lozsadi

Introduction

> "... for sleep is like epilepsy, and, in a sense, actually is a seizure of this sort.
> Accordingly, the beginning of this malady takes place with many during sleep, and
> their subsequent habitual seizures occur in sleep, not in waking hours. For when the
> spirit moves upwards ..."
> Aristotle, *On Sleep and Sleeplessness*, 350 BCE, tr. Beare JI.

Epilepsy is the commonest serious chronic neurological condition, affecting five individuals per 1,000 of the UK population. Patients will suffer unpredictable, unprovoked stereotyped seizures, causing symptoms and/or signs generated by abnormal synchronized neuronal network activity. Attacks may be subjective (e.g. sensory, limbic) experiences without evident behavioural change at mildest, and a generalized tonic–clonic seizure (convulsion) in its most severe form. Episodes typically last a few minutes, rarely more than five. Events are followed by a postictal refractory phase, during which individuals will appear drowsy and confused for typically less than 30 minutes. Thereafter, normal daytime behaviour and orientation or night-time sleep will be restored. Full recovery is expected in-between attacks, unless additional neurological problems are evident.

Epilepsy and sleep-related symptoms

Two-thirds of patients with epilepsy will remit on anti-epileptic drug treatment. Most with rare and/or subtle seizures, or in remission, are expected to lead a normal life. This group is likely to have normal sleep hygiene (habits and environmental factors influencing night-time sleep and daytime alertness) unless additional risk factors for sleep disturbance are present. These may include alcohol overuse, anxiety, depression, side-effects to anti-epileptic drugs, and associated sleep disorders, to name a few. Sleep is more likely to be disturbed in the remaining one-third, with neurological co-morbidity and poor seizure control. Key studies on this topic are summarized in Table 11.1. Most publications on sleep in patients with epilepsy rely on validated questionnaires, and less frequently on video-EEG (electroencephalography) monitoring or polysomnography.

Questionnaire-based studies on ambulant patients with epilepsy revealed that 21%–55% complained of daytime fatigue and somnolence. Both symptoms are known to reduce quality of life. Smaller case series with high proportions of seizure-free individuals

Table 11.1 Summary of larger studies on sleep disturbance in patients with epilepsy

Study	Sample size	Co-morbidity	Epilepsy	Control	Tools†	Results	Worse in patients with epilepsy (PWE)
Malow 1997	158	27 PWE also had polysomnography	68% focal 40% seizure free	68 'neurology' pts without epilepsy	ESS > 10 SA-SDQ symptoms of RLS	p < 0.05 predictors of raised ESS	In epilepsy BUT not significant (ns) when adjusted for OSA/RLS (!)
Manni 2000	244		78% focal 25.4% nocturnal 41% seizure free	205 healthy	ESS MCQ	not significant (ns)	
de Weerd 2004	486 all focal	Excluded those taking > 2 AEDs Posted questionnaires, 1183 screened	58% on single AED, No data on seizure control/nocturnal attacks	492 matched, pt selected	ESS SDL MOS-SS GSQ SF36-HS	ns p < 0.001 ns for snoring, awakening SOB	*Sleep disturbance worse in epilepsy: p < 0.0001, associated with QoL impairment; Mood not formally assessed
Khatami 2006	100	Cognitive, psychiatric neurological excluded	60% focal 62% seizure free	90 healthy not matched	ESS SA-SDQ UNS	ns, p = 0.01 when age correlated ns ns	Sleep complaints 30% vs10%
Piperidou 2008	124	Cognitive, psychiatric neurological excluded 28.2% OSA	71% focal 74% < 1/12; 41.7% nocturnal seizures	0	ESS>10 SA-SDQ AIS QOLIE-31	16.9% 24.6% insomnia EDS—low score p<0.05	Insomnia independent factor
Pizzatto 2013	140	Psychiatric excluded	64% symptomatic focal most with > 4 seizure /12	85 healthy matched	PSQI ESS SSS FLAQ	ns p < 0.003 p = 0.06 p < 0.001	Higher sleep disturbance & daytime dysfunction
Vendrame 2013	152	Sleep disorders excluded	48% suffered mood disorder 10.5% nocturnal seizures	0	ISI PSQI BDI-II QoLEI-31	51% affected reduced in poor sleep	70% reported poor sleep; linked to mood and AEDs

(continued)

Table 11.1 Continued

Study	Sample size	Co-morbidity	Epilepsy	Control	Tools[1]	Results	Worse in patients with epilepsy (PWE)
Ismayilova 2015	212; 208 analysed	Excluded sleep disorders, CVA, MS, CNS	47% nocturnal seizures 52% focal 21% seizure free	212 healthy matched	PSQI ESS > 10 BDS-PC Berlin Q	$p < 0.01$ ns $p < 0.01$ $p = 0.04$	$p \leq 0.05$ for Insomnia, EDS, sleep paralysis; Insomnia lower in seizure free; worse with epilepsy > 10 years
Unterberger 2015	200	Shiftwork, MMSE < 26, HADS > 10 excluded	50% focal 82% seizure free > 6 months	100	ESS PSQI BQ QOLIE-31	ns	Seizure rate was related to EDS; In 41% nocturnal seizures led to EDS
Im 2016	180	Pts off AED and with 'serious' medical conditions excluded	76% focal 37.8% seizure free	2836	ESS PSQI ISI GAS PHQ-9	$p = 0.012$ $p < 0.001$ $p < 0.001$ $p < 0.001$ $p < 0.001$ for depression	Adjusted for alcohol Sleep disturbance $p < 0.001$; Remission reduced risk

[1]Survey methods, questionnaires used to collect data. ESS: Epworth Sleepiness Scale; GSQ: Groningen Sleep Questionnaire (assessing sleep quality the previous night); PSQI: Pittsburgh Sleep Quality Index; SDL: Sleep Diagnosis List (derived from the Dutch Sleep Diagnosis Questionnaire),

Source: data from Malow BA, Bowes RJ, Lin X (1997). Predictors of sleepiness in epilepsy patients. *Sleep*, **20**(12), 1105–10; Manni R, Politini L, Ratti MT, et al. (2000). Sleep hygiene in adult epilepsy patients: a questionnaire-based survey. *Acta Neurol Scand*, **101**(5), 301-4; de Weerd A, de Haas S, Otte A, et al. (2004). Subjective sleep disturbance in patients with partial epilepsy: a questionnaire-based study on prevalence and impact on quality of life. *Epilepsia*, **45**(11), 1397-404; Khatami R, Zutter D, Siegel A, Mathis J, Donati F, Bassetti CL (2006). Sleep-wake habits and disorders in a series of 100 adult epilepsy patients—a prospective study. *Seizure*, **15**(5), 299-306; Piperidou C, Karlovasitou A, Triantafyllou N, et al. (2008). Influence of sleep disturbance on quality of life of patients with epilepsy. *Seizure*, **17**(7), 588-94; Pizzatto R, Lin K, Watanabe N, et al. (2013). Excessive sleepiness and sleep patterns in patients with epilepsy: a case-control study. *Epilepsy Behav*, **29**(1), 63-6; Vendrame M, Yang B, Jackson S, Auerbach SH (2013). Insomnia and epilepsy: a questionnaire-based study on prevalence. *J Clin Sleep Med*, **9**(2), 141-6; Ismayilova V, Demir AU, Tezer FI (2015). Subjective sleep disturbance in epilepsy patients at an outpatient clinic: A questionnaire-based study on prevalence. *Epilepsy Res*, **115**, 119-25; Unterberger I, Gabelia D, Prieschl M, et al. (2015). Sleep disorders and circadian rhythm in epilepsy revisited: a prospective controlled study. *Sleep Med*, **16**(2), 237-42; Im HJ, Park SH, Baek SH, et al. (2016) Associations of impaired sleep quality, insomnia, and sleepiness with epilepsy: A questionnaire-based case-control study. Epilepsy Behav, **57**(Pt A), 55-9. Reproduced courtesy of Dr D.A Lozadis.

and others who had experienced only a few attacks a month detected no significant difference in sleep hygiene when compared to controls. Polysomnography on patients with good seizure control showed subclinical abnormalities—increased sleep-onset latency, increased number of interictal epileptiform discharges, arousals, and cyclic alternating patterns—all leading to sleep fragmentation. The clinical significance of these changes remains to be established.

Twenty years ago, analysis using the Epworth Sleepiness Scale on 158 patients with epilepsy from the USA found that abnormal scores (> 10) were significantly more likely in this group than in 68 control neurology patients without epilepsy (Table 11.1; Malow, 1997). This difference was mainly caused by associated sleep disorders such as obstructive sleep apnoea, restless legs syndrome. Some years later, 244 patients with epilepsy, from Italy, failed to confirm these data (Table 11.1, Manni). Early results are inconsistent, as the Epworth Sleepiness Scale is not considered a suitably sensitive tool to screen sleep disturbance in patients with epilepsy.

Sleep quality and daytime sleepiness in adults have been the subject of numerous further publications. Somnolence in Swiss patients with epilepsy (Table 11.1, Khatami) was not significantly different to that in controls. The majority of patients studied were seizure-free at the time of the analysis. Sleep disturbance was found to be less frequent in this group than in those suffering frequent, particularly nocturnal, attacks.

A larger, Brazilian cohort (Table 11.1, Pizzatto) reported significantly worse daytime somnolence, significantly more frequent restless sleep, sleep-talking and -walking, bruxism, sleep paralysis, and abnormal dreams in patients with epilepsy than in healthy controls.

One Dutch study recruited adults with focal epilepsy treated with one or two anti-epileptic drugs. Data were collected on patients with epilepsy and compared to matched controls. The selection of a single and most common epilepsy type (localization related) produced informative data. Over 38% of patients with epilepsy reported sleep disturbances, compared to 18% of controls (Table 11.1, de Weerd). These findings were statistically significant. Using the SF36 Health Survey, patients with epilepsy scored worse than controls. This difference may be explained by associated depression, known to aggravate sleep problems. Reported sleep complaints were paralleled by reduced quality of life.

One well-designed study from Turkey (Table 11.1, Ismayilova) excluded patients with associated sleep disorders as well as other neurological diseases, such as stroke—conditions that all potentially impact on sleep. Results were compared to matched controls. In summary, patients with epilepsy experienced increased frequency of subjective sleep disturbance—most notably, sleep onset and maintenance insomnia, REM (rapid eye movement) sleep behavioural disorders, and sleep apnoea. Those with longstanding epilepsy were at higher risk, while others in remission were at lower risk.

A recent study from Korea reported increased incidence of sleep disturbance in those with epilepsy when compared to healthy controls. Researchers adjusted data for alcohol use, which in their sample was more commonly seen in the control group (Table 11.1, Im).

Insomnia, though commented on in some studies, is the focus of fewer publications. In a retrospective analysis of 152 epilepsy patients, using the Pittsburgh Sleep Quality

Index and Insomnia Severity Index, identified 78 (51%) with insomnia amongst patients with epilepsy (Table 11.1, Vendrame); insomnia was significantly increased in those prescribed multiple anti-epileptic drugs (particularly levetiracetam) and more likely to affect patients with symptoms of depression. Insomnia improved when patients with epilepsy entered remission.

Insomnia, a troublesome complaint, is also one of the commonest seizure triggers. This is particularly true for juvenile myoclonic epilepsy and generalized tonic–clonic seizures on awakening. Both of these syndromes are associated with a clear diurnal seizure pattern. Attacks typically occur: during drowsiness; within 2 hours of awakening; and, to a lesser degree, in late afternoon. Seizures are provoked by EEG synchronization associated with increased cyclic alternating patterns. Sleep deprivation exacerbates these diurnal EEG changes, worsening seizure control.

Sleep disturbances in children are more challenging to assess without polysomnography. A small study on 26 children with epilepsy found significantly more cases of excessive daytime sleepiness, sleep-disordered breathing, and parasomnias compared to controls. Future, larger trials on well-selected patients are expected to elucidate to what extent this is due to epilepsy, co-morbidity, or medication use.

In summary, we know that epilepsy is associated with over 100% increased sleep disturbances compared to control subjects. Factors known to contribute include poor seizure control, frequent seizures from sleep, associated sleep disorders (obstructive sleep apnoea, restless legs syndrome), mood and other psychiatric and neurological problems (mainly depression), and—to a lesser degree—prescribed medication and recreational toxins such as alcohol and nicotine. Regional variations (lifestyle, genetic, etc.) may also play a role. Most studies to date reported on small groups of patients with mixed epilepsy syndromes. Nevertheless, clear risk factors for sleep disturbance in patients with epilepsy have been identified. UK data on sleep quality and daytime sleepiness affecting adult patients with epilepsy is awaited. The results will guide screening and patient care in epilepsy out-patient clinics.

Nocturnal (sleep) seizures

The average person spends a third of his/her life sleeping. Gowers pointed out, over 100 years ago, that seizures generally followed a similar pattern, with one-third of attacks occurring during sleep. Twenty per cent of patients with epilepsy will experience exclusively night-time attacks. These are approximate numbers only. When epilepsy subtypes/syndromes are considered, there are marked diurnal differences. Frontal lobe seizures are far more likely to start from sleep (78%), while temporal lobe seizures are less so (only 20%). Some, mainly paediatric epilepsy syndromes, are exclusively associated with attacks from sleep.

Not only are particular epilepsies more common in sleep, but so are interictal epileptiform discharges. These are EEG spikes, polyspikes, sharp waves or spike and wave components occurring in isolation or in runs without clinical change, or subjective account of a seizure.

These abnormalities are more often seen in non-REM, particularly slow-wave, sleep than in wakefulness, and are virtually absent in REM sleep. Sleep induction is therefore often used as a provocation method during routine EEG recording.

Seizures arising from sleep show a similar predilection—more frequent in non-REM N1 and N2 sleep (Ng & Pavlova, 2013). Unless the patient is EEG monitored, mild seizures causing subjective experiences, or disturbance of consciousness, may remain unnoticed when occurring in sleep. The transition between nocturnal subclinical seizures and interictal epileptiform discharges is therefore gradual. In sleep, clinical distinguishing markers are often lost or missed. As the vast majority of patients with epilepsy do not undergo overnight EEG monitoring, the true impact of attacks (clinical and subclinical) from sleep is unknown. Daytime somnolence or increased sleep requirement may be indirect indicators of their presence.

The nocturnal variant of benign myoclonic epilepsy in infancy clinically may appear similar to sleep starts (hypnic jerks). This is a rare epilepsy syndrome, associated with EEG abnormalities, potential developmental delay (mainly language), and often a family history of epilepsy.

Childhood-onset nocturnal epilepsy syndromes include the rare electrical status epilepticus in slow-wave sleep. Children experience nocturnal focal and generalized seizures and daytime absences. EEG, by definition, shows generalized spike and wave discharges in 85%–100% of slow-wave sleep. Global cognitive regression ensues, or may be the presenting problem.

Landau–Kleffner syndrome, or acquired epileptic aphasia, is another rare childhood epilepsy syndrome associated with spike and wave discharges in slow-wave sleep and behavioural problems. EEG abnormalities are less prevalent than in electrical status epilepticus in sleep, and may be unilateral. Auditory agnosia (inability to interpret the nature and meaning of heard noises) is the primary deficit leading to language regression. Seizures may not affect all children. Some patients make a full recovery, though early-onset cases fare worse.

Atypical benign partial epilepsy (or pseudo-Lennox syndrome) is the mildest of the three conditions associated with spike and wave discharges in non-REM sleep. Learning difficulty often precedes the onset of generalized seizures at between 2 and 5 years of age. Though seizures remit by teens, developmental delay remains in over 50% of patients.

The commonest (up to 25%) childhood epilepsy syndrome is benign focal epilepsy with centrotemporal spikes, or benign rolandic epilepsy, and affecting children from 3 years of age. Sixty per cent of seizures occur from sleep. Attacks start as facial paraesthesia, evolving into lower facial muscle contractions and dysarthria (speech disturbance caused by weakness or loss of muscle control). Children may experience sleep disturbance and cognitive deficit as a consequence.

The above selected epilepsy syndromes have been summarized; all are associated with seizures predominantly or exclusively from sleep. The childhood epilepsies characterized by spike and wave discharges in non-REM sleep confirm that frequent/continuous interictal epileptiform discharges in sleep also have a significant impact on daytime cognition and development. Daytime somnolence and fatigue have not been studied in these children.

Epilepsy syndromes in adults are predominantly focal in onset. The second most prevalent of these are frontal lobe seizures, occurring in up to 30% of adults with epilepsy. An estimated 78% will experience seizures from sleep. Unfortunately, studies exploring sleep-related complications of epilepsy do not analyze subgroups (i.e. individual epilepsy syndromes). As expected, those diagnosed with active frontal lobe epilepsy are at high risk of sleep disturbances. Furthermore, case reports indicate that several healthy relatives of patients with cryptogenic (cause remains elusive) nocturnal frontal lobe epilepsy are also prone to increased number of nocturnal arousals when compared to controls.

An alarming complication is sudden unexpected death in epilepsy. This occurs in over 500 patients a year in the UK alone, and 7,000 in the United States and Europe combined. By definition, death is not caused by co-morbidity or seizure-related injury, status epilepticus. Fifty-eight per cent of deaths from epilepsy occur in sleep. Individuals are usually found dead, supine in bed, often with indirect evidence of a seizure (petechial haemorrhages, tongue bites, etc.). Events, when captured during EEG monitoring, are suggestive of death due to postictal cardiorespiratory suppression. Sleep-related autonomic changes are thought to increase risk. Treatment with selective serotonin uptake inhibitors (antidepressant) reduces the probability of sudden unexpected death in epilepsy (Maguire et al., 2016).

Epilepsy and associated neurological conditions affecting sleep

Epilepsy is often caused by underlying neurological disease such as head injury, tumour, or stroke on a background of additional genetic susceptibility. Many of these conditions will be associated with sleep disturbance whether or not accompanied by epilepsy. At present, it is unknown whether additional symptomatic epilepsy further increases the risk of sleep disturbance or whether genetic factors and the underlying neurological condition entirely account for this. It is not the scope of this chapter to discuss this further.

Depression is common in the general population. Chronic disease further increases prevalence. Epilepsy increases the risk of associated depression out of the proportion of chronic diseases in general. Prevalence is quoted at 23.1% (Fiest et al., 2013). Depression in patients with epilepsy is often undetected and untreated. When co-existent, however, it will aggravate sleep disturbance, thus worsening seizure control.

Not only are mood and psychiatric conditions more common in patients with epilepsy. A US audit of 480 patients with epilepsy reported an over 100% increased prevalence of liver conditions, migraine or severe headache, facial pain, emphysema and stroke in those with a diagnosis of epilepsy (Centres for Disease Control and Prevention, 2010). When several chronic conditions are present (no data for epilepsy), insomnia is exacerbated, suggesting a supra-additive effect (Koyanagi et al., 2014). The relationship is reciprocal, as insomnia itself increases the risk of cardiovascular disease and also leads to aggravation of several other chronic diseases including epilepsy.

Epilepsy and sleep disorders

Sleep disorders are more common in patients with epilepsy than in the general population (van Golde et al., 2011). The prevalence of obstructive sleep apnoea is up to one-third in this group. Among 39 treatment-resistant candidates assessed for epilepsy surgery, five otherwise asymptomatic patients were diagnosed with severe obstructive sleep apnoea requiring treatment. A larger study on 283 patients with epilepsy identified 10.2% with obstructive sleep apnoea via screening with a questionnaire. When individuals with excessive daytime sleepiness were selected, 70% of 63 patients with epilepsy had an Apnoea Hypopnoea Index score > 10, and 16% scored over 50. Risk increases in older males with high BMI (body mass index) and epilepsy onset late in life. Muscle relaxant, sedative anti-epileptic drugs (i.e. benzodiazepines) and the vagal nerve stimulator further aggravate obstructive sleep apnoea. Nocturnal seizures may also contribute via postictal respiratory suppression. When nocturnal hypoxia is treated, seizure control also improves.

Central apnoea in patients with epilepsy has been less extensively studied. It is a documented feature of several epilepsy syndromes (e.g. Rett syndrome). In case series of patients with epilepsy assessed with polysomnography (n = 719), 15 (3.7%) experienced central sleep apnoea and 33 (7.9%) combined (obstructive and central) sleep apnoea (Vendrame et al., 2014). Neither nocturnal seizures nor seizure frequency appeared different between groups. Two out of three seizures were focal. None of the monitored episodes of desaturation were related to seizures. It is unclear whether patients prone to central/combined apnoea are at higher risk of sudden unexpected death in epilepsy.

Restless legs/periodic limb movement in sleep is not associated with arousal in all cases. Therefore, reported sleep disturbance may vary. Studies quote a prevalence of 17%–18% in selected epilepsy patients. Data is conflicting on whether numbers are significantly higher in patients with epilepsy than in controls.

REM sleep behavioural disorder is commonly seen in the elderly with a diagnosis of neurodegenerative disease. Epilepsy is also known to be more frequent amongst these patients (Lozsadi & Larner, 2006). Prevalence is reported to be 12.5% in patients over 60 years of age admitted for diagnostic video-EEG telemetry for nocturnal events.

Circadian rhythm sleep disorders and non-REM (NREM) sleep parasomnias remain to be studied in patients with epilepsy. There is an association between NREM parasomnia and nocturnal frontal lobe epilepsy.

Anti-epileptic drugs and sleep

Earlier sections discussed how epilepsy is associated with altered sleep architecture. These alterations in untreated patients include increased number of stage shifts, reduced REM sleep, and increased sleep fragmentation. Changes improve with chronic treatment. Anti-epileptic drugs, on the one hand, will reduce nocturnal seizures and interictal epileptiform discharges, while on the other hand will cause side-effects, such as somnolence, insomnia, and altered sleep (micro) architecture (Jain & Glauser, 2014).

Na channel blockers

This group of anti-epileptic drugs is most commonly prescribed in developed countries. One informative study on carbamazepine recruited ten patients with temporal lobe epilepsy; whilst on carbamazepine they had higher REM arousal indices than healthy controls. Cyclic alternating pattern parameters during polysomnography showed low rate and cycle/sequences in controls; this increased in patients with epilepsy and yet further in those treated with carbamazepine. It is difficult to comment as to what extent these changes resulted in clinical benefit.

Studies are scarcer on other members of this anti-epileptic drug group. Both lamotrigine and phenytoin affected sleep differently in newly diagnosed patients with epilepsy when compared to treatment-resistant and chronic application.

Nayak et al. (2015) combined polysomnography and questionnaires in 20 patients with juvenile myoclonic epilepsy (the commonest primary generalized epilepsy syndrome) and 20 matched controls in a well-designed study. Ten patients with epilepsy were anti-epileptic drug naive, and ten were prescribed sodium valproate. REM sleep duration was found to be significantly higher in the sodium valproate treated group. REM sleep arousals and rates of cyclic alternating patterns (during N1 and N2, but not N3) were significantly higher in patients with epilepsy than in controls. Cyclic alternating pattern rates during N3 were highest in drug-naive patients with epilepsy, suggesting a beneficial effect of sodium valproate lowering rates of N3-stage cyclic alternating patterns. Questionnaire-based data indicate that those changes are accompanied by improved sleep quality in sodium valproate treated patients. In sodium valproate treated healthy adults, no change was seen on visual scoring of sleep. Another publication shows reduced daytime naps in children after sodium valproate withdrawal.

Barbiturates and benzodiazepines

Medications in this group are prescribed as sedatives, anaesthetic agents, and anti-epileptic drugs. Clobazam, a benzodiazepine, in a randomized placebo-controlled trial on healthy individuals, reduced sleep latency, N1, slow-wave sleep and wake after sleep onset, while increasing N2 sleep. This is to be expected, as other benzodiazepines are often prescribed as sleeping tablets. Phenobarbital, most often prescribed in developing countries, has been studied in healthy adults as well as patients with epilepsy. It reduces sleep latency, arousals, and REM sleep in a dose-dependent manner. At the same time, N2 sleep is increased.

GABAergic drugs

The two most commonly prescribed GABAergic medications, gabapentin and pregabalin, are not only anti-epileptic drugs, but are also licensed for neuropathic pain and used off label as anxiolytics. Gabapentin increases slow-wave sleep and REM sleep, and reduces awakenings as well as N1 sleep in patients with epilepsy. This coincides with improved seizure control in most. Pregabalin in healthy adults increases slow-wave sleep and sleep efficiency, while reducing awakenings and REM sleep. Other studies on patients with epilepsy and insomnia found increased slow-wave sleep and improved daytime attention with adjunctive application.

Melatonin

Though melatonin has not been licensed for use in patients with epilepsy, some specialists will recommend acute treatment if sleep deprivation is the cause of sudden deterioration of seizure control. There is no data to support its long-term use as an anti-epileptic drug.

Non-medical treatment of epilepsy

A third of patients with epilepsy will continue to experience seizures despite taking anti-epileptic drugs. A selected few of these (estimated 1:105 per annum in the UK) will be suitable candidates for surgical treatment. A ketogenic (low carbohydrate) diet is predominantly used as adjunctive therapy with anti-epileptic drugs in children with refractory epilepsy. Insomnia is a common side-effect. In keeping with this, the diet reduces total sleep time and N2 sleep, increasing REM sleep. Vagal nerve stimulator (implanted device attached to cranial nerve X) is known to aggravate obstructive sleep apnoea, though other data on its effect on sleep are conflicting. Respective epilepsy surgery is described to increase total sleep time and reduce arousals in those with improved postoperative seizure control (Engel class I and II).

Summary

- Epilepsy is an episodic and the commonest serious chronic neurological condition affecting 5 in 1,000 individuals in the UK.
- Up to 50% of patients complain of daytime fatigue or somnolence.
- Sleep disturbance is twice as common in those with epilepsy than in healthy controls.
- Insomnia, excessive daytime somnolence, or altered sleep architecture is more likely when epilepsy is associated with:
  - co-morbidity: depression, learning difficulty, stroke, etc.
  - sleep disorders: obstructive sleep apnoea, central sleep apnoea, restless legs syndrome, periodic limb movement in sleep
  - toxins/medications: barbiturate, benzodiazepine or alcohol use
  - poor seizure control, mainly active night-time seizures
- Improving screening and treatment of reversible factors will benefit sleep hygiene, seizure control, as well as quality of life.

References

Centres for Disease Control and Prevention (CDC). 2010. Comorbidity in adults with epilepsy—United States 2010. *Morbidity and Mortality Weekly Report*, **62**, pp. 849–53.

Fiest, K. M., Dykeman, J., Patten, S. B., Wiebe, S., Kaplan, G. G., Maxwell, C. J., Bulloch, A. G. & Jette, N. 2013. Depression in epilepsy: a systematic review and meta-analysis. *Neurology*, **80**, pp. 590–99.

Im H. J., Park S. H., Baek S. H., Chu M. K., Yang K. I., Kim W. J., Yun C. H. 2016. Associations of impaired sleep quality, insomnia, and sleepiness with epilepsy: A questionnaire- based case-control study. *Epilepsy Behavior*, **57**(Pt A), pp. 55–9.

Ismayilova V., Demir A. U., Tezer F. I. 2015. Subjective sleep disturbance in epilepsy patients at an outpatient clinic: A questionnaire-based study on prevalence. *Epilepsy Research*, **115**, pp. 119–25.

Jain, S. V. & Glauser, T. A. 2014. Effects of epilepsy treatments on sleep architecture and daytime sleepiness: an evidence-based review of objective sleep metrics. *Epilepsia*, **55**, pp. 26–37.

Khatami R., Zutter D., Siegel A., Mathis J., Donati F., Bassetti C. L. 2006. Sleep-wake habits and disorders in a series of 100 adult epilepsy patients—a prospective study. *Seizure*, **15**(5), pp. 299–306.

Koyanagi, A., Garin, N., Olaya, B., Ayuso-Mateos, J. L., Chatterji, S., Leonardi, M., Koskinen, S., Tobiasz-Adamczyk, B., Haro, J. M. 2014. Chronic conditions and sleep problems among adults aged 50 years or over in nine countries: a multi-country study. *PLoS ONE*, **9**(12), e0114742.

Lozsadi, D. A. & Larner, A. J. 2006. Prevalence and causes of seizures at the time of diagnosis of probable Alzheimer's disease. *Dementia and Geriatric Cognitive Disorders*, **22**, pp. 121–4.

Maguire, M. J., Jackson, C. F., Marson, A. G. & Nolan, S. J. 2016. Treatments for the prevention of sudden unexpected death in epilepsy. *The Cochrane Database of Systematic Reviews*, **7**, CD011792.

Malow B. A., Bowes R. J., Lin X. 1997. Predictors of sleepiness in epilepsy patients. *Sleep*, **20**(12), pp. 1105–10.

Manni R., Politini L., Ratti M. T., Marchioni E., Sartori I., Galimberti C. A., Tartara A. 2000. Sleep hygiene in adult epilepsy patients: a questionnaire-based survey. *Acta Neurologica Scandinavica*, **101**(5), pp. 301–4.

Nayak, C. S., Sinha, S., Nagappa, M., Kandavel, T. & Taly, A. B. 2015. Effect of valproate on the sleep microstructure of juvenile myoclonic epilepsy patients—a cross-sectional CAP based study. *Sleep Medicine*, **17**, pp. 129–33.

Ng, M. & Pavlova, M. 2013. Why are seizures rare in rapid eye movement sleep? Review of the frequency of seizures in different sleep stages. *Epilepsy Research and Treatment*, Article ID 932790.

Piperidou C., Karlovasitou A., Triantafyllou N., Terzoudi A., Constantinidis T., Vadikolias K., Heliopoulos I., Vassilopoulos D., Balogiannis S. 2008. Influence of sleep disturbance on quality of life of patients with epilepsy. *Seizure*, **17**(7), pp. 588–94.

Pizzatto, R., Lin K., Watanabe, N., Campiolo, G., Bicalho, M. A. H., Guarnieri, R., Claudino, R., Walz, R., Sukys-Claudino, L. 2013. Excessive sleepiness and sleep patterns in patients with epilepsy: a case-control study. *Epilepsy Behavior*, **29**(1), pp. 63–6.

Unterberger I., Gabelia D., Prieschl M., Chea K., Hofer M., Högl B., Luef G., Frauscher B. 2015. Sleep disorders and circadian rhythm in epilepsy revisited: a prospective controlled study. *Sleep Medicine*, **16**(2), pp. 237–42.

van Golde, E. G., Gutter, T. & de Weerd, A. W. 2011. Sleep disturbances in people with epilepsy; prevalence, impact and treatment. *Sleep Medicine Reviews*, **15**, pp. 357–68.

Vendrame M., Yang B., Jackson S., Auerbach S. H. 2013. Insomnia and epilepsy: a questionnaire-based study. *J Clin Sleep Medicine*, **9**(2), pp. 141–6.

Vendrame, M., Jackson, S., Syed, S., Kothare, S. V. & Auerbach, S. H. 2014. Central sleep apnea and complex sleep apnea in patients with epilepsy. *Sleep and Breathing*, **18**, pp. 119–24.

de Weerd A., de Haas S., Otte A., Trenité D. K, van Erp G., Cohen A., de Kam M., van Gerven J. 2004. Subjective sleep disturbance in patients with partial epilepsy: a questionnaire-based study on prevalence and impact on quality of life. *Epilepsia*, **45**(11), pp. 1397–404.

Chapter 12

Sleep, inflammation, and disease

Michelle A. Miller

Introduction

This chapter briefly examines the relationship between sleep and the immune system and how changes in sleeping patterns may contribute to disease. It looks at some of the possible mechanisms and pathways that may be responsible, as well as potential treatment options and public health importance.

Sleep behaviour

Sleep is a fundamental and natural process. Whilst its exact purpose remains to be elucidated, it is clear that it is important in the maintenance and restoration of health-related pathways in the body. This is achieved through a number of processes, including energy regulation, cellular repair, and infection control, and may occur during either non-rapid-eye movement (NREM) sleep or rapid-eye movement (REM) sleep. Individuals cycle between the two phases during the night, with dreaming occurring in the REM phase.

Sleeping habits within our society are constantly changing. In the past 100 years there has been a decrease in the number of hours people claim they sleep. These changes are partly due to a decreased dependency on daylight hours and partly due to an increase in shift work and changes in lifestyle and home environments. It is important that we understand the importance of sleep and the effect these changes may have on health and disease.

There are over 70 known sleep disorders. One of the most common, obstructive sleep apnoea (OSA), is caused by a physical obstruction of the airway. It is estimated that 12 million Americans may have this potentially life-threatening disorder. Breathing is interrupted during sleep and this condition is characterized by chronic sleep deprivation and excessive daytime sleepiness (EDS). It is normally treated by the application of continuous airway pressure (CPAP), which maintains an open airway.

Sleep and inflammation

Sleep and the immune system appear to have a reciprocal relationship. Anecdotally, sleep is reported to be an early response to acute infections such as the cold and influenza virus. Early Greek writings noted that sleepiness often accompanied infection. This is now believed to be the result of the activation of the immune system and amplification of physiological sleep regulator mechanisms, including increased production of inflammatory cytokines (Zielinski & Krueger, 2011). Short sleep duration and poor sleep quality may affect one's susceptibility to, and ability to fight off, infection.

The body responds to infectious materials, unknown objects, tumours, and transplanted material by way of the evolutionary conserved innate immune system. Activation of this pathway occurs via Toll-like receptors (TLRs) and nuclear factor-kappaB (NF-κB). This in turn leads to increased activation of more than 200 genes, including those which are involved in the production of cytokines and inflammatory markers. Activation of these host defence and immune mechanisms not only leads to an increase in inflammatory cytokines but also to an increase in body temperature, longer periods of slow-wave sleep (SWS), and reduced wakefulness. In advanced stages of inflammation, the sleep-promoting effects are diminished and reduced NREM and increased wakefulness may result.

The influenza virus has been associated with large increases in NREM sleep and increased production of interleukin-1 (IL-1), which is one of the first inflammatory cytokines to be implicated in sleep regulation. Viruses have been implicated in a number of conditions that involve sleep disorders, including chronic fatigue syndrome and sudden infant death syndrome. Sleep deprivation can also alter the immune response to a viral challenge, with reduced antibody responses to hepatitis A vaccination being reported in sleep-deprived young adults.

Bacterial infection activates the innate immune system and affects sleep, but the route of administration, as well as the bacterial species involved, can alter the timing of the sleep response. Furthermore, both killed bacteria and components of the bacterial cell wall can induce NREM sleep changes.

Sleep deprivation and inflammation

Regular daily fluctuations in the level of various cytokines have been reported in normal individuals. These diurnal variations may also be related to the sleep–wake cycle, with circulating levels being affected by sleep deprivation (Irwin et al., 2016; Miller & Cappuccio, 2010). After a period of sleep deprivation the body tries to recover lost sleep, suggesting that sleep is not a passive activity and that prolonged sleep loss may have devastating consequences on the immune system. It is therefore important to establish, at the population level, the optimum amount of sleep required to remain healthy and safe. At the individual level, it is also important to determine what factors determine this need and to recognize that not everyone may require the same amount of sleep. Studies on animals indicate that prolonged sleep deprivation leads to the death of the animal possibly as a result of the failure of the host defence mechanisms.

Work pressure, social and domestic demands and responsibilities, lifestyle, or the presence of a medical or sleep disorder may all contribute to chronic sleep restriction. It has been proposed that the function of sleep is to maintain the integrity of the neuroendocrine system, such that if the integrity of this system is disrupted by disease or inflammation, the organism will respond by modulating sleep so as to restore the balance (Hurtado-Alvarado et al., 2013). Accumulated evidence suggests that chronic restriction of sleep below 7 hours per night leads to significant adverse health outcomes. The level of circulating pro-inflammatory mediators depends on the intensity and duration of sleep loss. Whereas acute sleep loss may stimulate the innate immune system, chronic sleep loss may affect the adaptive immune system.

A recent meta-analysis and systematic review, which included both cohort and experimental sleep deprivation studies (n = 72), found that sleep disturbance and long sleep duration (but not short sleep duration) were associated with markers of systemic inflammation (Irwin et al., 2016). Some gender differences were observed; women showed greater increases in high-sensitivity C-reactive protein (hs-CRP) and IL-6 than men, suggesting that women may be more vulnerable to the effects of sleep disturbances. Studies conducted to date, however, have had some limitations. For example, sleep is often measured using questionnaires as opposed to using objective sleep-measuring devices, and sleep is often only recorded at a single, as opposed to multiple, time points. Prospective studies, which address these limitations, are required.

Sleep, inflammation, and disease

Sleep disruption (quality and quantity) affects immune function, and as many chronic conditions have an underlying inflammatory component, it is not surprising that sleep deprivation is associated with disease morbidity and mortality. Emerging evidence suggests that the combination of both poor sleep quality and short sleep may be particularly detrimental to health.

Inflammatory processes are important in the development of cardiovascular disease (CVD) and the major risk factors, including obesity, type 2 diabetes, and hypertension (Miller & Cappuccio, 2013). There is a U-shaped relationship between sleep duration & all-cause mortality, and CVD, with a greater risk in long sleepers (see Chapter 8). Similarly, circulating inflammatory cytokines can be altered by short and long sleep (Irwin et al., 2016).

Obesity is becoming a global epidemic in both adults and children. A recent meta-analysis of longitudinal studies in children suggests that there is an increased risk of overweight/obesity among short-sleeping children (Fatima et al., 2015). Obesity leads to a change in an individual's metabolic profile and an accumulation of adipose tissue (fat), which produces inflammatory cytokines and hormones such as resistin and leptin. Leptin plays a key role in appetite regulation. It also has profound inflammatory effects and is affected by sleep.

There is a bi-directional relationship between glucose regulation and sleep. Diabetes can lead to the development of sleep abnormalities and short sleep can lead to a decrease in glucose tolerance. Both quantity and quality of sleep predict the risk of developing type 2 diabetes (see Chapter 8). Furthermore, activation of inflammatory signalling pathways contributes to insulin resistance.

In healthy subjects, acute sleep deprivation leads to an increase in blood pressure and activation of the sympathetic nervous system. Short sleep has been shown to be associated with a significantly increased risk of hypertension, which in turn is associated with an increase in inflammatory markers (Miller & Cappuccio, 2013).

Metabolic syndrome (MetS), which has an increased prevalence in OSA patients, is characterized by a clustering of cardiovascular and metabolic risk factors in a given individual and has been associated with an increase in pro-inflammatory markers. More recently, short sleep duration has been shown to be an independent risk factor for incident metabolic syndrome in a population-based longitudinal study (Kim et al., 2015).

Sleep disorders, including insomnia, contribute to the development of depression. Depressed patients have a significant nocturnal increase in circulating inflammatory markers as compared with controls (Motivala et al., 2005).

Inflammation in the central nervous system is associated with cognitive impairment and the development of neurodegenerative disorders such as Alzheimer's disease (AD). Sleep disturbances may contribute to the development of inflammation in these conditions.

Clinically unrelated conditions such as rheumatoid arthritis, systemic lupus erythematous, and Crohn's disease have similar immune dysregulation. An affected individual may often have more than one of these conditions. An imbalance in inflammatory cytokines is central to the development and progression of these immune-mediated disorders, in which an association between disease activity and sleep disturbances is often reported. Sleep disturbances are not always associated with the concomitant pain, and some studies using TNF-α antagonists to treat joint inflammation have reported a concomitant reduction in daytime sleepiness (Ranjbaran et al., 2007).

Various cytokines show daily variations in normal individuals, but at given time points may be higher in people with asthma than in controls. Indeed, asthma attacks that require emergency assistance often occur at night, when cytokines may be at their most elevated. Many asthmatics report being awakened by sleeping difficulties, and sleep disorders exacerbate this condition (Majde & Krueger, 2005).

Sleep and its effect on inflammation may be important in the development of, and recovery from, cancer. Many cancer patients also report both sleeping problems and depression.

Sleep disorders, inflammation, and disease

In many different ethnic populations, the prevalence of OSA is relatively high. It affects at least 1%–5% of middle-aged individuals, although men are twice as likely as women to have OSA (Lam & Ip, 2007).

The link between sleep disorders such as OSA and serious health problems, including CVD, is well established. NREM sleep is normally accompanied by a decrease in metabolic rate, sympathetic nerve activity, and heart rate. This pattern of cardiovascular quiescence is interrupted by OSA, which triggers a cascade of acute haemodynamic, autonomic, chemical, metabolic, and inflammatory effects. Long-term exposures to such effects can lead to the development, or exacerbation, of existing CVD (Miller & Cappuccio, 2010). A recent report has recommended not only that OSA be considered in all resistant hypertensive patients, but also that any hypertensive patients with a BMI in excess of 27 kg/m^2 should be examined for the presence of sleep disorders (Chobanian, 2003). Long-term

CPAP treatment improves daytime and nocturnal blood pressure control in these patients and is associated with a decrease in markers of inflammation (Miller & Cappuccio, 2010).

Evidence from studies in children is of particular interest as the results in children are less likely to be confounded by the presence of co-morbidities. Children with sleep-disordered breathing (SDB) have higher levels of the inflammatory marker hs-CRP than children with no SDB. Those children with elevated markers were also reported to have EDS or learning difficulties (Tauman et al., 2004). Likewise, levels of inflammatory markers were reported to be higher in non-obese children with OSA aged 4–9 years than in children without OSA matched for age, gender, ethnicity, and BMI. These levels returned to the level of the controls after the children with OSA had had an adenotonsillectomy, indicating that perturbations of inflammatory mechanism occur in very young children, even in the absence of obesity. If left unchecked, these effects could lead to the activation of further downstream pathways and may lead to an increased risk of end-organ damage (Miller & Cappuccio, 2010).

In some individuals, the daytime sleepiness associated with OSA is not always eliminated by CPAP treatment. It is therefore important to consider other treatment regimes, some of which may address the underlying inflammatory component. These include weight reduction and exercise, which, by reducing adipose tissue, may reduce the production of inflammatory cytokines. Results from a pilot study have indicated that treatment with etanercept, which acts on the inflammatory molecule TNF-α, leads to an improvement in both the frequency of airway closure and the associated sleep latency (Vgontzas, 2008). This adds to the evidence that suggests that pro-inflammatory cytokines contribute to the pathogenesis of OSA and sleepiness, and also indicates that anti-inflammatory medications may be a beneficial treatment for this disorder. Further large randomized trials with sufficient follow-up periods are required to determine causal relationships and the possible treatment benefits associated with anti-inflammatory treatment regimes in the treatment of OSA.

Summary

- Sleeping 7–8 hours per night appears to be optimal for health, but there is a need for improved measurements of sleep quantity and quality.
- The temporal relationship between acute and short-term chronic deprivation and disease may, in part, be mediated by inflammation.
- Inflammation plays an important underlying role in disease development.
- The prevalence of many such inflammatory-based diseases has risen in the last decade in both children and adults.
- Sleep curtailment may lead to an increase in the inflammatory processes underlying these diseases. It remains to be determined whether biologically restorative sleep can reverse or halt such disease progression.
- Future research is required to address some of these issues and to elucidate the role of sleep in public health, which may be of particular importance in preventing disease development and progression in children.

References

Chobanian, A. V., Bakris, G. L., Black, H. R., Cushman, W. C., Green, L. A., Izzo, J. L. Jr, Jones, D. W., Materson, B. J., Oparil, S., Wright, J. T. Jr, Roccella, E. J.; Joint National Committee on Prevention, Detection, Evaluation, and Treatment of High Blood Pressure; National Heart, Lung, and Blood Institute; National High Blood Pressure Education Program Coordinating Committee. 2003. Seventh report of the Joint National Committee on Prevention, Detection, Evaluation, and Treatment of High Blood Pressure. *Hypertension*, **42**(6), pp. 1206–52.

Fatima, Y. & Doi, S.A. 2015. Longitudinal impact of sleep on overweight and obesity in children and adolescents: a systematic review and bias-adjusted meta-analysis. *Obesity Reviews*, **16**(2), pp. 137–49.

Hurtado-Alvarado, G., Pavón, L., Castillo-García, S. A., Hernández, M. E., Domínguez-Salazar, E., Velázquez-Moctezuma, J. & Gómez-González, B. 2013. Sleep loss as a factor to induce cellular and molecular inflammatory variations. *Clinical and Developmental Immunology*, **80**, p. 1341.

Irwin, M. R., Olmstead, R. & Carroll, J. E. 2016. Sleep disturbance, sleep duration, and inflammation: a systematic review and meta-analysis of cohort studies and experimental sleep deprivation. *Biological Psychiatry*, **80**(1), pp. 40–52.

Kim, J. Y., Yadav, D., Ahn, S. V., Koh, S. B., Park, J. T., Yoon, J., Yoo, B. S. & Lee, S. H. 2015. A prospective study of total sleep duration and incident metabolic syndrome: the ARIRANG study. *Sleep Medicine*, **16**(12), pp. 1511–15.

Lam, J. C. & Ip, M. S. 2007. An update on obstructive sleep apnea and the metabolic syndrome. *Current Opinion in Pulmonary Medicine*, **13**(6), pp. 484–9.

Majde, J. A. & Krueger, J. M. 2005. Links between the innate immune system and sleep. *The Journal of Allergy and Clinical Immunology*, **116**(6), pp. 1188–98.

Miller, M. A. & Cappuccio, F. P. 2010. Sleep, inflammation, and disease. In: Cappuccio, F. P., Miller, M. A. & Lockley, S. W. eds. *Sleep, Health and Society: from aetiology to public health*. Oxford: Oxford University Press, pp. 239–68.

Miller, M. A. & Cappuccio, F. P. 2013. Biomarkers of cardiovascular risk in sleep-deprived people. *Journal of Human Hypertension*, **27**(10), pp. 583–8.

Motivala, S. J., Sarfatti, A., Olmos, L. & Irwin, M. R. 2005. Inflammatory markers and sleep disturbance in major depression. *Psychosomatic Medicine*, **67**(2), pp. 187–94.

Ranjbaran, Z., Keefer, L., Stepanski, E., Farhadi, A. & Keshavarzian, A. 2007. The relevance of sleep abnormalities to chronic inflammatory conditions. *Inflammation Research*, **56**(2), pp. 51–7.

Tauman, R., Ivanenko, A., O'Brien, L. M. & Gozal, D. 2004. Plasma C-reactive protein levels among children with sleep-disordered breathing. *Pediatrics*; **113**(6), e564–e569.

Vgontzas, A.N. 2008. Does obesity play a major role in the pathogenesis of sleep apnoea and its associated manifestations via inflammation, visceral adiposity, and insulin resistance? *Archives of Physiology and Biochemistry*, **114**(4), pp. 211–23.

Zielinski, M. R. & Krueger, J. M. 2011. Sleep and innate immunity. *Frontiers in Bioscience (Scholar Edition)*, **1**(3), pp. 632–42.

Chapter 13

Sleep and pregnancy

Michele L. Okun

Introduction

Sleep disturbance is a common complaint of pregnancy. Beginning almost immediately at conception, pregnant women complain of disrupted nocturnal sleep and daytime fatigue. Although considered to be ubiquitous throughout normal pregnancy, emerging evidence indicates that the degree to which sleep is disturbed throughout pregnancy is highly variable among women. Recent data suggest that about 25% of pregnant women report significant sleep complaints in the first trimester, whereas up to 75% report some form of sleep disruption by the third trimester. Interestingly, some women indicate that sleep is improved following conception. Many endogenous and exogenous factors, including pregnancy-related physiological, hormonal, and anatomical changes, as well as lifestyle changes, can impact the degree and chronicity of sleep disturbance. Regrettably, there is still much to learn in terms of what women can/should expect with regards to the *timing, degree, frequency,* and/or *severity* of a specific pregnancy-related sleep disturbance(s), despite the number of published studies evaluating what sleep during pregnancy encompasses. Clinically, this research is important. With the rates of adverse pregnancy outcomes increasing, such as preterm birth and postpartum depression, exploring risk factors that are modifiable and amenable to intervention may prove exceptionally beneficial. Although only just emerging, investigators are examining the role that pregnancy-related sleep disturbances may play in increased risk for adverse pregnancy and infant outcomes.

Common pregnancy-related sleep disturbances

There are various methods of classifying and measuring sleep disturbances. Sleep disturbances relevant to pregnancy are typically classified as: disturbed sleep quality, poor sleep continuity, short/long sleep duration, restless legs syndrome, and sleep-disordered breathing (SDB). The subjective perception of poor sleep is the most commonly assessed sleep disturbance during pregnancy, with sleep quality typically declining as pregnancy progresses. Interestingly, the assessment of SDB (see 'Sleep-disordered breathing during pregnancy') during pregnancy is on the rise. Likely a consequence of the soaring overweight/obesity epidemic, SDB is presenting as a troublesome pregnancy-related sleep problem. Sleep continuity, another measure of sleep, is the degree of fragmentation in a sleep period. Several indices describe sleep continuity, including sleep latency, number of awakenings, and total minutes spent awake. Pregnancy is often characterized by poor sleep continuity. A frequent need to urinate, physical discomfort, leg and back pain, and heartburn are cited as reasons for poor sleep quality and poor continuity.

Understanding and relaying information about the dynamic changes in sleep that occur during pregnancy require an acceptance of two (somewhat contradictory) premises. First, several sleep patterns are unique to each trimester of pregnancy. Many changes often occur in conjunction with temporal physiological changes, so clinicians can generally inform women as to what they can expect in each trimester. However, there is also the idea that sleep progressively worsens across pregnancy, with many of the sleep disturbances augmented with the ongoing pregnancy. This poses a challenge for clinicians to accurately determine which women will have significant sleep disturbance, when, and to what degree. Supplement these events with the extreme variability noted across women and the ability to generalize is further reduced. Current investigations are exploring how sleep patterns change within a trimester, and whether these changes are relevant to maternal or fetal outcomes. In spite of these limitations, and often for the sake of simplicity, sleep is typically described separately for each of the three trimesters.

Sleep by trimester

Initially in the first trimester, women complain of increased fatigue and report taking more naps; however, both objectively assessed (polysomnography (PSG) or actigraphy) and subjectively assessed sleep indicate that women also experience an increase in total sleep time, take longer to fall asleep once they turn off the lights, and have poorer sleep efficiency (defined as the total amount of time a person sleeps divided by the total amount of time spent in bed) during the nocturnal sleep period. An increase in the frequency of napping behaviour is also reported in the first trimester (Lee, 2006). However, the published and accepted generalizations often miss the inherent variability known to occur in sleep. Sleep data from 160 pregnant women in early pregnancy (10–20 weeks) support this hypothesis (Okun et al., 2013). Sleep deficiency, defined as short sleep duration, insufficient sleep, or insomnia, suggests extreme variability in sleep even at 10 weeks' gestation (Figure 13.1).

Over a 2-week period, persistent sleep deficiency (observed at all time points) was reported in 17% of women by diary and 15% from actigraphy. However, sleep efficiency, marked by regular sleep duration, sufficient sleep, or no insomnia, was reported by 49.4% of women by diary and 46.9% by actigraphy. Hence, it is likely that for a percentage of women, sleep deteriorates in the first trimester, while for others sleep is improved or at least only modestly impaired. Unfortunately, the bulk of the studies do not have pre-pregnancy, prospective sleep data from which to make accurate postulations.

During the first trimester, sleep disturbances and their variability are likely the result of increases in the steroid hormones oestrogen and progesterone, and their subsequent effects on other relevant systems and behaviour (Teran-Perez et al., 2012). Physical effects

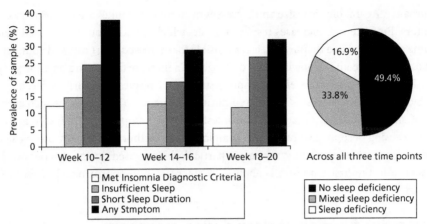

Fig. 13.1 Prevalence of diary-defined sleep deficiency criteria at each individual time point and its pattern across all three time points.

Reproduced with permission from Okun ML et al. Prevalence of sleep deficiency in early gestation and its associations with stress and depressive symptoms. *Journal of Women's Health*, Volume 22, Issue 12, pp. 1028–37.
Copyright © 2013, Mary Ann Liebert, Inc.

resultant of intense fluctuations in these hormones are often experienced very early on in gestation. For example, even before the uterus begins compressing the bladder and reducing bladder capacity, women experience an increased need to urinate. This results from the inhibitory effects of progesterone on the smooth muscles of the bladder. Similarly, progesterone has soporific effects which may contribute to the increase in daytime sleepiness and fatigue. Other physical symptoms that may increase sleep disturbance and daytime fatigue include nausea and vomiting, physical discomfort (tender breasts or back pain), and mood changes.

During the second trimester, sleep patterns improve slightly compared to the first trimester. This is likely a result of acclimation and stabilization of hormones. However, it must be noted that very little attention has been paid to this period in pregnancy. Women report an improvement in energy and less fatigue. The increase in time spent awake after sleep onset (known as 'WASO'—wake after sleep onset) and the number of awakenings observed in the first trimester, for instance, wanes in the second trimester, but never reaches pre-pregnancy sleep patterns (Okun et al., 2009). Interestingly, sleep quality and other subjective perceptions of sleep remain disturbed owing to continued physiological changes. The discrepancy between subjective and objective sleep steadily increases during the second trimester, as suggested by our data (Figure 13.1) (Okun et al., 2013). Although the exact nature of the discrepancy is unknown, during the latter half of the second trimester women become more aware of the changing physiology, such as fetal movements, increased heartburn, and more frequent snoring, all of which can impact subjective perception of sleep.

It is during the third trimester that the majority of sleep disturbances occur, with an increase in spontaneous night-time awakenings compounding physiological sleep disturbance. Again, physical size and increases in steroid hormones are the primary contributors. Progesterone increases respiratory rate, which, in addition to increased blood volume and a restricted diaphragm, is responsible for increased heart rate and complaints of shortness of breath. Meanwhile, low oestrogen can increase fatigue and daytime sleepiness. Despite the protective effects of progesterone on respiration, various mechanical and biochemical mechanisms are altered during pregnancy. These changes increase the risk of sleep-disordered breathing. The intestines and oesophageal sphincter are displaced, causing oesophageal reflux and complaints of heartburn, especially during sleep. Lastly, the risk of restless legs syndrome is particularly increased during this period. The prevalence in the first trimester is about 12%, increasing to approximately 25% in the third trimester.

Restorative function of sleep during pregnancy

One would be hard-pressed to dismiss the notion that sleep has restorative functions, especially during pregnancy. It is advocated that there must be an evolutionary function to sleep. Thus, there are various hypotheses regarding the purpose or role of sleep, and all of these maintain empirical support (Kim et al., 2015; Krueger et al., 2015). Some hypotheses include saving calories, immune enhancement, brain connectivity, performance restoration, and metabolism regulation. Put simply, sleep is thought to promote physical and mental restoration. Knowledge of the alterations in metabolism and arousal that occur as a result of pregnancy is also an important consideration. Pregnancy is a high metabolic effort situation and much of the maternal energy is directed towards the fetal–placental component in a time-dependent manner. There is a shift towards anabolic activity, beginning with the mother and ending with the fetus. This physiological shift is timed to facilitate the appropriate growth and maturation of the fetus, as well as to be protective. Additionally, expectant mothers describe their activity levels as more passive. This may serve to conserve energy at a time of high expenditure. Augmenting this theory, despite the evidence that sleep disruption does occur, much of the pre-existing sleep architecture is left fairly intact during the course of pregnancy, although there have been some studies showing alterations in slow-wave sleep (SWS) and in Stage 1 at various points of gestation. This suggests that there may be an adaptive process in response to the increased wake-after-sleep onset observed during pregnancy. The mother becomes more adept at acquiring consolidated, albeit shorter, sleep periods, which may be conducive to the pending newborn's requirements.

Frequent pregnancy-related sleep disorders

Insomnia during pregnancy

Insomnia—a symptom complex consisting of difficulty in falling asleep, or maintaining sleep, or non-refreshing sleep despite adequate opportunity for sleep, in combination with some daytime dysfunction—is a frequent complaint in the general population. Often it transpires following life events, stress, or physical disruptions, which are usually transient. It can be acute, abating in a short period of time, or it can endure and become a chronic condition. Epidemiological studies have described the prevalence of insomnia without restrictive criteria, such as frequency or severity, to be approximately 33% worldwide (Buysse, 2013). This suggests that a third of the adult population has experienced some difficulty in falling asleep or maintaining sleep, or had early morning awakenings. When additional criteria are utilized with these same individuals, the number drops to approximately 10%. Insomnia is therefore not a rare sleep disorder.

The American Academy of Sleep Medicine (AASM) acknowledges sleep during pregnancy as an associated sleep disorder. The bulk of the literature corroborates the notion that sleep experienced by pregnant women, particularly in the third trimester, meets the diagnostic criteria for insomnia. However, insomnia that presents for the first time during pregnancy is often dependent on the gestational week and can therefore present differentially across the gestational period. In spite of this, very little empirical data exist on how to address this from a clinical perspective. Furthermore, only a few epidemiological studies recognize pregnancy as a status that can contribute to insomnia symptoms. There are six major diagnostic categories that have been established for chronic insomnia: medical, psychiatric, circadian, behavioural, pharmacological, and primary sleep disorder. While some may argue that pregnancy is a 'medical condition', it is not often defined as a medical condition with respect to insomnia. The initiation and perpetuation of sleep problems may arise as a result of pregnancy-associated changes such as the increased need to urinate, altered hormones, back pain, or RLS (restless legs syndrome). It is when the symptoms persist and begin to disrupt the daytime functioning of the mother that further evaluation should be sought. Recently published data indicate that 12.6% of pregnant women with no self-reported history of insomnia met diagnostic criteria for insomnia in early gestation (~12 weeks) (Okun et al., 2015). Given the increasing evidence that insomnia increases risk for various adverse health outcomes, including depression and cardiovascular disease, the evaluation and treatment of insomnia during pregnancy should not be ignored.

Restless legs syndrome during pregnancy

RLS is acknowledged by the AASM and is classified as a sleep disorder in the International Classification of Sleep Disorders. The symptoms associated with RLS involve unpleasant leg sensations that are most often bilateral and often described as a creeping or crawling sensation; motor restlessness and relief with movement; worsening or exclusive presence of symptoms at rest; and symptoms worsening at night. They are distinctly different from the intense leg cramps that also arise during pregnancy. About 7%–10% of the general population experience RLS. This number has been shown to reach up to 26% in the months before delivery. The data describing the frequency of RLS during pregnancy originated from four dated epidemiological studies that applied varying definitions of RLS. It was not until 1995 that a standard definition for RLS was adopted and incorporated into practice.

The diagnosis is based primarily on clinical criteria; however, hypotheses regarding the cause of RLS, particularly in pregnancy, have ranged from psycho-hormonal, to psychomotor-behavioural, to iron metabolism. There is often an associated anaemia, low iron or folate levels, and genetic or familial problems with iron metabolism and dopamine generation and possibly receptivity. Recently, a significant association was reported between elevated oestrogen concentrations in the third trimester and rates of RLS. At this time, there are no data to indicate that oestrogen (hormone) contributes (similarly or differentially) to RLS development in early pregnancy.

Despite the inconsistency in the prevalence rates, pregnant women are considered at a 2- to 3-fold risk of developing RLS compared to non-pregnant women, particularly in the third trimester. Anecdotal evidence suggests that 1–2 days prior to delivery, RLS dissipates and/or disappears. It is also noted to drastically decrease in the early postpartum period, particularly for women who developed it during pregnancy. Although the exact aetiology is unknown, researchers and clinicians advocate pre-pregnancy counselling about adequate dietary intake of iron and folate, the importance of prenatal vitamins, and other changes in relevant health behaviours (i.e. caffeine intake) so that women understand RLS and possible solutions. Additional research is still very much needed to understand the possible consequences of RLS during pregnancy as well as how to prevent it.

Sleep-disordered breathing during pregnancy

Immense physiological, physical, and hormonal changes imminent with pregnancy can lead to SDB. SDB, characterized by abnormal respiratory patterns (e.g. apnoeas, hypopnoeas) or ventilation (e.g. hypoxia), is associated with cardiovascular morbidity, including incident hypertension, inflammation, and sympathetic activation. Snoring and SDB in pregnancy increase 2- to 4-fold compared to the pre-pregnancy state (~4%–5%). Current evidence suggests that up to 14% of non-pregnant women snore, with that number doubling to ~ 28%–59% for women in their third trimester. Rates for SDB are estimated to be ~10% at 14 weeks' gestation, climbing to 15%–40% by 28–29 weeks. Not surprisingly, rates dramatically decline in the postpartum period.

Although the exact mechanisms for this dramatic increase are unclear, several physiological changes are noted to predispose a woman to increased airway resistance and SDB. These include excessive weight gain, decreased functional residual capacity due to mass displacement of the diaphragm, and pharyngeal oedema of pregnancy. Recent investigations show that third-trimester women have narrower upper airways than non-pregnant and postpartum women. This may occur as a result of weight gain and fat deposition that infiltrates pharyngeal muscle tissue or soft tissue deposition in the neck. Although increasing levels of progesterone counteract and increase respiratory effort, it is clear that a significant percentage of women are at risk for SDB during pregnancy. Among pregnant women, SDB is associated with increased rates of hypertension, preeclampsia, and intrauterine growth restriction. All of these are linked to poor outcomes for the infant. Moreover, there is also emerging evidence suggesting that women with SDB during pregnancy are at greater risk for developing future cardiovascular disease. Thus, assessing and treating SDB during pregnancy is of high clinical importance.

Factors that may contribute to disrupted sleep during pregnancy

Psychosocial factors

Various psychosocial factors may mediate how sleep is disrupted during pregnancy. These factors include the age of the mother, her initial and subsequent BMI, ethnicity, and health behaviours such as nutritional practices, exercise practices, smoking or consumption of alcohol, and prenatal stress. Unfortunately, few studies examining sleep in general have reported on these factors, and only one study assessing sleep during pregnancy has commented on any of these variables. Studies considering gender and/or age differences have provided some of the information. Increasing age, for instance, was found to be associated with less time asleep, poorer sleep efficiency, and more minutes awake in the last 2 hours of sleep. Similarly, women aged 30–40 years had less SWS percentage than women aged 20–30 years. Extrapolation and comparison from most of the studies examining gender and/or age are difficult because a majority of the individuals in these studies are beyond childbearing years and subsequently may have age-associated sleep changes, such as hormonal changes. Other factors such as BMI are associated with poorer sleep efficiency and more wake time. Preliminary data from my lab indicate that pregnant women who exercise modestly (0–500 metabolic equivalent (MET) minutes a week) have better actigraphy-assessed sleep than sufficient exercisers (> 500 MET minutes per week) or non-exercisers. Interestingly, there were no differences in subjectively assessed sleep parameters. Since most pregnant women are told not to smoke or drink alcohol during pregnancy, there is little evidence about how these behaviours affect sleep during pregnancy. Lastly, stress is an important correlate of sleep, particularly during pregnancy. There is a clear bi-directional relationship between stress and sleep which can exacerbate each other. While it is clear that stress negatively impacts sleep, we have also shown that poor sleep in early gestation leads to higher self-reported symptoms of stress and depression (Okun et al., 2013). The role of chronic sleep loss in pregnancy, and its role as a chronic stressor, and relevant outcomes, has been recently reviewed by Palagini et al. (2014). Taken together, it is clear that various psychosocial and behavioural factors have pregnancy-specific consequences for sleep during pregnancy.

Immunological factors—cytokines

Immunological factors, and cytokines in particular, are extremely important in all phases of gestation, including the success or failure of implantation, placental development, and timing of labour. They are also key aspects in the initiation and progression of sleep. Evaluation of the effects of sleep deprivation upon immune function has generally focused on people with disorders of excessive daytime sleepiness, healthy adult men, or depressed populations. A consistent finding is that pro-inflammatory cytokines are elevated in these cohorts. Experimentally induced sleep deprivation has been found to alter the diurnal pattern of cellular and humoral immune functions and possibly decrease overall immune function in normal adults. More recently, support for the hypothesis that sleep improves immune function comes from a meta-analysis on sleep and inflammation

(Irwin et al., 2016). Pregnancy-related sleep disturbance is associated with a cytokine profile that favours a dominance of pro-inflammatory cytokine production, particularly IL-6, IL-8, IFN-γ, and TNF-α (Okun et al., 2009). While this has been observed primarily in the second half of pregnancy, a dysregulated cytokine milieu is linked to adverse pregnancy and infant outcomes (Okun et al., 2009).

Endocrinological factors—hormones

Once conception occurs, numerous endocrine changes take place on an almost-daily basis. The bi-directional communication between the mother and the fetal–placental unit relies on a host of hormonal factors. Recent work intimates that oestrogen enhances the total time spent in rapid eye movement (REM) sleep and reduces the latency period prior to REM sleep. Progesterone is secreted in high amounts by the placenta and increases non-REM (NREM) sleep, shortens sleep latency, and reduces wakefulness after sleep onset. Both sex steroids have recognized downstream effects on sleep-moderating cytokines (e.g. IL-1 and TNF-α) and components of the hypothalamic pituitary adrenal (HPA) axis (e.g. corticotropin-releasing hormone (CRH), cortisol) (Irwin et al., 2015). Cortisol, the end result of the HPA axis, is not only a hormone released in stressful situations, but it is also known as the hormone of awakening because the release peak occurs in the morning, although this may be altered in certain sleep disorders such as insomnia and mood disorders. Finally, neurosteroids such as pregnanolone, allopregnanolone, and pregnenolone are involved in the generation of slow-wave sleep (Teran-Perez et al., 2012). Similar to sleep and immune function, sleep and the endocrine system have a bi-directional relationship which facilitates the regulation of different physiological processes during pregnancy, including sleep.

Summary

+ Sleep disturbances during pregnancy have been identified, yet only modestly described.
+ During a snapshot of time during each trimester, pregnant women will likely complain of fatigue, poor sleep quality, and nocturnal sleep disturbances.
+ Sleep loss, sleep restriction, and sleep deprivation have been correlated with cytokine and hormone alterations in various populations and are beginning to be addressed in pregnant women.
+ Research on stress and pregnancy concludes that there are negative pregnancy consequences from high stress, particularly as it pertains to sleep.
+ There is an urgent need to collect sleep data during pregnancy and understand how sleep can interact with other pregnancy-related factors to heighten adverse outcomes.
+ Implementing cognitive-behavioural education interventions will improve not only maternal sleep, but also the health and sleep habits of the mother's offspring.

References

Buysse, D. J. 2013. Insomnia. *JAMA*, **309**, pp. 706–16.

Irwin, M. R., Olmstead, R. & Carroll, J. E. 2016. Sleep disturbance, sleep duration, and inflammation: a systematic review and meta-analysis of cohort studies and experimental sleep deprivation. *Biological Psychiatry*, **80**(1), pp. 40–52.

Kim, T. W., Jeong, J. H. & Hong, S. C. 2015. The impact of sleep and circadian disturbance on hormones and metabolism. *International Journal of Endocrinology*, Article ID 591729. doi: 10.1155/2015/591729

Krueger, J. M., Frank, M. G., Wisor, J. P. & Roy, S. 2015. Sleep function: toward elucidating an enigma. *Sleep Medicine Reviews*, **28**, pp. 42–50.

Lee, K. A. 2006. Sleep during pregnancy and postpartum. In: Lee-Chiong, T. ed. *Sleep: a comprehensive handbook*. Hoboken, NJ: Wiley-Blackwell, pp. 629–35.

Okun, M. L., Buysse, D. J. & Hall, M. H. 2015. Identifying insomnia in early pregnancy: validation of the Insomnia Symptoms Questionnaire (ISQ) in pregnant women. *Journal of Clinical Sleep Medicine*, **11**, pp. 645–54.

Okun, M. L., Kline, C. E., Roberts, J. M., Wettlaufer, B., Glover, K. & Hall, M. 2013. Prevalence of sleep deficiency in early gestation and its associations with stress and depressive symptoms. *Journal of Women's Health*, **22**, pp. 1028–37.

Okun, M. L., Roberts, J. M., Marsland, A. L. & Hall, M. 2009. How disturbed sleep may be a risk factor for adverse pregnancy outcomes. *Obstetrical & Gynecological Survey*, **64**, pp. 273–80.

Palagini, L., Gemignani, A., Banti, S., Manconi, M., Mauri, M. & Riemann, D. 2014. Chronic sleep loss during pregnancy as a determinant of stress: impact on pregnancy outcome. *Sleep Medicine*, **15**, pp. 853–9.

Terán-Pérez, G., Arana-Lechuga, Y., Esqueda-Leon, E., Santana-Miranda, R., Rojas-Zamorano, J. Á. & Velázquez Moctezuma, J. 2012. Steroid hormones and sleep regulation. *Mini Reviews in Medicinal Chemistry*, **12**, pp. 1040–48.

Chapter 14

Sleep in children: A permanently evolving set of challenges

David Gozal and Leila Kheirandish-Gozal

Introduction

> If sleep doesn't serve an absolutely vital function, it is the biggest mistake evolution
> ever made.
> Alan Rechtschaffen, The University of Chicago.

Studies have clearly shown that children in our society are frequently not getting sufficient sleep on a stable and regular schedule. Many studies have also evaluated the potentially adverse impact of poor sleep on health outcomes. Whilst poor sleep may affect a child's ability to learn, their mood status, and their health, the focus of this chapter is on sleep duration and its determination in children.

The sleeping child: sleep duration

In 2004, the 'Sleep in America' poll surveyed parents about their children's sleep habits, behaviour, problems, and disorders in association with their daily schedules, and 2 years later the same approach was pursued in teens and adolescents. Both polls indicated that we actually overestimate the amount of time our children sleep, and that our children sleep much less than what we thought was appropriate for their stage of development. It is noteworthy that the tools employed to estimate sleep using questionnaires exhibit intrinsic unreliability that precludes more accurate pinpointing of how much sleep children get in any given environment (Nascimento-Ferreira et al., 2015). However, despite the limitations of most survey-based inquiries, it is estimated that we sleep ~ 1 hour less than what we used to sleep one century ago, and the trends in such direction appear to have accelerated more recently, likely related to the introduction of a variety of electronic devices into the bedroom, and obviously in the unlikely absence of significant genetic changes (Falbe et al., 2015; Keyes et al., 2015). Lately, increasingly more studies have been published on sleep duration in children, with most of these studies aiming to evaluate the potentially adverse impact of poor sleep on health outcomes. A number of studies have looked at sleep duration in children, but few of these publications actually applied objective measurements of sleep or inquired about differences in sleep during weekdays or at the weekend (Spruyt et al., 2011). Although these studies are methodologically heterogeneous, they reflect marked changes taking place in our rapidly evolving 24/7 society. These studies, and the data in Figure 14.1, should further provoke critical reflection, and more importantly should lead to a call for national longitudinal studies on sleep–wake patterns in children, particularly if we want to address the impact on health from a valid ecological standpoint. Indeed, few longitudinal studies have been carried out that have primarily focused on sleep–wake patterns in children, and fewer still have investigated sleep behaviours. As such, what constitutes normal sleep patterns during childhood, and even what constitutes normal sleep behaviour, remain open questions. This relative absence of objectively recorded data is all the more surprising considering that a child engages in sleep more than in any other activity during the 24-hour cycles, and parents and health professionals have meticulously delineated, observed, and quantified normal patterns of activities such as eating or playing, and yet not traditionally done so for sleeping patterns (Buxton et al., 2015). Therefore, the most forgotten, overlooked, or even actively ignored behaviour of this century is undoubtedly childhood sleep. However, modern life trends that impose further reductions in sleep in children have emerged, and regrettably continue to gain momentum.

Acknowledging that both parents and professionals working with children take particular pleasure and pride at their accomplishments, such as the first steps, the first words, the good grades, extracurricular activities, and so forth, it becomes apparent that our society places most emphasis on daytime functioning, and in doing so, all too often we forget the critically important role of sleep in this context. It is now quite well established that sleep plays a vital role in brain maturation, somatic growth, information processing, memory consolidation, learning, and other important cognitive functions. Since sleep subserves so many aspects of overall wellbeing, it likewise can exert multi-organ impact on functioning, as will become clear throughout this book. A multitude of environmental factors and daytime activities tend to intrude into our life, and potentially rob children of their sleep needs. Moreover, parental awareness of these intrusions is relatively weak, while the tools for assessing such awareness are also in need of further development and validation (McDowall et al., 2016). For example, according to polls of the National Sleep Foundation, 43% of school-aged children and 57% of adolescents have a TV in their bedroom. As many as 42% have a mobile phone in their bedroom, and many other electronic devices, such as computers, video games, and others, are pre-eminently and frequently present in children's bedrooms (Li et al., 2007). Denigration of the night and the dark as an adverse period has also become pervasively communicated to children, such that 60%–72% of children routinely have a night light in their bedroom. Moreover, continued urge for sustained uninterrupted social e(electronic)-contact is increasingly observed in youngsters, and at increasingly younger ages. In summary, historical trends point to increasing reductions in the opportunity for sleep in children and also to the 'pollution' of that sleep opportunity by a variety of intrusionary elements that may further lead to reduced sleep duration.

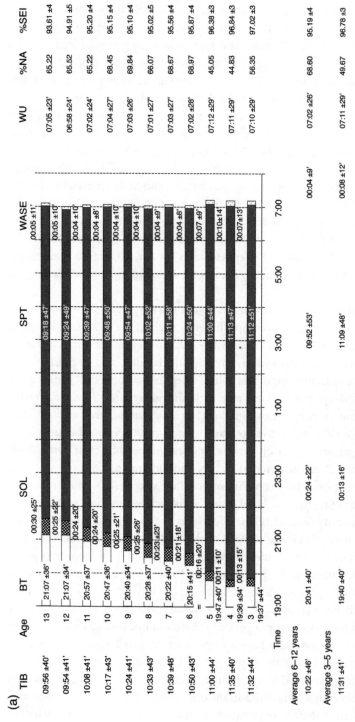

Fig. 14.1a Parent report of sleep duration on school nights in Flemish children.

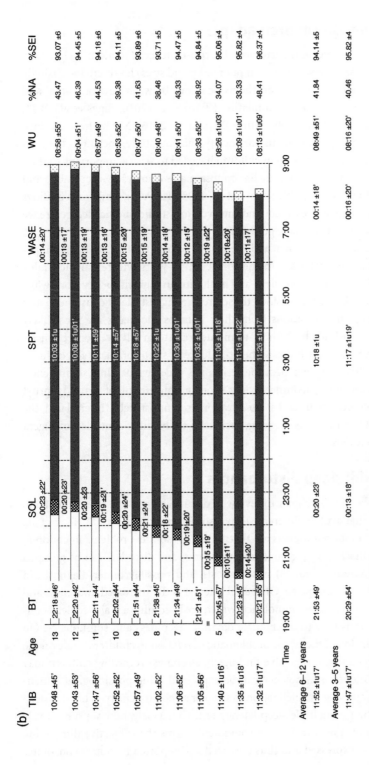

Fig. 14.1b Parent report of sleep duration on weekend nights in Flemish children.

Abbr.: TIB, time in bed; BT, bedtime; SOL, sleep-onset latency; SPT, sleep period time; WASE, wakefulness after sleep end; WU, wake-up time; %NA, % children not spontaneously awake; % SEI, Sleep Efficiency Index in %.

During weekend BT shifts on average 1 hour, SOL is shorter, WU shifts also ~ 1 hour, yet children slept only ~ 30 minutes more. In spite of an extra hour the majority of children still needed to be awakened during the weekend. Furthermore, 1 in 12 children has an irregular sleep–wake pattern.

Reproduced with permission from Spruyt K, O'Brien LM, Cluydts R, Verleye GB, and Ferri R. Odds, prevalence and predictors of sleep problems in school-age normal children. *Journal of Sleep Research*, Volume 14, Issue 2, pp. 163–176, Copyright © 2005 John Wiley and Sons.

The sleeping child: do children adapt?

If an ephemeral lifestyle emerges as the irremediable consequence of modern society, how well do children adapt? Associations between poor sleep and stress levels are increasingly being reported, and, likewise, findings on the associations between environmental and societal changes and sleep are also accumulating (Baird et al., 2016; Biggs et al., 2011; Brand et al., 2009; El-Sheikh et al., 2008; Sayin & Buyukinan, 2016). Not in the least, since the familial context is rapidly changing in our society, the potential associations between family structure and function and sleep in children have led to several important studies, all of which suggest that changes in family life impose major changes in sleep habits and duration in children (Brand et al., 2009; Simard et al., 2008). However, while such findings clearly raise a red flag, further assessment and intervention studies are needed before we can formulate and implement adequate guidelines.

The collective observational evidence and the results of intervention trials that hope-fully will be performed and collected in the forthcoming years will reveal the multi-directional relationships between poor sleep and health in our current society worldwide, and particularly among the children, since those are the biggest 'sleep consumers', and therefore, perturbations and deviations from their homeostatic needs are most likely to carry an incremental risk for both short-term and long-term adverse consequences. Notwithstanding, surveys already indicate the prevalence of sleep complaints in children to be in the range of 20%–60% (e.g. bedtime resistance, excessive daytime somnolence, co-sleeping, delayed sleep onset, bedtime anxiety, snoring, enuresis, night terrors) (Spruyt et al., 2005). Since sleep behaviour and sleep duration are unmistakably interrelated, the need for more empirical evidence is pressing, such as to enable the delineation of cogent and efficacious interventions.

The sleeping child: sleep disturbances

While it is not the scope of this chapter to review in detail each possible sleep complaint, we should emphasize that over 50 different sleep disorders are described (Sheldon et al., 2015), of which three important aspects are that: (1) sleep, and its problems in children, differ from that in adults; (2) sleep complaints, problems, and disorders can be grouped into psychological or physical; and (3) misdiagnosis, and possibly under-diagnosis, of most sleep problems is commonplace. Of special interest is the increased awareness and reporting of disorders of excessive somnolence, which are becoming a major societal con-cern. The difficulty here is how to disentangle daytime sleepiness and somnolence. On the one hand, the definition of the two is problematic in relation to children, while on the other hand, both subjective and objective findings of sleepiness regarding children may not always converge. Indeed, somnolence can be expressed using physiological dimen-sions such as those comprising the inclination to sleep or sleep propensity—that is, a sleep drive, often assessed by the multiple sleep latency test. Conversely, how we subjectively experience sleepiness, or how it feels to be somnolent, forms the subjective dimension, and how somnolence is expressed and thus observed and reported by others constitutes the behavioural dimension. In a developing child, the somnolence phenotype can be quite challenging to unravel, since it may encompass externalizing and internalizing behaviours. Furthermore, these three dimensions of somnolence are often interchanged, and are 'de facto' interchangeable. Nonetheless, more explicit and systematic use of these measures, or of other measures that are more objective and better suited for the paediatric age range, should serve as a guide to diagnosing sleep duration and behaviour problems in the child. In fact, sleepiness and alertness are perceived as correlates of the sleep–wake system. However, the variety of causes and pathways leading to low quantity and poor quality of sleep in children may co-exist, and therefore pose a formidable challenge to recognizing and treating such sleep-related problems (Spruyt et al., 2005).

In contrast to such assumptions, our clinical and educational practice has shown that parental and child education and increased awareness on appropriate sleep and hygiene, along with small modifications to the bedroom environment, are accompanied by a relatively high degree of success in improving many of the presenting complaints. A valuable rule of thumb regarding optimal amount of sleep has been: more than 12 hours for preschoolers, about 12 hours for the school-aged child, and about 9 hours thereafter. More specifically, when school 'learning load' increases (i.e. at age 6), the child should sleep for at least 11 hours, and from then onwards ~ 15 minutes less per subsequent birthday. However, a recent consensus document can also be used as a generic guide, since substantial inter-individual variability exists across the age and population spectrum (Hirshkowitz et al., 2015).

Sleep in children is rarely, if ever, optimal, and bedtime has especially shifted to later hours, which converges with presenting complaints by parents, such as bedtime reluctance and excessive daytime fatigue, tiredness, lack of energy, poor attention span, irritability, mood swings, and somnolence. Moreover, findings in some of those sleep duration or behaviour studies suggest that especially those children raised in disadvantageous situations are at increased risk of chronic poor sleep (Wong et al., 2013). In his textbook, Stores (2001) assigned a role to the caregiver in the majority of sleep problems in children by stating that 'the caregiver(s) play a role in *defining, causing, or maintaining* their child's sleep problems'. Indeed, poor sleep is one of the most reported complaints by caregivers, but children seldom, if ever, complain about their own sleep. As such, in research and in clinical practice, one needs to be conscious of the different perceptions on sleep by the complainant, the sufferer, and the observer (e.g. clinician or schoolteacher). From aforementioned considerations, it becomes apparent why poor sleep remains a very common, and yet markedly under-recognized, health problem.

The sleeping child: sleep loss and health outcomes

Animal studies consistently suggest an adverse impact on health by sustained sleep loss; for instance, sleep loss may trigger generalized inflammatory and stress responses in the brain (Esumi et al., 2011). Although substantive causative relationships between sleep loss and end-organ dysfunction are missing in relation to children, it is widely assumed that when sleep is reduced either acutely or chronically, it is not without changes in brain and behaviour (Cirelli, 2006). Collective evidence increasingly points to disruptions of endocrine and metabolic functions as well as lower self-esteem, mood symptoms, and somnolence and inattentiveness at school, and suggests a link between insufficient or short sleep and obesity. Therefore, studies on the impact of poor or insufficient sleep in a developing child foregoing sleeping time to accommodate a highly media overloaded life are critically needed. Hence, defining in a first stage what normal sleep behaviour and habits are in a child is the first step in the process. The delineation of normative sleep should encompass the wide range of normal developmental, physical, and maturational changes across childhood, as well as cultural, environmental, and social influences, finally leading to the determination and characterization of potential sleep phenotypes that allow for more personalized estimates of sleep need, sleep quality, and impact of sleep on other physiological systems. This approach subsequently summates the multitude of relationships with sleep duration.

The sleeping child: in practice

A more comprehensive account of these aspects can be found elsewhere (Spruyt & Gozal, 2010). Schematically, findings discussed in this chapter potentially reflect five variables that may vary with respect to sleep (Figure 14.2 and Box 14.1):

1. Bedtime
2. Total sleep time, which can be shortened or fragmented/disrupted by endogenous or exogenous factors
3. Rise time
4. Occurrence of the sleep phase within the circadian rhythm
5. Variability of the sleep phase within the circadian rhythm for weekdays and weekend days (irregular sleep).

See also Figure 14.2 and Box 14.1.

Bedtime is an extremely crucial and daily turning point in the lives of many families. It is rather apparent that many, if not most, children will do their best to postpone their bedtime with varying degrees of success, the latter depending, for instance, on parenting style. Unequivocally, shifts in bedtime will also affect total sleep times, since during school weekdays, rise time is quite rigid owing to the standard and rather consistent school start times. During weekends, both bedtime and rise time can shift drastically, and this can either happen sporadically or can assume a more chronic and consistent pattern. Shifts are much more likely to arise in adolescence, and during weekends the sleep phase rhythm can be seriously disrupted. Of importance to the changes in bedtime is the interrelation between bedtime and the other variables, such that it becomes very arbitrary when a certain degree of irregularity in bedtime leads to changes in sleep and wake that are considered dysfunctional. An additional, potentially forgotten, marker of poor sleep is spontaneous awakening despite the 'mandatory' rise time.

One difficulty regarding the interpretation of results emanating from research on sleep deprivation and disruption in children is that laboratory and naturalistic environment

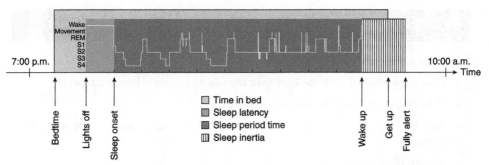

Fig. 14.2 The construct of sleep duration: five variables that would be pertinent for screening in primary care settings.

Reproduced with permission from Spruyt K, O'Brien LM, Cluydts R, Verleye GB, and Ferri R. Odds, prevalence and predictors of sleep problems in school-age normal children. *Journal of Sleep Research*, Volume 14, Issue 2, pp. 163-176, Copyright © 2005 John Wiley and Sons.

conditions may differ substantially regarding these variables, and this problem therefore impedes generalization of findings. The acquisition of reliable evidence is furthermore hampered by the ongoing search for accurate methodologies that allow for the objective collection of information on sleep–wake pattern data in the home environment, and by the lack of clear definitions for sleep problems and disorders in childhood as to what is normal or pathological pertaining to certain developmental ages, and the research is further challenged by the confounding factors related to baseline sleep duration. Notwithstanding, complaints of poor sleep being voiced by parents should be taken seriously, and attempts to quantify them should be undertaken, despite these methodological issues (Box 14.2).

Box 14.1 Practice points

- Inquire about sleep quantity and quality.
- Evaluate sleep environment and hygiene (habits, potential disruptors), and determine regularity.
- Critically reflect on behavioural signs (e.g. physical complaints, learning difficulties, somnolence, emotional difficulty) in terms of poor or insufficient sleep.
- Embed poor/insufficient sleep in context (e.g. exams, stress, anxiety, traumatic experience, depression, rumination, cultural setting, parenting).
- Compare subjective and objective measures from several respondents in the child's environment (parents, siblings and friends, teachers, other).
- Establish sleep duration needs and formulate realistic expectations to correct sleep-related deficiencies.

Box 14.2 Questions a healthcare provider can ask

- What is the usual bedtime?
- How many times is bedtime later than the usual bedtime? How much later?
- How long does it usually take to fall asleep?
- Are there night awakenings? How often? And how long does it take to return to sleep?
- What is the usual rise time?
- How many times is rise time later than the usual rise time? How much later?
- Is awakening occurring spontaneously or does the child need to be awakened?

As mentioned earlier, a promising research field is the impact of family functioning on sleep (Brand et al., 2009; Meltzer & Mindell, 2007), such that discerning the common threads linking family environment and its adverse impact on sleep, and therefore the impact of poor sleep on children, should generate clusters of aggregate data that enable formulation of initial strategies regarding effective management of poor sleep in children. Hence, in the future, we will have to incorporate measures of familial functioning and of the fast-changing community functioning into the evaluation of sleep in children, particularly regarding parameters such as bedtime and variability of sleep phase. Since societal and family behaviours are undoubtedly important modifiers and critical determinants of sleep habits in children, tools to quantify such aspects of sleep will have to be developed. This will then enable us to determine with increased accuracy the important effect of sleep on cognition, child development, and health.

Summary

- The impact of poor sleep on the developing child is underrated and virtually unexplored.
- The normative, age-appropriate sleep needs during a child's development remain largely undefined.
- Insufficient or disrupted sleep leads to increased daytime somnolence, which can manifest in multiple and diverse ways.
- Sleep in the child might serve both as a reliable reporter of multiple settings, such as parental characteristics, psychopathology, education, and parenting skills, as well as an indicator of psychosocial stress and trauma, and cultural and social demands, and sleep disorders ultimately lead to increased health-related burden.
- Healthcare providers should periodically monitor any condition that may affect the amount of sleep in a developing child.
- Healthcare providers need to use history taking and objective sleep assessments to assess bedtime, rise time, total sleep duration, variability of sleep over time, and alignment of sleep with other circadian factors (Box 14.2).

◆ Fine attunement between the social rhythms and the biological rhythm throughout an individual's lifespan should be a priority, and this principle applies also to sleep.

◆ Sleep measures need to be included *a priori* in research studies.

◆ Further studies are needed to explore the effects of sleep on cognition and affective functioning in children.

References

Baird, J., Hill, C. M., Harvey, N. C., Crozier, S., Robinson, S. M., Godfrey, K. M., Cooper, C., Inskip, H.; SWS Study Group. 2016. Duration of sleep at 3 years of age is associated with fat and fat-free mass at 4 years of age: the Southampton Women's Survey. *Journal of Sleep Research*, **24**(4), pp. 412–18.

Biggs, S. N., Lushington, K., van den Heuvel, C. J., Martin, A. J. & Kennedy, J. D. 2011. Inconsistent sleep schedules and daytime behavioral difficulties in school-aged children. *Sleep Medicine*, **212**, pp. 780–86.

Brand, S., Gerber, M., Hatzinger, M., Beck, J. & Holsboer-Trachsler, E. 2009. Evidence for similarities between adolescents and parents in sleep patterns. *Sleep Medicine*, **10**, 1124–31.

Buxton, O. M., Chang, A. M., Spilsbury, J. C., Bos, T., Emsellem, H., Knutson, K. L. 2015. Sleep in the modern family: protective family routines for child and adolescent sleep. *Sleep Health*, **1**, pp. 15–27.

Cirelli, C. Cellular consequences of sleep deprivation in the brain. *Sleep Medicine Reviews*, **10**, pp. 307–21.

El-Sheikh, M., Buckhalt, J. A., Keller, P. S. & Granger, D. A. 2008. Children's objective and subjective sleep disruptions: links with afternoon cortisol levels. *Health Psychology*, **27**, pp. 26–33.

Esumi, L. A., Palma, B. D., Gomes, V. L., Tufik, S. & Hipólide, D. C. 2011. Inflammatory markers are associated with inhibitory avoidance memory deficit induced by sleep deprivation in rats. *Behavioural Brain Research*, **221**, pp. 7–12.

Falbe, J., Davison, K. K., Franckle, R. L., Ganter, C., Gortmaker, S. L., Smith, L., Land, T. & Taveras, E. M. 2015. Sleep duration, restfulness, and screens in the sleep environment. *Pediatrics*, **135**(2), e367–e375.

Hirshkowitz, M., Whiton, K., Albert, S. M., Alessi, C., Bruni, O., DonCarlos, L., Hazen, N., Herman, J., Katz, E. S., Kheirandish-Gozal, L., Neubauer, D. N., O'Donnell, A. E., Ohayon, M., Peever, J., Rawding, R., Sachdeva, R. C., Setters, B., Vitiello, M. V., Ware, J. C. & Adams Hillard, P. J. 2015. National Sleep Foundation's sleep time duration recommendations: methodology and results summary. *Sleep Health*, **1**, pp. 40–43.

Keyes, K. M, Maslowsky, J., Hamilton, A. & Schulenberg, J. 2015. The great sleep recession: changes in sleep duration among US adolescents, 1991-2012. *Pediatrics*, **135**, pp. 460–68.

Li, S., Jin, X., Wu, S., Jiang, F., Yan, C. & Shen, X. 2017. The impact of media use on sleep patterns and sleep disorders among school-aged children in China. *Sleep*, **30**, pp. 361–7.

McDowall, P. S., Galland, B. C., Campbell, A. J. & Elder, D. E. 2017. Parent knowledge of children's sleep: a systematic review. *Sleep Medicine Reviews*, **31**, pp. 39–47.

Meltzer, L. J. & Mindell, J. A. 2007. Relationship between child sleep disturbances and maternal sleep, mood, and parenting stress: a pilot study. *Journal of Family Psychology*, **21**, pp. 67–73.

Nascimento-Ferreira, M. V., Collese, T. S., de Moraes, A. C., Rendo-Urteaga, T., Moreno, L. A. & Carvalho, H. B. 2015. Validity and reliability of sleep time questionnaires in children and adolescents: a systematic review and meta-analysis. *Sleep Medicine Reviews*, **30**, pp. 85–96.

Sayin, F. K. & Buyukinan, M. 2016. Sleep duration and media time have a major impact on insulin resistance and metabolic risk factors in obese children and adolescents. *Childhood Obesity*, **12**(4), pp. 272–8.

Sheldon, S. H, Kryger M. H, Ferber, R. & Gozal, D. 2015. *Principles and Practice of Pediatric Sleep Medicine*. USA: Elsevier Saunders.

Simard, V., Nielsen, T. A., Tremblay, R. E., Boivin, M. & Montplaisir, J. Y. 2008. Longitudinal study of preschool sleep disturbance: the predictive role of maladaptive parental behaviors, early sleep problems, and child/mother psychological factors. *Archives of Pediatrics & Adolescent Medicine*, **162**, pp. 360–67.

Spruyt, K. & Gozal, D. 2010. Sleep in children: the evolving challenge of catching enough and quality Zzz's. In: Cappuccio, F. P., Miller, M. A. & Lockley, S. W. eds. *Sleep, Health and Society: from aetiology to public health*. Oxford: Oxford University Press, pp. 215–38.

Spruyt, K., Molfese, D. L. & Gozal, D. 2011. Sleep duration, sleep regularity, body weight, and metabolic homeostasis in school-aged children. *Pediatrics*, **127**(2), e345–e352.

Spruyt, K., O'Brien, L. M., Cluydts, R., Verleye, G. B. & Ferri, R. 2005. Odds, prevalence and predictors of sleep problems in school-age normal children. *Journal of Sleep Research*, **14**(2), pp. 163–76.

Stores, G. 2001. *A Clinical Guide to Sleep Disorders in Children and Adolescents*. New York: Cambridge University Press.

Wong, W. W., Ortiz, C. L., Lathan, D., Moore, L. A., Konzelmann, K. L., Adolph, A. L., Smith, E. O. & Butte, N. F. 2013. Sleep duration of underserved minority children in a cross-sectional study. *BMC Public Health*, **13**, p. 648.

Chapter 15

Loss of sleep or loss of dark? (Answer: both are threats to optimum health)

Richard G. Stevens

Introduction

As the world has become increasingly industrialized and modernized, the maladies of infectious diseases have waned while new burdens of chronic diseases such as cancer and heart problems have surged. The transition from hunter/gatherer and agrarian culture to the modern, industrial life has accelerated in the last hundred years. One hallmark of this transition has been how we light our environment. Up until the late 1800s, light inside buildings and at night was from burning wood or oil; such light is relatively dim and dominated by long wavelengths of orange and red. The sun during the day is bright, and rich in short wavelengths (i.e. blue light). With the invention of the electric light bulb, illumination during the night can be much brighter than a fire, and also rich in short wavelengths.

The question is to what extent this new bright/blue artificial light accounts for some of the chronic disease burden in the modern world.

Electric light—the enabler

Electric light has changed our world. We can now work and play at any time of day or night. Electric light enables us to do anything we want to do when we want to do it, like eat. Eating was once virtually confined to daytime, and part of our circadian adaptation to life on earth has been to avoid the feeling of hunger during night-time hours. This important fact relies on the daily ebb and flow of the hormones of appetite controlled by our endogenous circadian rhythmicity. To our ancestors in the jungle, wanting food at night would mean wandering around in the dark, without much in the way of weaponry, with small teeth and no claws, and thereby at imminent threat of death by predation. And if not being eaten, then falling into a ditch, or stumbling on a log and hitting a rock head-first. So it's better to be quiet and still at night, whether awake or asleep, and not be hungry.

Circadian rhythmicity

Life on the planet started 3 billion years ago, or maybe 4 billion depending on how one interprets the evidence. One thing does seem clear: all life descends from a common ancestry, because how else can the ubiquity of the genetic code of DNA be explained? The same codon sequence with very little variation determines the same amino acid in cyanobacteria, saguaros, and humans. Since the Beginning, there has been in each day about 12 hours of dark and 12 hours of sunlight (with dusk and dawn transitions). This has repeated for countless days, and will presumably continue until the end of days. The impact on how we have all evolved is undoubtedly tremendous.

Almost all life has adapted to the 24-hour light–dark cycle of the sun by development of an endogenous circadian rhythmicity in physiology. For humans, this takes the form of a 'daytime physiology' and a 'night-time physiology'. In constant dark, with no temporal cues, we will cycle, on average, at a little longer than 24 hours in body temperature, activity, sleep, melatonin levels, and many other biological markers, in perpetuity. The daily light–dark cycle resets this clock to the 24-hour day. This endogenous rhythmicity is orchestrated by the core circadian genes, of which there are only about ten (Stevens et al., 2014). These genes also control the expression of many other genes which, in turn, control metabolic processes that, if disrupted, could provide potential links to many of the maladies of modern life, such as poor sleep, obesity, diabetes, cancer, and mood disorders (Stevens et al., 2007).

For tests of a circadian link to specific ailments, many researchers focus on shift workers. People whose jobs require work outside of daytime hours almost, by definition, experience circadian disruption to a greater extent than the typical daytime worker. For example, Hansen et al. (2016) examined the Danish Nurse Cohort of about 20,000 nurses who were disease-free in 1993 and were then followed to 2013. They found that by the end of follow-up, those nurses who reported working primarily night shift on the baseline questionnaire in 1993 were at a 58% higher risk of developing diabetes than daytime nurses. Nurses who reported working evenings at baseline were at an intermediate risk—22% higher than daytime nurses.

Obayashi et al. (2013) took a different approach to examining depression. They conducted a cross-sectional study of elderly people in Japan. Light measurements were taken at night with the room lights turned off in the bedrooms of each of 516 subjects. Each subject was also asked a series of questions, some of which were to assess depression. Based on the questionnaire responses, the subjects were defined as 'depressed' (n = 101) or 'non-depressed' (n = 415). The light level in the bedroom at night among the depressed individuals was higher than that among the non-depressed individuals, although averages remained at about 1 lux—below what is thought to have substantial effects on melatonin production, even with eyes wide open. This study tackles an interesting question: do humans need absolute dark at night during sleep time to function at their best? If not, how dark is dark enough?

Transition to night-time physiology

During daytime, we are active and hungry, and have low circulating melatonin and high body temperature. During night, our body temperature drops, melatonin rises, hunger abates, and sleep pressure builds. The transition to night-time physiology in the absence of electric lighting begins at about dusk (Wright et al., 2013); light from fire (e.g. wood or candle) is long wavelength and apparently has little or no impact on transition to night-time physiology in the evening. From a circadian perspective, this long-wavelength light is interpreted as 'dark' (Stevens, 2015a). Several recent reports describe sleep duration in the few remaining pre-electric societies of indigenous peoples, and some surprising findings have been made: people don't begin sleep until well into the night, and attain actual sleep for only about 7 hours over the 11 or 12 hours of night (Stevens, 2015b). It turns out that dark is required for transition to night-time physiology, but sleep is not.

In the modern world, the transition to night-time physiology is delayed on account of electric light in the evening coming from room-light as well as the increasingly prevalent use of personal electronic devices which are rich in the short wavelengths that signal 'daytime' to our physiology. When bright, short wavelength (e.g. blue) light hits the retina, our endogenous rhythmicity cannot overcome this signal, and so we remain in daytime physiology often until late into the evening, when we finally turn out the lights for sleep. Even after lights off, the alerting effects of light can persist several hours into sleep, reducing sleep quality. Seven hours of sleep embedded within 11 hours of night-time physiology, as in pre-electric peoples, may be far more restorative than 7 hours embedded within only 7 hours of night-time physiology, as often occurs in the modern world.

Sleep disruption versus dark disruption

Increasing numbers of both observational epidemiological studies and laboratory experiments in humans are documenting the adverse metabolic and disease effects of what is called 'restricted sleep'. Sleep is crucial to health, but these studies in almost no cases actually distinguish between lack of sleep and lack of dark (Stevens et al., 2014). The distinction is extremely important. The idea that one must be asleep during all hours of dark belies our evolutionary past as embodied in those pre-electric societies mentioned earlier (see 'Transition to nighttime physiology'). Before electricity, sleep was fragmented over the dark period, but nighttime physiology was not interrupted by the sleep–wake transitions. If, during those natural periods of wakefulness at night, people are instructed to turn on lights and leave the bedroom, however, then an anomalous transition to daytime physiology begins. This has been the wrong-headed recommendation from official bodies for far too long.

Breast cancer

In the mid-1980s, a prominent conundrum was the 'mystery of breast cancer'—that is to say, why was breast cancer risk so much higher in the industrialized countries than in the developing ones, and why was risk rising fast in the developing world? There was a greater than 5-fold difference after taking account of the age structures of the populations, and there was no scientific consensus on why this was happening.

The conventional wisdom (i.e. conjecture) was that it must be diet; the high-fat western diet accounted for the high risk in westernized countries, and as developing countries adopted this toxic food, breast cancer risk was surging. Then, in the 1980s, results were published from several large cohort studies of diet and breast cancer that showed absolutely no relationship between dietary fat consumption and later risk. This was baffling for a couple reasons: first, it was very clear that countries with the highest breast cancer rates were also on the highest fat diets, and second, it was also very clear that rats fed a high-fat diet had many more breast cancers after receiving a chemical initiator than rats fed a low-fat diet.

If diet is not the answer, then what else changes as societies industrialize? Answer: many things, one of which is the increasing use of electricity to light the night. So, maybe light-at-night explained a portion of the breast cancer pandemic (Stevens, 2009). Another way to put it is that loss of the natural dark period of about 12 hours each night might increase risk.

The biological rationale was that loss of dark would lead to a reduced duration of melatonin production over the night; melatonin is one of the most potent agents in inhibiting the development of chemically induced breast cancer in Sprague-Dawley rats, a model widely used in cancer toxicology assays (Stevens et al., 2014). The rationale was later broadened considerably to become: electric lighting can lead to circadian disruption, of which melatonin suppression is one aspect; other aspects include alterations in circadian gene expression, which in turn affect cell cycle regulation, metabolism, DNA damage response, and hormone production (Stevens & Zhu, 2015).

Though easy to state, the idea is very difficult to test in humans, in part because nowadays everyone is exposed, at least to some extent, to electric light during the night. From the basic idea, a series of specific predictions (hypotheses) were made. Direct human evidence must rely on observational epidemiology because randomized trials are logistically untenable as well as being unethical for any intervention that may cause harm. Unfortunately, observational epidemiology can almost never actually examine the exposure or real interest, and must therefore rely on surrogates for the real exposure. To wit, the exposure of interest is ill-timed electric light exposure—particularly at night—that may cause circadian disruption over an extended period of time. The following predictions are based on a variety of candidate surrogates for this chronic exposure to light-at-night.

***

Caveat: One of the most serious shortcomings of observational epidemiology is the potential for exposure misclassification. That is to say, if the exposure surrogate chosen for a study is poorly related to the actual exposure of interest, then it becomes more likely that the study will deliver a null result. This can lead to a conclusion of 'no effect' of the true exposure based on a lack of association of the surrogate with the disease outcome, even when a strong effect of true exposure actually exists. In addition, the greater the measurement error of the surrogate, the more likely there will be a null result even if the surrogate itself is strongly associated with risk.

***

The predictions are as follows:

◆ Shift workers will be at higher risk of breast cancer.

The most studied question is whether non-day work hours increase risk. This was the first prediction of the light-at-night idea, and is based on the assumption that night workers are exposed to more night-time light, and thereby experience greater circadian disruption, than day workers. Of course, day-working people do use electric light in the evening, which can delay transition to night-time physiology, so they are not unexposed, but the night workers have even greater exposure. Or so the reasoning goes.

So far, more than 20 studies have been published, and they seem to be converging on the result that shift-working women are at modestly greater risk of breast cancer. These findings do not prove that light at night or circadian disruption is the cause, however, even though that possibility was the initial reason why these studies were conducted.

It is again important to stress that almost all persons in the modern world are exposed to electric light-at-night, so the shift-worker studies have relevance for everyone. Shift workers are something like the canary in the coal mine (Stevens, 2016); if they suffer elevated disease risk due to circadian disruption caused by ill-timed electric lighting, then that is a caution to all segments of society.

♦ Short sleep duration would increase risk.

The idea was to use reported hours of sleep by study subjects as a surrogate for hours of dark each night; the focus was not on the length or quality of actual sleep (Stevens, 2002). The first study published by Pia Verkasalo (2005) was conducted in Finland. The results were provocative and did show an association in the direction predicted: short sleep was found to be associated with elevated risk, and long sleep duration with a lower risk. Since this first study, however, a half dozen other studies have been published and no clear pattern has emerged; some studies report elevated risk with short sleep, while others do not.

This leaves the question in an uncomfortable state: either there is no effect of sleep duration on cancer risk, or duration of dark does matter but the sleep questions used in studies are rife with error so that no conclusion can be drawn.

♦ Blind women would be at lower risk.

In 1990, not long after the light-at-night idea was published (Stevens, 1987, Am J Epidemiol), Robert Hahn published the first study to report lower breast cancer risk in blind women (in the journal *Epidemiology*). He reasoned that if light-at-night increased breast cancer risk in sighted women, then blind women should be at lower risk because they cannot perceive light. Since then, another half dozen epidemiological studies of various designs, including controlling for the absence or presence of light perception, have reported findings consistent with Hahn's result, for example in the study by Flynn-Evans et al. (2009). Given the small number of studies, and modest risk estimates, however, there is insufficient evidence to convince a panel of experts of cause and effect. In addition, blind women may be different from sighted women in other ways that affect risk, although attempts were made to adjust for this possibility.

♦ Higher ambient light level of the bedroom during sleep time would increase risk.

This prediction has been tested in a couple of case-control studies and supported. The exposure assessment was particularly dicey, however: asking a woman to accurately assess the relative light level in her bedroom at night after the lights had been turned out, in a period of her life before her diagnosis of breast cancer, is close to futile. The only hope here is to conduct a prospective study of many thousands of disease-free women by asking specific questions about bedroom light level, or even making photometric measurements, and then following these women for breast cancer outcome. Obviously, this kind of study is hugely expensive and will take a long time.

◆ Indigenous far-north populations would have a lower risk of breast cancer.

In 1999, a German researcher named Thomas Erren predicted that indigenous populations of the far north should have lower breast cancer incidence than more southern populations. His reasoning was that during the winter, when dark was near constant, such people would use wood fire only so long as necessary during the 'day' for food and survival; they would thereby have maximum melatonin production over 24 hours. Conversely, during the summer, with near constant sunlight, they would still take dark cover each 'night' for 7 or 8 hours of sleep. Over the span of the year they would have greater total melatonin production than southern peoples. It is very difficult to determine breast cancer incidence in far-north indigenous populations such as the Sami people of Finland, but those few studies that have been done support Erren's prediction.

◆ Community night-time light level as measured from satellite images would be associated with breast cancer incidence among those communities (or countries).

Several studies by different research groups in different parts of the world have published results that support this prediction. These are called 'ecological studies' and are limited by the fact that there is no individual-level data on people. So an association at the population level may be an artefact of some other attribute of each society's make-up that goes along with industrialization that is the actual cause. Ecological analyses do provide an upper limit on the impact of an exposure on a disease outcome, however; if light-at-night accounts for any substantial portion of the breast cancer burden, then it should be apparent at the population level.

Animal evidence

There are many studies examining the effects of altered lighting on physiology and on disease outcomes in rats and mice. For breast cancer, the evidence is very strong: light exposure at night increases breast cancer in rats and mice. In fact, David Blask and his colleagues have taken the animal model to its limit of relevance to humans by implanting a human-derived breast cancer in a nude rat, and then infusing this human tumour with human blood taken in the middle of the night. Blood taken in the dark stops the growth of the tumours, whereas blood taken at night after a light exposure does not slow the tumour development at all.

Another approach has recently been published that examined the effect of simulated rotating shifts on the development of a mouse tumour that is an analogue of a known genetically determined breast cancer in humans called Li–Fraumeni syndrome. Kirsten Van Dycke and colleagues (Current Biology, 2015) subjected a group of these genetically susceptible mice to a 12-hour dark:12-hour light protocol for their entire lives; another group had the light and dark switched each week. The 'night-working mice' developed their cancers much earlier in their lives than the 'day-working' mice.

The impact of altered lighting on metabolic disorders and weight gain is also being investigated. Laura Fonken and colleagues have made several interesting findings, including that the body mass of mice is increased and glucose tolerance reduced when they are exposed to light during the night, despite similar caloric intake and activity as mice on a 12:12 light–dark cycle. The role of timing of food intake on circadian health is an important topic that is now coming to the fore. Members of the same lab headed by Randy Nelson at Ohio State University have also published intriguing findings on the role of altered lighting on depressive-like symptoms in mice and hamsters. This, too, is an important area of inquiry.

Wrap-up

And what of the deep sea? Among the minority of organisms found not to have the genes driving an endogenous circadian rhythmicity are those found at the ocean vents several miles below the surface, where nary a photon of sunlight can penetrate. Evidently, they just don't need the circadian apparatus to cope successfully in that environment. Elsewhere, the vast majority of life exploits a robust endogenous circadian physiology for optimum health and a survival advantage.

For us, the terrestrial king of beasts, electric light is compromising that advantage. Yet it doesn't have to. As the basic biology of phototransduction from the retina to the circadian system, and of the functioning of the endogenous circadian apparatus, is being elucidated, it is becoming clear that the technology of lighting can adapt to provide illumination yet also accommodate circadian health. In the simplest terms, strong blue-enriched light in buildings in the morning (e.g. bright compact fluorescent) is optimum, as is dimmer, blue-depleted redder light in the evening (e.g. low-wattage incandescent). Just as we have too much light in the evening, we also are deprived of the strong light signal from the sun during the day given that most of us now work inside buildings. This can lead to a sort of circadian fog in which our physiology doesn't know when night ends and day begins, nor the obverse.

The latest lighting technologies can accomplish visual stimulation while remaining circadian friendly by changing wavelength and intensity to suit the time of day of human activity. It is 'artificial' (human-made) light, yet admits the new reality: very few of us are going to give up electric lighting.

Summary

- Life evolved on earth with bright full-spectrum days and dark nights.
- In response, an endogenous circadian physiology has emerged that is crucial to our health and wellbeing.
- Light at night from burning wood or oil does not upset this circadian rhythmicity.

◆ However, electric lighting in the typical human environment at home or in the office is often capable of disrupting circadian physiology, at least to some extent.

◆ On this basis, overuse of electric lighting may account for a portion of some of the international burden of common maladies of the industrialized world, such as breast cancer, obesity, diabetes, and mood disorders.

References

Blask D.E., Brainard G.C., Dauchy R.T., Hanifin J.P., Davidson L.K., Krause J.A., Sauer L.A., Rivera-Bermudez M.A., Dubocovich M.L., Jasser S.A., Lynch D.T., Rollag M.D., Zalatan F. 2005. Melatonin-depleted blood from premenopausal women exposed to light at night stimulates growth of human breast cancer xenografts in nude rats. *Cancer Research*, 1, **65**(23), 11174–84.

Flynn-Evans, E. E., Stevens, R. G., Tabandeh, H., Schernhammer, E. S. & Lockley, S. W. 2009. Total visual blindness is protective against breast cancer. *Cancer Causes & Control*, **20**, pp. 1753–6.

Fonken L.K., Lieberman R.A., Weil Z.M., & Nelson R.J. 2013. Dim light at night exaggerates weight gain and inflammation associated with a high-fat diet in male mice. *Endocrinology*. **154**(10), 3817–25.

Hansen, A. B., Stayner, L., Hansen, J. & Andersen, Z. J. 2016. Night shift work and incidence of diabetes in the Danish Nurse Cohort. *Occupational and Environmental Medicine*, **73**, pp. 262–8.

Obayashi, K., Saeki, K., Iwamoto, J., Ikada, Y. & Kurumatani, N. 2013. Exposure to light at night and risk of depression in the elderly. *Journal of Affective Disorders*, **151**, pp. 331–6.

Stevens, R. G. 1987. Electric power use and breast cancer: a hypothesis. *American Journal of Epidemiology*, **125**(4), 556–61.

Stevens R.G. 2002. Lighting during the day and night: possible impact on risk of breast cancer. *Neuroendocrinology Letters*, **23**(Suppl 2), 57–60.

Stevens, R. G. 2009. Electric light causes cancer? Surely you're joking, Mr. Stevens. *Mutation Research*, **682**, pp. 1–6.

Stevens, R. G. 2015a. *A dark night is good for your health*. [Online]. [Accessed 1 January 2018]. Available from: https://theconversation.com/a-dark-night-is-good-for-your-health-39161

Stevens, R. G. 2015b. *Are we sleep-deprived or just darkness deprived?* [Online]. [Accessed 1 January 2018]. Available from: http://www.huffingtonpost.com/the-conversation-us/are-we-sleep-deprived-or_b_8389340.html

Stevens, R. G. 2016. Circadian disruption and health: shift work as a harbinger of the toll taken by electric lighting. *Chronobiology International*, **33**(6), pp. 589–94.

Stevens, R.G. & Zhu, Y. 2015. Electric light, particularly at night, disrupts human circadian rhythmicity: is that a problem? *Philosophical Transactions of the Royal Society of London. Series B, Biological Sciences*, 5, **370**(1667), pii: 20140120. doi: 10.1098/rstb.2014.0120

Stevens, R. G., Blask, D. E., Brainard, G. C., Hansen, J., Lockley, S. W., Provencio, I., Rea, M. S. & Reinlib, L. 2007. Meeting report: the role of environmental lighting and circadian disruption in cancer and other diseases. *Environmental Health Perspectives*, **115**, pp. 1357–62.

Stevens, R. G., Brainard, G. C., Blask, D. E., Lockley, S. W. & Motta, M. E. 2014. Breast cancer and circadian disruption from electric lighting in the modern world. *CA: A Cancer Journal for Clinicians*, **64**, pp. 207–18.

Van Dycke, K. C., Rodenburg, W., van Oostrom, C. T., van Kerkhof, L. W., Pennings, J. L., Roenneberg, T., van Steeg, H. & van der Horst G. T. 2015. Chronically alternating light cycles increase breast cancer risk in mice. *Current Biology*, **25**(14), pp. 1932–7.

Verkasalo, P. K., Lillberg, K., Stevens, R. G., Hublin, C., Partinen, M., Koskenvuo, M. & Kaprio, J. 2005. Sleep duration and breast cancer: a prospective cohort study. *Cancer Research*, **65**(20), pp. 9595–600.

Wright Jr, K. P., McHill, A. W., Birks, B. R., Griffin, B. R., Rusterholz, T. & Chinoy, E. D. 2013. Entrainment of the human circadian clock to the natural light-dark cycle. *Current Biology*, **23**, pp. 1554–8.

Chapter 16

Circadian rhythms, sleep, and anti-cancer treatments

Pasquale F. Innominato and David Spiegel

Introduction

Our physical environment is imprinted on our biology at the neural, endocrine, and cellular level. Solar and lunar cycles are reflected in all of our patterns of sleep and wakefulness and oestrogen and progesterone levels in women. Expression of clock genes in cells varies with clock-like precision across the 24-hour cycle. The suprachiasmatic nucleus (SCN) in the brain is the master regulator of circadian hormones such as melatonin and cortisol. Our bodies adapt to external cycles of light and dark from the inside-out as well as the outside-in.

The circadian timing system, circadian rhythms, and sleep

Aberrations in sleep–wake cycles, rest–activity rhythms, and genetic or suprachiasmatic control of circadian rhythms engender endocrine abnormalities, especially flattened diurnal cortisol rhythms, that affect cancer risk and progression. In mice, surgical ablation of the central biologic clock, the SCN, or chronic exposure to the equivalent of transmeridian long-haul flights over several time zones (resulting in jet lag), both of which blunt the circadian cortisol, temperature, and activity rhythms, resulted in a 2-fold increase in the rate of growth of implanted cancers (Innominato et al., 2010). Variations in cortisol throughout the 24-hour cycle provide available energy for activity during the day and metabolic respite at night. There is robust circadian variation in the release of cortisol from the adrenal cortex such that levels begin to rise prior to habitual wake time and reach a trough in the evening. The underlying 24-hour pattern of cortisol is primarily driven by the SCN, the central circadian pacemaker in mammals. Altered diurnal slope of cortisol has been reported in association with a variety of cancers, including, but not limited to, breast, ovarian, and lung cancer, as well as coronary artery disease, fibromyalgia, depression, early-life abuse, and disrupted sleep (Sephton & Spiegel, 2003). Circadian disruption increases disease risk and offers opportunities for more effective administration of treatment. Sleep disturbance in particular is common among both cancer patients and their family caregivers and is linked to morbidities and mortality (Spiegel, 2008). Patterns of rest and activity are closely linked to hormonal variation, and quality and quantity of life.

Circadian biomarkers and inter-individual variability

To evaluate the functioning status of the circadian timing system, we need to measure a circadian rhythm whose pattern can inform us on the behaviour of the system. One issue concerns the need to assess this marker rhythm throughout at least 24 hours, usually for 72 hours or longer, but definitely including measures through the night. As a consequence, the assessment method ought to be as minimally invasive as possible, especially if used in cancer patients, who are required to undergo several invasive and frequent procedures for the management of their neoplastic disease. Thus, repeated blood samples used to measure circulating levels of hormones or other soluble factors would not be the optimal choice in the oncological setting. However, the measurement of substances in other biological fluids, such as the saliva, could be considered, even though night-time sampling would impact on the subject's sleep.

One hormone that can be measured in the saliva, with a rhythm fittingly mirroring that in the blood, is cortisol, whose relevant variation physiologically occurs mostly during diurnal hours. Indeed, in normal conditions, cortisol, synthetized and released by the cortex of the adrenal gland, under circadian control from both the central pacemaker and the local peripheral molecular clock, peaks in blood and saliva early in the morning, to prepare our body and mind for the stress of the day, then regularly decreases throughout late morning and afternoon, to reach low values during evening and night, thereby availing sleep. Therefore, diurnal measures could allegedly be sufficient to assess cortisol rhythm, in order to minimize patient discomfort. Diurnal salivary cortisol rhythm was first used in cancer patients by the team at Stanford, USA (Sephton et al., 2000), to assess circadian function in relation to immune parameters, psychosocial variables, and cancer prognosis. Notwithstanding its clinical relevance, detailed hereinafter, since erratic fluctuations or abnormal diurnal-flattened or consistently high profiles of salivary cortisol can be found in cancer patients, information about its levels during the night could be essential to fully monitor circadian function, and supposedly sleep as well.

Another biomarker of circadian function, notably connected to the sleep–wake cycle, is the circadian rhythm in rest and activity. This rhythm can be evaluated non-invasively with the use of an accelerometer—usually worn on the wrist, but seldom elsewhere, such as on the hip or ankle—which records and stores the number of limb or body movements per unit of time, throughout the whole monitoring duration. The most widely used of such devices (the actigraph) is a watch-sized one, which can be continuously worn on the wrist, throughout day and night. The analysis of its recordings can provide objective information about both the function of the circadian timing system, and about sleep quality and quantity. The initial demonstration of the clinical relevance of actigraphy monitoring in cancer patients for cancer prognosis and patient wellbeing (described hereinafter) was provided by a team in Villejuif, France (Mormont et al., 2000). Actigraphy monitoring in cancer patients could be easily performed over long periods of time, with almost any intervention from the patient and minimal nuisance, even at home. Moreover, recent technological advancement has rendered the device smaller, lighter, and capable of seamlessly tele-transmitting data in real time to health practitioners. Elucidative and depictive examples of robust and disrupted circadian rhythms in cortisol and rest–activity are shown in Figure 16.1.

Other biomarker rhythms relating to circadian function include body temperature and melatonin. For the former, recent wireless devices can be used to measure core body temperature (with more difficulties and discomfort), and proximal or distal skin temperature (more easily and for a longer duration). For the latter, since melatonin levels are usually high at night and low throughout the day, the same issues of sleep perturbation for night-time measures and the need for repeated sampling hinder the clinical implementation of such measures in cancer patients. Nonetheless, both biomarker rhythms have been evaluated in small groups of cancer patients, and can therefore be used if specific clinical questions need to be answered (Innominato et al., 2014).

Altogether, the monitoring of circadian biomarkers in cancer patients in free-living ambulatory conditions, mainly rest–activity and cortisol rhythms, has shown that circadian function can be profoundly altered, sleep can be perturbed, and a large inter-patient variability in circadian and sleep processes occurs, likewise to that in the general population.

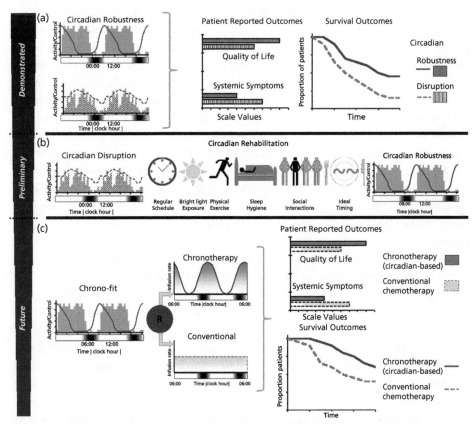

Fig. 16.1 Examples of robust and disrupted circadian rhythms in cortisol and rest–activity, and therapeutic implications in the oncological setting.

Reproduced courtesy of Pasquale F. Innominato.

The implications for anti-cancer treatments are that we have to take into account not only the global functioning status of the circadian timing system (i.e. whether it is robust or disrupted), but also its phase (i.e. the internal timing in reference to the external cues). Thus, in cancer patients as well as in the general population, the preferred sleep timing, for example, spans over several hours, with subjects who like to go to bed at the same time while others prefer to stay awake for longer and vary their bedtime. As expected, a therapeutic intervention developed to optimize treatment timing ought to account not only for altered circadian function, but also for individual chronotype—that is, the internal propensity for optimal sleep timing, in real-world conditions.

Circadian rhythms, sleep, and cancer

There is accumulating evidence that disruption of circadian cycles, including rest–activity rhythms and hormonal patterns, is associated with cancer and indeed predicts more rapid progression of it. Sufficient evidence has been acquired to prompt the International Agency for Research on Cancer of the World Health Organization to conclude that, 'shift work that involves circadian disruption' is a probable human carcinogen.

Epidemiological studies have linked increased risk of cancer incidence and progression with disruption of the circadian clock, for example among people engaged in overnight shift work and those who undertake frequent long-distance air travel. While the exact mediating physiological mechanism in these studies is unclear, the authors consider circadian disruption to be at least partially responsible. Given cortisol's marked circadian variation, immunosuppressive effects, and role in mediating stress, a number of studies have examined the relationship between cortisol and cancer. Early work suggested that women with metastatic breast cancer had relatively flattened diurnal patterns of cortisol. As stated previously, a number of studies have examined within-patient population differences in loss of normal diurnal cortisol variation in relation to subsequent survival outcome. Flattened diurnal cortisol rhythms predict shorter survival with breast, lung, renal cell, and ovarian cancer. A similar, but non-significant, trend has been found between cortisol rhythm and overall survival in patients with metastatic colorectal cancer. Depression is associated with loss of normal diurnal variation in cortisol and a blunted waking rise. Depression, especially severe and chronic, also predicts shorter survival with breast and lung cancer. One possible mechanism linking abnormal cortisol levels and cancer progression stems from the observation that higher mean diurnal cortisol as well as depression are associated with lower levels of cell-mediated immunity (Sephton & Spiegel, 2003).

Sleep and cortisol abnormalities are related. Flattened diurnal cortisol rhythms are associated with the number of patient-reported awakenings during the night. Many cancer patients with advanced disease spend a significant amount of time awake during the night and also asleep during the day. These behavioural abnormalities are also associated with immune dysregulation, including pro-inflammatory cytokine effects on brain function, which induce depressive symptomatology (Miller et al., 2008; Lutgendorf et al., 2010). Poor sleep related to shift work is associated with night-time light exposure and therefore reduced melatonin levels. Melatonin has both anti-oxidant and free radical scavenger properties, so its suppression with exposure to night-time light pollution may contribute to the increase in cancer incidence among shift workers. Sleep disruption is also associated with decrements in the functioning of natural killer cells, which are crucial to breast cancer surveillance and control. In addition, disrupted sleep among cancer patients is associated with loss of vagal tone during the day, restricting the person's ability to self-soothe physiologically in the face of stress. This reduction in heart-rate variability (which primarily reflects vagal rather than sympathetic activity) predicts shorter cancer survival. Disrupted sleep can also cause or worsen fatigue, and increase susceptibility to developing depressive and anxiety disorders, and may also reduce social support from spouses/partners. Consequently, sleep problems are associated with poorer quality of life and shorter cancer survival times (Palesh et al., 2014; Innominato et al., 2015).

Iatrogenic circadian entrainment and circadian and sleep disruption

The circadian timing system features a peculiar flexibility to the changing environment, in order to adapt to, and anticipate, the external changes around 24 hours. This characteristic is particularly helpful after transmeridian travel, as we are then capable of synchronizing our rhythms to the new time zone after a certain amount of time, on those occasions when we experience symptoms of jet lag. Hence, this adaptive behaviour of our circadian timing system implies that the central clock connects with multiple afferent and efferent connections to other systems that convey information regarding environmental changes. An obvious and foremost change that takes place when travelling to a new time zone is the shift in the time of natural daylight and darkness, with paramount implications for social life and sleep. Indeed, the SCN receives direct information about external lighting conditions through a specific neuronal trait from the retina in the eye. Thus, the central clock can constantly adapt to the modifications of the timing of dawn and dusk, and shift accordingly the whole array of physiological rhythms, so as to accustom our sleep and hunger, for example, to the new local time. This process of entrainment—that is, of adjustment of our internal time so that it is synchronized with external cycles—can be accelerated and better fine-tuned by the concomitant transmission of various coherent signals about the temporal environment to the central clock, including, for instance, sleep timing, social interactions, physical activity, and meal timing, among others. It appears clear, then, that several external factors, processed by different brain areas or other peripheral tissues, can impact on the function and coordination of the circadian timing system, at the level of both the central pacemaker and the peripheral molecular clocks, through bi-directional, redundant, and complex networks. This sensitivity to exterior stimuli and internal processes further links the circadian timing system to the sleep–wake cycle, which itself is endogenous, entrainable, and affected by external and internal factors. Among these elements, drugs administered to treat, palliate, or prevent other conditions, such as cancer and treatment side-effects, can alter circadian and sleep functions (Innominato et al., 2010, 2014).

Indeed, chemotherapy drugs are fundamentally required to be toxic, in order to kill and/or inhibit proliferating cancer cells. As such, they have an impact not simply on cancer cells, but on healthy cells as well. As a consequence, toxicity occurs in tissues whose cells have a higher than usual proliferation rate, such as bone marrow, digestive tract mucosa, or hair follicles, manifesting in cytopenia, stomatitis, diarrhoea, and alopecia, for instance. Nevertheless, other systemic side-effects can occur as well. These general symptoms include most frequently fatigue (both physical and mental) and anorexia, but sleep alterations and circadian disruption likewise occur. Moreover, fatigue and anorexia complaints, encompassing somatic and psychological distress, tend to more commonly manifest together in patients undergoing chemotherapy (Innominato et al., 2010). This clustering supports the hypothesis that a common pathogenic mechanism is responsible for their occurrence. Given the circadian temporal control on physical and mental performance and appetite, the impact of sleep on such functions, and the intrinsic pliancy and receptivity of circadian and sleep functions to external stimuli, it is plausible that anti-cancer treatment-induced fatigue and anorexia could be a consequence, at least partly, of circadian disruption. Whilst abundant research efforts are made to better understand the mechanisms behind fatigue and anorexia, hitherto with scant therapeutic options attained, circadian and sleep alterations have been mostly overlooked, with a present dearth of data on their incidence, severity, duration, and underlying processes. Nevertheless, studies conducted on rather small groups of patients, but employing multi-functional, repeated assessments of objective parameters and subjectively reported outcomes, have demonstrated the impact of chemotherapy on circadian and sleep functions, and the association between disruption of circadian rhythms and sleep and systemic symptoms. These studies, albeit still limited in number and size, have been possible thanks to the recent technological developments, enabling enduring tele-monitoring from the patient's home, as well as a systems medicine analytical approach. Thus, the current model assumes a complex and multi-layered psycho-neuro-immunological network influencing the reactions of the body and mind to chemotherapy, engendering circadian disruption and sleep alteration (Sephton & Spiegel, 2003). This hypothesis also applies to other forms of anti-cancer treatment, such as molecular-targeted agents, immunomodulators, radiotherapy, and surgery. Moreover, in addition to chemotherapeutic agents, drugs administered for supportive care, too, can affect the circadian timing system and sleep. This is the case for several anti-emetic drugs, acting on the central nervous system, whose modification of brain biochemistry can directly—or via relevant encephalic nuclei—alter the functioning of the central pacemaker, hence of the circadian timing system and of sleep and arousal functions. Similar effects on circadian and sleep processes occur with the administration of glucocorticoids, especially if at high dose and violating circadian rhythm, and with psychotropic drugs, both widely used in supportive care. Therefore, it is complicated to distinguish between circadian and sleep disruption induced by chemotherapy itself, or by supportive drugs. Nonetheless, the curtailment of iatrogenic circadian and sleep alterations in cancer patients requires an improvement in the administration scheduling of both chemotherapeutic agents and supportive drugs. Chemotherapy acutely impairs rest–activity rhythms, accounting for both sleep disruption and fatigue during the day, and the effect is cumulative with successive courses. These disruptions in sleep architecture impair not only physical activity but also cognitive function. In animal models, cytotoxic chemotherapy induces sleep fragmentation via stimulation of inflammatory processes. Cytokines induce 'sickness behaviour' that includes fatigue and insomnia through direct effects on the brain. Thus, not only cancer, but also anti-cancer treatments, can contribute to the alteration of the normal function of our body clock and our sleep and wake cycle (Innominato et al., 2010).

Nevertheless, sometimes a sought-after effect of a medication can be the modification of circadian and/or sleep functions. This is the concept of a chronobiotic agent—that is, a substance capable of phase-adjusting and re-entraining a desynchronized circadian timing system, as its main therapeutic effect. Albeit several drugs have a sometimes desirable chronobiotic repercussion, to date no concrete use of chronobiotics is implemented in cancer clinical practice. However, exogenous melatonin has been tested in several studies on patients with different cancer types and stages, at various doses and for disparate durations, as a supportive drug, given the lack of evident side-effects. The observed results have often been inconclusive, and its use in the oncological setting remains very limited. Evidently, the heterogeneity of drug prescriptions and patient populations, alongside a maybe sub-optimal pharmacokinetic profile of the used fast-release melatonin, has played a role in these findings. Indeed, a more recent sustained-release formulation of melatonin, which more fittingly mimics the endogenous hormone profile rather than induces a short-lasting peak, is under investigation as a chronobiotic agent in cancer patients. Nevertheless, the results in cancer patients and in subjects with primary sleep problems indicate that melatonin has an overall hypnotic effect. Therefore, in selected cases, melatonin could be preferred to other sedative hypnotics commonly prescribed to cancer patients, because of its wider therapeutic index; in addition, it could help to retain or restore circadian function, thanks to its chronobiotic properties. So, it is possible that analogous effects could occur in cancer patients with novel selective melatonin receptors agonists, indicated for circadian rhythm sleep disorders (non-24-hour). Still, the posology and likely pharmacology ought to be improved to fully exploit its therapeutic potential in the oncological setting.

In addition to pharmacological interventions targeting circadian and sleep processes, the circadian timing system can be re-entrained through behavioural actions (Figure 16.1). Likewise, sleep can be improved by hypnotic drugs, but probably more effectively and more safely by cognitive-behavioural therapy. Indeed, this therapeutic approach aims to improve improper habitudes, assumptions, and mindsets involving sleep through cognitive and behavioural changes. Despite the assortment of procedures through which this intervention can be delivered, altogether cognitive-behavioural therapy for insomnia has displayed statistically significant and clinically meaningful amelioration in subjective sleep outcomes in patients with cancer, and is recommended as the upfront treatment of insomnia in this setting. Additionally, and presumably through sleep regulation and circadian resynchronization, this approach may also improve vigour, mood, and overall health-related quality of life. Hence, improved sleep hygiene and regular daily routine are the starting point for a robust circadian function. Temporal habits can be further regularized through an integrated, interpersonal-psychotherapy approach aimed at reducing circadian disruptive triggers, at establishing and maintaining an orderly schedule of sleep, physical activity, and meals, and simultaneously at improving the performance of interpersonal and social relationships. This so-called interpersonal and social rhythm therapy has proven efficacy in pharmaco-resistant relapsing psychiatric conditions, but has not yet been tested in the oncological setting (Innominato et al., 2014). Nevertheless, a positive impact of this therapeutic approach on cancer patients can be arguably assumed, based on the common features of vulnerability to circadian disruption and sleep problems and the associated psychological and somatic distress found in patients with severe psychiatric illness and in those with cancer. Moreover, circadian function, as well as sleep process, can be phase-shifted by timed exposure to bright light. Thus, light therapy is a straightforward practice employed to cope with jet lag, but can also have beneficial activity in certain types of psychiatric conditions and sleep disorders, and is completely exempt from toxicity. Initial reports in small cohorts suggest a positive effect of bright light therapy in cancer patients undergoing chemotherapy in preventing fatigue and circadian rhythm desynchronization. The full beneficial potential of these behavioural interventions can be attained allegedly through their integration within a multidisciplinary, patient-centred systems approach to medicine. This requires an accurate identification and selection of patients and of corresponding personalized behavioural interventions and the sequential delivery of appropriate induction and maintenance treatments, whose duration and reiteration depend upon constant and dynamic monitoring of circadian biomarkers and sleep. Despite this complexity, a restoration of robust circadian and sleep functions would conceivably result in an improvement in the severity of systemic symptoms in cancer patients, and in general health-related quality of life, as well as in the survival and tolerance of such patients to treatments, particularly when chemotherapy is administered according to the circadian clock.

Cancer chronotherapy

Cancer chronotherapy consists of the delivery of anti-cancer drugs at the optimal circadian time, when circadian physiology and the molecular clock create the conditions for a minimal toxicity on healthy cells and a maximal activity against cancer cells (Innominato et al., 2010). This scientific elaboration of this kind of chemotherapy administration is founded on the numerous circadian rhythms temporally governing the whole-body and intracellular pharmacokinetic and pharmacodynamic profiles of a drug, hence its efficacy and toxicity, whose magnitude can vary by several fold according to the time of medicine intake. This has been demonstrated for numerous anti-cancer agents in models, from cell culture, though experimental rodents, to humans. For intravenous injection, still the most common administration route for cytotoxic chemotherapy agents, the clinical implementation of cancer chronotherapy depends on programmable-in-time pumps that can infuse several drugs at any time of the day or the night, with a versatile profile according to the clinical requisites. Hence, the progress of cancer chronotherapy depends on solid basic experimental information, technologically advanced devices, and expressly designed clinical trials with compelling associated translational research, as well as on a befitting education of the patient, related caregivers, and healthcare personnel, and on devoted mathematical computational modelling within the frame of an exhaustive systems biology and systems medicine approach (Innominato et al., 2010 and 2014). It follows that a wide array of multidisciplinary expertise is required to bring forth cancer chronotherapy in everyday clinical practice. Thus, notwithstanding the soundness of its scientific rationale and the clinical evidence, timing medical treatment to circadian rhythms remains an unusual practice. Besides the added complexity of timing optimization to the indication, combination, and posology of a drug, a presumable hurdle to the general endorsement of cancer chronotherapy is the misconception that the timing of administration has trivial impact on the therapeutic index of a medication. Yet, a plethora of evidence substantiates the relevance of circadian timing on tolerability and anti-tumour activity, to an extent comparable to dose modifications and inter-individual variability. Given the inter-individual differences in circadian and sleep timing and functional status, as well as treatment-induced alterations of circadian and sleep processes, upcoming trials in cancer chronotherapy ought to adopt a personalized and a dynamic approach so as to continually refine the delivery pattern, with ambulatory monitoring of circadian rhythms and sleep, and with the employment of pre-emptive and pro-active response actions. Expectedly, this individualization and real-time fine-tuning would improve the outcomes of cancer patients in comparison with current conventional chemotherapy schedules, resulting in a safe administration within the patient's home environment; an increased tolerance, with less frequent and severe side-effects and symptoms; a better subjectively perceived health-related quality of life; and a greater anti-cancer efficacy, ensuing longer overall and cancer-specific survival (Figure 16.1).

Summary

- Cancer is a disruption of cellular control mechanisms leading to poorly controlled growth, turning the building blocks of the body into an invasive enemy.
- Cancer leads to disruption of the circadian timing system that temporally coordinates the body's neural, endocrine, and immune systems. Chemotherapy can also disrupt circadian function.
- Dysregulated patterns of sleep and activity, and hormones such as cortisol and melatonin, result from, and contribute to, poor outcomes in cancer.
- These circadian alterations provide opportunities for more effective cancer treatment by improving rest and activity cycles, enhancing sleep efficiency, normalizing hormone patterns, and employing chronomodulated chemotherapy.
- With cancer treatment, timing is everything.

References

Innominato, P. F., Lévi, F. A. & Bjarnason, G. A. 2010. Chronotherapy and the molecular clock: clinical implications in oncology. *Advanced Drug Delivery Reviews*, **62**(9-10), pp. 979–1001.

Innominato, P. F., Roche, V. P., Palesh, O. G., Ulusakarya, A., Spiegel, D. & Lévi, F. A. 2014. The circadian timing system in clinical oncology. *Annals of Medicine*, **46**, pp. 191–207.

Innominato, P. F., Spiegel, D., Ulusakarya, A., Giacchetti, S., Bjarnason, G. A., Lévi, F. & Palesh, O. 2015. Subjective sleep and overall survival in chemotherapy-naïve patients with metastatic colorectal cancer. *Sleep* Medicine, **16**, pp. 391–8.

Lutgendorf, S. K., Sood, A. K. & Antoni, M. H. 2010. Host factors and cancer progression: biobehavioral signaling pathways and interventions. *Journal of Clinical Oncology*, **28**, pp. 4094–9.

Miller, A. H., Ancoli-Israel, S., Bower, J. E., Capuron, L. & Irwin, M. R. 2008. Neuroendocrine-immune mechanisms of behavioral comorbidities in patients with cancer. *Journal of Clinical Oncology*, **26**, pp. 971–82.

Mormont, M. C., Waterhouse, J., Bleuzen, P., Giacchetti, S., Jami, A., Bogdan, A., Lellouch, J., Misset, J. L. & Touitou, Y., Lévi, F. 2000. Marked 24-h rest/activity rhythms are associated with better quality of life, better response, and longer survival in patients with metastatic colorectal cancer and good performance status. *Clinical Cancer Research*, **6**, pp. 3038–45.

Palesh, O., Aldridge-Gerry, A., Zeitzer, J. M., Koopman, C., Neri, E., Giese-Davis, J., Jo, B., Kraemer, H., Nouriani, B. & Spiegel, D. 2014. Actigraphy-measured sleep disruption as a predictor of survival among women with advanced breast cancer. *Sleep*, **37**, pp. 837–42.

Sephton, S. E., Sapolsky, R. M., Kraemer, H. C. & Spiegel, D. 2000. Diurnal cortisol rhythm as a predictor of breast cancer survival. *Journal of the National Cancer Institute*, **92**, pp. 994–1000.

Sephton, S. & Spiegel, D. 2003. Circadian disruption in cancer: a neuroendocrine-immune pathway from stress to disease? *Brain, Behavior, and Immunity*, **17**, pp. 321–8.

Spiegel D. 2008. Losing sleep over cancer. *Journal of Clinical Oncology*, **26**, pp. 2431–2.

Chapter 17

Sleep and pain

Nicole K. Y. Tang, Esther F. Afolalu,
and Fatanah Ramlee

Introduction

To many people, pain is an unpleasant sensory and emotional experience. Whilst it alerts
us to (potential) danger, its occurrence during sleep can negatively affect the quality and
quantity of sleep. In fact, sleep disturbance is a common feature of chronic painful conditions. This interrelationship has troubled clinicians and fascinated scientists.

Pain and sleeplessness are issues that undermine quality of life and are two of the commonest reasons for medical appointments. The prevalence and chronicity of both problems increase with age, presenting a major public health challenge to our ageing society.
A timely integration of the epidemiological knowledge of sleep and pain will offer insights
into the state of the nation's health and will inform treatment development and early prevention initiatives.

Co-occurrence of pain and sleep disturbance

The extent of co-occurrence is most evident at the clinical end of the spectrum, where
50%–80% of patients seeking treatment from hospital pain clinics report clinical insomnia of moderate to high severity (McCracken et al., 2011). Nevertheless, a link between pain and sleep disturbance has also been detected in large-scale surveys, using
samples representative of the general population as a whole. In an international telephone
survey involving 18,980 people aged 15 years or above, living in the UK, Germany, Italy,
Portugal, and Spain, respondents were asked to report their pain experience. Chronic
painful physical conditions (CPPCs) were defined as pain conditions lasting for at least
6 months, and were classified into five broad categories: joint/articular, limb, back,
gastro-intestinal, and headaches. Four main insomnia symptoms aligned with diagnostic
criteria were assessed for prevalence, and these were difficulty initiating sleep, disrupted
sleep, early morning awakening, and non-restorative sleep. Of the respondents, 17% reported at least one CPPC, and the prevalence of each individual insomnia symptom
ranged from 4.5% to 7.5%. The rate of insomnia differed by the presence or absence of
a CPPC: 23% of those with a CPPC reported at least one insomnia symptom, compared
with only 7.4% of those with no CPPC. Conversely, the rate of CPPCs differed by insomnia status: more than 40% of those with insomnia symptoms reported at least one

CPPC, compared with only 15% of those with no insomnia symptoms. Similar findings have been reported in other health surveys. For instance, in Norway, among 47,700 respondents aged 20–89 years, those with insomnia were more than twice as likely to report a co-occurring CPPC with uncertain organic aetiology such as fibromyalgia (FM), musculoskeletal pain, and headache. Reporting of insomnia was also associated with an increased risk of other CPPCs with known organic aetiology such as osteoporosis, rheumatoid arthritis, and migraine. In the 2003 US National Sleep Foundation 'Sleep in America' poll, daily bodily pain was a serious issue among community-dwelling older people (aged 55–84 years). Daily bodily pain was reported by 35% of all interviewees and by 50% of those interviewees with arthritis. The presence of pain was associated with an increased risk of not only insomnia symptoms (difficulty initiating sleep and waking from sleep, early morning awakening, non-restorative sleep, short nightly sleep duration), but also symptoms linked to other sleep disorders such as sleep apnoea (daytime sleepiness, snoring, and periodic limb movement disorder).

Together, these population-based surveys reveal that insomnia and pain are risk factors of each other even at the non-clinical end of the spectrum. Despite differences in samples and assessment methodologies, the findings are consistent across studies, suggesting some universality in the pain–sleep association among western developed countries. However, the cross-sectional nature of the analysis precludes inferences about causality. While we can be confident that insomnia symptoms and CPPCs often co-occur, it is unclear whether insomnia is a cause or effect of CPPCs. Possibilities remain that they are epiphenomenal to each other or they are both conditions manifested by one or more common underlying factors, which may or may not have been studied.

Pain is a risk factor of sleep disturbance/insomnia onset

Surveys with repeated measures of sleep and pain over time can help establish the temporal order of events. Utilizing a well-defined insomnia-free sample at baseline, several longitudinal studies have provided sound evidence that pain contributes to the subsequent development of insomnia.

LeBlanc et al. (2009), in Canada, followed up 464 good sleepers over a year with three postal surveys at 6-monthly intervals. They found that 1-year incidence rates for insomnia syndrome and symptoms were 7.4% and 30.7%, respectively. Bodily pain at baseline was one of five most significant predictors of an insomnia syndrome onset (odds ratio (OR) = 0.98). Bodily pain was measured using the SF-12 (Short Form Health Survey), with a higher score representing less pain. The OR suggested that each increase of 1 point on the SF-12 bodily pain subscale (i.e. reduction in pain) was associated with a 2% decrease in the risk of developing a case of insomnia within 1 year.

Apparently, the type, spread, and frequency of pain experienced can make a difference in the course of insomnia development. Ødegård et al. (2013) utilized two waves of data drawn from the HUNT study to evaluate the relative and joint influence of headache and chronic musculoskeletal complaints (CMSCs; referring to pain and/or stiffness in muscles and joints) on the risk of insomnia onset 11 years later. Of the 27,185 adults (aged

≥ 20 years) who completed a health survey at both assessments, 19,271 were insomnia-free at baseline. For this subgroup, both baseline headache and CMSCs independently predicted insomnia onset at follow-up, but having both types of pain (OR = 2.0) predisposed respondents more strongly to insomnia onset than having headache (OR = 1.5) or CMSCs (OR = 1.6) alone. Moreover, there was a dose–response relationship: headache occurring 7 days or more per month (OR = 2.2) and widespread CMSCs meeting the 1990 American College of Rheumatology (ACR) criteria (OR = 2.0) carried a higher risk of insomnia incidence than headache of lower frequency and CMSCs affecting fewer body areas.

A similar dose–response relationship was also observed in a prospective study (Tang et al., 2015) involving 6,676 insomnia-free older adults (aged ≥ 50 years) residing in Staffordshire, UK. Compared to respondents without pain, the risk of incident insomnia 3 years from baseline was 2.31 times greater for those reporting widespread pain and 1.57 times greater for those reporting some pain, but did not meet the American College of Rheumatology (ACR) criteria. The risk of incident insomnia remained robust even when a large number of potential confounds were adjusted for, including age, gender, education, occupational class, anxiety, depression, co-morbidity, and sleep disturbance at baseline. Of particular interest was the finding that physical limitation and restricted social participation were significant mediators of the pain–sleep relationship, explaining up to 66% of the total effect of widespread pain on insomnia onset. This illuminated the potential behavioural mechanism underpinning the prospective pain–insomnia relationship. A possible interpretation of this finding is that pain increases the risk of insomnia by interfering with the regulation of sleep homeostasis and circadian rhythm through altering/restricting the pattern of physical and social activity and exposure to zeitgebers (e.g. sunlight).

The temporal order of pain and insomnia can be a 'chicken or the egg' issue, but findings of the above studies suggest an aetiological role of pain in the development of insomnia and the investigation of potential mediators at the population level is an exciting new trend to watch. Between studies, the length of the follow-up period varied from 1 to 11 years, with stronger effects of pain being detected in studies measuring insomnia onset at a later follow-up. A lengthy follow-up is both a blessing and a curse. While it helps establish an association over time, temporal resolution of the relationship established depends on the frequency and quality of the measurement and can be vulnerable to biases introduced by selective attrition. The studies reviewed above varied in their assessment interval and frequency, but similar levels of care were applied in measuring the effect of pain of different types and spread and adjusting for potential confounds. They have generated some neat evidence of specificity, temporality, and a biological gradient of the pain–insomnia relationship.

Sleep disturbance/insomnia is a risk factor of pain disorders

The aetiological role of pain in insomnia onset does not preclude the role of sleep disturbance in the development of CPPCs. In fact, the pain–sleep relationship is likely to be reciprocal, analogous to what has been shown in experimental research, where the induction of acute sleep deprivation or fragmentation in healthy young adults can lead to greater pain report, higher pain sensitivity, and lower pain tolerance.

Several prospective studies have provided convincing evidence that sleep problems are a trigger or an aggravator of pain disorder. Mork & Nilsen (2012) tracked the development of widespread pain (a key diagnostic criterion for FM) in 12,350 pain-free women between 1984–6 and 1995–7. While the analysis was based on the same HUNT dataset, Mork & Nilsen (2012) conceptualized sleep problems as an exposure rather than an outcome and restricted the sample's gender composition to female only, given the higher prevalence of FM in women. Compared to women who 'never' experienced sleep problems, those who reported having sleep problems 'often' or 'always' at baseline were 3.4 times more likely to report physician-diagnosed FM 11 years later. The risk was adjusted for age, frequency of physical exercise, body mass index, psychological wellbeing, smoking, and education. Further, an age-stratified analysis revealed that the association between sleep problems and FM was stronger in older women (aged > 45 years; adjusted RR = 5.41) than in younger women (aged 20–44 years; adjusted RR = 2.98).

It must be noted that although age is a moderator of the relationship, young people with problems sleeping are not immune to the risk of pain disorders. In one of the very few studies that examined the prospective impact of sleep on pain in adolescents, Auvinen et al. (2010) found that, among the 1,773 15- to 19-year-old Finns who responded to both the baseline and 6-month follow-up questionnaires, insufficient sleep quantity or quality at baseline was an independent risk factor for neck pain (adjusted RR = 3.2) and low back pain (2.41) in girls at follow-up. Also, the development of widespread pain is not exclusive to women. Morphy et al. (2007) followed up 1,589 adult men (44%) and women (56%) over 12 months and found that insomnia at baseline was significantly associated with subsequent incidence of widespread pain (adjusted RR = 1.45). The association remained significant after adjusting for the effects of age and gender.

The prospective studies reviewed above primarily evaluated the development of pain in healthy individuals with problems sleeping. The extent to which insomnia onset would aggravate pain in those who are already living with chronic pain remains to be determined. A number of clinical studies have found a strong positive correlation between pain intensity and insomnia severity in patients. Carefully designed time-lagged analyses that examine the impact of insomnia onset on *change* in pain among patients will help to address this question.

Directions forward

The longitudinal association between insomnia and pain has thus far only been painted in broad strokes. Figure 17.1 provides a schematic summary of the evidence reviewed, the simplicity of which probably does not reflect the complexity of the pain–sleep relationship. Continual methodological innovations in prospective study design, measurement, and analysis are required to deepen and broaden our understanding. Several approaches may be considered, as described below.

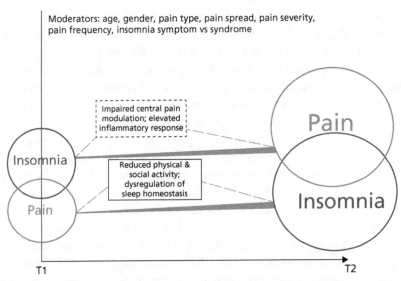

Moderators: age, gender, pain type, pain spread, pain severity, pain frequency, insomnia symptom vs syndrome

Impaired central pain modulation; elevated inflammatory response

Reduced physical & social activity; dysregulation of sleep homeostasis

Pain

Insomnia

Insomnia

Pain

T1   T2

Fig. 17.1 A schematic summary of the chapter. The figure summarizes the evidence on the prospective relationship between pain and insomnia, and vice versa, as revealed by the population-based studies reviewed. T1 stands for Time 1 (baseline), and T2 stands for Time 2 (follow-up). Predictors at T1 and predicted variables at T2 are represented by circles. The increasing size of the circle symbolizes the increasing prevalence with age and time, while the overlap represents the interrelationship/co-occurrence of the two conditions. Potential mediators of the relationships are presented in rectangles. The dotted line of the top rectangle expresses uncertainty in relation to the mediating role of central pain modulation and inflammatory response in the insomnia–pain relationship, given a lack of direct epidemiological evidence. Moderators of the overlap and prospective relationships are listed at the top of the figure. Reproduced courtesy of the authors.

Evaluating theoretically driven mediators that translate pain into sleep problems, and vice versa

Such evaluation can be facilitated by prospective cohort studies with multiple waves of assessment. Aided by appropriate analytical techniques, the time-specific structure of the data provides an excellent platform for examining the processes mediating the pain–sleep relationship. Identification of mediators reveals novel targets for treatment and prevention. For example, Tang et al. (2015b) found empirical evidence to suggest that pain-related dysregulation of physical and social activity is an important behavioural pathway to sleep disruption. Promoting physical and social participation in older people with pain may buffer co-morbid insomnia and help improve quality of life in general.

Improving the precision, range, pattern of sleep, and pain measurement

Self-report measures of sleep and pain are most popular among cohort studies for their ease of use, accessibility, and affordability. Although they provide unique insights into the sleepers' perception of their sleep, they do not provide physiological information about sleep processes. Recall and reporting biases aside, it is well recognized that there are systematic discrepancies between subjectively and objectively estimated sleep. Compared to normal sleepers, people with insomnia have a tendency to overestimate wake and underestimate sleep, and a range of cortical, physiological, and psychological factors have been proposed to account for this tendency (Harvey & Tang, 2012). However, sleep misperception is a phenomenon often overlooked in epidemiological studies. Likewise, pain is a multidimensional experience that demands precision and specificity in measurement. While self-reported presence, spread, and intensity of pain are valid and clinically relevant, they do not provide much information about the type of pain and the underlying central and peripheral pain modulating mechanisms.

Future population-based studies should consider incorporating objective sleep assessment and diversifying pain measures. Although there will be time and cost implications, proportionate use of technologies combined with appropriate sampling methods can help demonstrate the biological plausibility of the suggested sleep–pain link and open up new horizons for future research and treatment development. In recent years, we have witnessed an increased application of actigraphy for sleep assessment in micro-longitudinal studies examining the day-to-day association between sleep and pain (Tang et al., 2012) and randomized controlled trials (RCTs) evaluating interventions of insomnia co-morbid with pain. However, polysomnography—the 'gold standard' of sleep measurement—is still rarely used in cohort studies. In terms of pain assessment, it is encouraging to note that a couple of recent population-based studies have diversified the measurement of pain and found evidence for (i) a cross-sectional relationship of pain tolerance during a cold pressor task with sleep onset latency, sleep efficiency, and insomnia frequency and severity, and (ii) the prospective association between a reduction in typical sleep duration over a period of 5 years and a higher average level of circulating pro-inflammatory markers such as C-reactive protein (CRP) and inter-leukin-6 (IL-6) over the subsequent 5 years (Ferrie et al., 2013). These findings corroborate with experimental studies that suggest a role for central pain modulation and inflammation in explaining increased pain responses following sleep disturbance. Note, however, that sleep/insomnia was measured in both studies using self-report questionnaires. There is still some way to go in terms of building a multi-faceted understanding of sleep and pain, both as overlapping living experiences and as measurable physiological phenomena.

Investigating the combined effect of pain and insomnia on future health and wellbeing

If pain contributes to the development of insomnia over time and insomnia aggravates existing pain, a question that logically follows would be: 'What is the additive and synergistic effect of pain and insomnia on health and wellbeing in the long term?' An interesting study by Campbell et al. (2013) tested whether people with chronic pain who then went on to develop sleep problems have an increased risk of incident depression.

These investigators utilized three waves of data (baseline, 3-year, and 6-year) drawn from the North Staffordshire Osteoarthritis Project, a prospective cohort study with 13,986 adults aged ≥ 50 years. To provide a well-defined baseline sample, they restricted the analysis to 2,622 participants who had pain across all three assessment points but were free from insomnia and depression at baseline. The incidence rate of probable cases of depression at 6 years was found to be 4.7%. Compared to those who did not report problems sleeping at 3 years, those who did were associated with an increased risk of probable depression at 6 years (RR 2.85, 95% CI 1.62–5.02). Adjusting for potential confounds (e.g. baseline age, gender, marital status, employment status, alcohol intake, smoking status, body mass index), incident insomnia at 3 years trebled the risk of incident depression at 6 years in people with pain at baseline (RR 3.47, 95% CI 1.97–6.03). These findings highlight the potential benefit of treating sleep problems early for those with persistent pain. Provision of sleep interventions alongside traditional pain management may lead to better physical and mental health outcomes.

Better sleep, better health?

In closing, studies on the association between sleep and pain have focused to date on the negative effects on each other, i.e., either pain causing bad sleep or sleep disturbances worsening pain. Very few studies have examined the effect of improvement in sleep and/ or pain at the population level outside of the context of RCTs.

Davies et al. (2008) made a notable attempt to address the balance and to identify factors that precede and predict a reduction in pain. Their study involved 679 adults (aged 25–65 years) with chronic widespread pain who responded to two waves of assessments 15 months apart. While 56% of these individuals continued to report widespread pain at follow-up, 44% no longer met the ACR criteria of widespread pain. Interestingly, the likelihood of reporting a 'resolution' of widespread pain was doubled in those who reported 'restorative sleep' at baseline compared to those who did not. These findings suggest that restorative sleep may be a characteristic of those who report an improvement in pain, and allude to a possible therapeutic effect of sleep that could be exploited to improve outcomes for chronic pain patients with concomitant insomnia.

The tantalizing prospect that improved sleep is followed by improvement in pain is not without empirical support. One secondary analysis of a CBT-I trial among older adults with osteoarthritis pain and insomnia showed that short-term improvement in insomnia (occurring within 2 months of treatment) predicts long-term improvement in sleep, pain, and fatigue at 9–18 months after treatment. Furthermore, a meta-analysis of 11 eligible RCTs evaluating the efficacy of CBT-I on pain and other physical and psychosocial functioning outcomes has revealed that in chronic pain patients, completing a course of CBT-I was associated with a large improvement in sleep quality, a small improvement in pain, and a moderate improvement in fatigue at post-treatment, compared to those receiving a control intervention. The effects on sleep quality and fatigue were well maintained at follow-up (3–12 months), when a moderate therapeutic effect on depression also emerged (Tang et al., 2015a).

Taken together, these findings outline the positive side of the reciprocal relationship between sleep, pain, and other mental and physical health outcomes. This positive association is minimally understood in the context of public health, but could be fruitfully exploited for the prevention and management of long-term health conditions.

Summary

+ Everyone sleeps and most of us experience pain at some point in our lives.

+ The overlapping experience of pain and sleeplessness is not exclusive to a select few, but shared to various degrees across the whole population.

+ The interrelationship between pain and sleep can be studied at the population level, to further our understanding of the nature of the association and the factors moderating and mediating the relationship.

+ Knowledge gained from population-based studies will provide insights into the state of the nation's health and will inform treatment development and early prevention initiatives.

References

Auvinen J. P., Tammelin, T. H., Taimela, S. P., Zitting, P. J., Järvelin, M. R., Taanila, A. M. & Karppinen, J. I. 2010. Is insufficient quantity and quality of sleep a risk factor for neck, shoulder and low back pain? A longitudinal study among adolescents. *European Spine Journal*, **19**(4), pp. 641–9.

Campbell, P., Tang, N. K. Y., McBeth, J., Lewis, M., Main, C. J., Croft, P. R., Morphy, H. & Dunn, K. M. 2013. The role of sleep problems in the development of depression in those with persistent pain: a prospective cohort study. *Sleep*, **36**(11), pp. 1693–8.

Davies, K .A., Macfarlane, G. J., Nicholl, B. I., Dickens, C., Morriss, R., Ray, D. & McBeth, J. 2008. Restorative sleep predicts the resolution of chronic widespread pain: results from the EPIFUND study. *Rheumatology*, **47**(12), pp. 1809–13.

Ferrie, J. E., Kivimäki, M., Akbaraly, T. N., Singh-Manoux, A., Miller, M. A., Gimeno, D., Kumari, M., Davey Smith, G. & Shipley, M. J. 2013. Associations between change in sleep duration and inflammation: findings on C-reactive protein and interleukin 6 in the Whitehall II Study. *American Journal of Epidemiology*, **178**(6), pp. 956–61.

Harvey, A. G. & Tang, N. K. Y. 2012. (Mis) perception of sleep in insomnia: a puzzle and a resolution. *Psychological Bulletin*, **138**(1), pp. 77–101.

LeBlanc, M., Mérette, C., Savard, J., Ivers, H., Baillargeon, L. & Morin, C. M. 2009. Incidence and risk factors of insomnia in a population-based sample. *Sleep*, **32**(8), pp. 1027–37.

McCracken, L. M., Williams, J. L. & Tang, N. K. Y. 2011. Psychological flexibility may reduce insomnia in persons with chronic pain: a preliminary retrospective study. *Pain Medicine*, **12**(6), pp. 904–12.

Mork, P. J. & Nilsen, T. I. 2012. Sleep problems and risk of fibromyalgia: longitudinal data on an adult female population in Norway. *Arthritis and Rheumatism*, **64**(1), pp. 281–4.

Morphy, H., Dunn, K. M., Lewis, M., Boardman, H. F. & Croft, P. R. 2007. Epidemiology of insomnia: a longitudinal study in a UK population. *Sleep*, **30**(3), pp. 274–80.

Ødegård, S. S., Sand, T., Engstrøm, M., Zwart, J. A. & Hagen, K. 2013. The impact of headache and chronic musculoskeletal complaints on the risk of insomnia: longitudinal data from the Nord-Trøndelag health study. *The Journal of Headache and Pain*, **14**(1), p. 24.

Tang, N. K. Y, Goodchild, C. E., Sanborn, A. N., Howard, J., & Salkovskis, P. M. 2012. Deciphering the temporal link between pain and sleep in a heterogeneous chronic pain patient sample: a multilevel daily process study. *Sleep*, **35**(5), pp. 675–87.

Tang, N. K. Y., Lereya, S. T., Boulton, H., Miller, M. A., Wolke, D. & Cappuccio, F. P. 2015a. Nonpharmacological treatments of insomnia for long-term painful conditions: a systematic review and meta- analysis of patient-reported outcomes in randomized controlled trials. *Sleep*, **38**(11), pp. 1751– 64.

Tang, N. K. Y., McBeth, J., Jordan, K. P., Blagojevic-Bucknall, M., Croft, P. & Wilkie, R. 2015b. Impact of musculoskeletal pain on insomnia onset: a prospective cohort study. *Rheumatology*, **54**(2), pp. 248–56.

Part 3

Society

Chapter 18

Sleep in western culture: A historical perspective

A. Roger Ekirch

Introduction

Although a universal necessity, sleep, as the past powerfully indicates, is not a biological constant. Rather than sharing a common set of characteristics, sleep has varied over both time and space in duration, structure, environment, and quality, owing principally to cultural imperatives and technological advances. Western sleep surfaces have themselves ranged from piles of straw to modern mattresses costing two thousand pounds. In light of the diverse patterns of behaviour that distinguish our waking lives, it seems naive, in retrospect, ever to have expected a rigid consistency in human sleep.

Historians and sleep

To a degree, historians are hindered in analyzing human sleep by an absence of scientific data of the sort available to modern researchers. Lacking actigraphs (wearable instruments that measure our movements and record our sleep–wake cycles) and other sensitive instruments central to sleep medicine, historians are forced to rely upon less precise evidence that is predominantly literary rather than quantitative—the random remains of the past rather than hard data generated by live human subjects in closely monitored clinics. As resurrectionists, we are left to gather information from a variety of written sources: early medical texts and religious treatises, poems, plays, and other forms of imaginative literature, as well as personal documents, from diaries and letters to memoirs. As for newspapers and periodicals, only in the 1700s did those in Britain and America begin to print more than a smattering of letters and essays, much less any on the subject of sleep. Even so, historians of sleep do enjoy two major advantages. Pre-industrial families, even more than today, attached great significance to their slumber, making it a topic of widespread interest and concern. 'Nothing is holesomer', a sixteenth-century Dutch physician observed, 'than sounde and quiet sleep' (Ekirch, 2005). Equally important, though evidence relating to sleep is sparse for western societies prior to the late Middle Ages, historians are blessed, after the fifteenth century, with having a span of more than five hundred years in which to distinguish, as best they can, enduring patterns in sleep behaviour from short-term trends.

Segmented sleep in pre-industrial western cultures

Before the Industrial Revolution, sleep in western households, let alone that in other cultures, differed in a variety of respects from that of today. Most obviously, by the late Middle Ages, if not earlier, a medical consensus had evolved regarding the source of human sleep. Physicians, for the most part, accepted the Aristotelian conviction that the impetus for sleep originated in the stomach by means of 'concoction'—a process by which fumes arising from the digestion of food ascended to the brain, where, after cooling, they congealed to facilitate sleep by smothering the senses (Dannenfeldt, 1986; Ekirch, 2015a). Not only did sleep restore exhausted minds and weary bodies, but it also afforded troubled souls an escape from life's hardships. According to an English writer in 1607, sleep 'strengtheneth all the spirits', 'comforteth the body', 'taketh away sorrow', and 'asswageth furie of the mind'. Or, as a popular saying emphasized, falling asleep was to 'forget the world'. 'Sleep hab no massa', attested a Jamaican slave proverb (Ekirch, 2005).

The predominant form of sleep, very likely from time immemorial, was segmented, consisting of two intervals of roughly 3 to 4 hours apiece ('first sleep' and 'second sleep'), bridged by up to an hour or so of wakefulness usually originating after midnight, depending upon the time of sleep onset. In *The Canterbury Tales*, Princess Canacee slept 'soon after evening fell' and subsequently stirred from 'her first sleep', whereas her companions, retiring much later, first awakened closer to dawn (Ekirch, 2001, 2005). The earliest known reference to biphasic sleep lies in Homer's *Odyssey*, written in either the late eighth or early seventh century BC. Virgil in the *Aeneid* (first century BC) described the chore of spinning flax performed after the 'first sleep' by the 'careful housewife' who makes 'night itself contribute to her thrift' (Ekirch, 2015b).

Besides other mundane activities—tending to fires, caring for livestock, or filching fruit from a neighbour's orchard—individuals of myriad faiths—Protestants, Catholics, and Jews—employed this nightly hiatus as a sacred time for prayer and meditation when, according to an English moralist, the soul has 'the least encumbrance' from profane distractions. When confronted by Satan instead, Martin Luther claimed to 'instantly chase him away with a fart' (Ekirch, 2005, 2015b; Garnier, 2013). Then, too, centuries before the modern study of chronopharmacology, ill patients imbibed potions and elixirs advised by physicians for the dead of night. In medical texts, this was also a favoured interlude to conceive children. A sixteenth-century French doctor claimed that 'after the first sleep' well-rested couples 'do it better' and 'have more enjoyment'. Few individuals, however, appear to have remained awake for good (Ekirch, 2005). Among other singular qualities, it was said, for instance, that Thomas Ken, an English Bishop, 'rose generally very early, and never took a second sleep' (Ekirch, 2005).

Often, persons awoke from a dream during their first sleep. In addition to its other benefits, sleep, by virtue of nocturnal visions, afforded not only a source of prophecy and divine instruction but also a well-travelled path to better understanding one's character. Well before Sigmund Freud and the Romantic philosophers of the nineteenth century, early modern Europeans valued the personal insights acquired from dreams. According to Thomas Tryon, a seventeenth-century sceptic of the prophetic qualities of dreams, 'Let the night teach us what we are, and the day what we should be' (Ekirch, 2005). Further, for many persons, from African-American slaves to upper-class Europeans, visions offered a means to visit distant or dead loved-ones, a source of considerable solace in times of high mortality. Far from being ridiculed, persons reported such visits to friends and family. A Venetian rabbi, Leon Modena, wrote of reunions with both a revered teacher and his mother. 'Very soon, you will be with me', she told him (Ekirch, 2005).

The 'light' revolution

Biphasic sleep arose principally from a dearth of artificial illumination within pre-industrial households. To relieve the darkness, families relied upon the meagre light afforded by candles (more often tallow than wax), oil lamps, and such primitive sources as candlewood (resinous pine knots) and rushlights (dried reeds coated in fat). In the view of sleep scientists, modern lighting, or in turn its absence, has a profound impact on the circadian pacemaker (suprachiasmatic nucleus), a tiny bundle of cells in the hypothalamus at the base of the brain. Arguably the most important function that the pacemaker regulates is the sleep–wake cycle. Charles A. Czeisler has written, 'Every time we turn on a light, we are inadvertently taking a drug that affects how we will sleep' (Ekirch, 2005). Notably, in the early 1990s, when a team led by Thomas Wehr at the National Institute of Mental Health deprived human subjects at night of artificial illumination, their sleep after 3 weeks adopted a biphasic pattern nearly identical to that of pre-industrial households. Moreover, like their forebears, Wehr's subjects often awakened from dreams during rapid eye movement (REM) sleep around midnight (Ekirch, 2005).

Not surprisingly, anthropologists in the late nineteenth and twentieth centuries discovered this pattern of segmented sleep among non-western cultures deprived of modern lighting. Of the Tiv population of subsistence farmers in central Nigeria, one study concluded in 1953, 'At night, they wake when they will and talk with anyone else awake in the hut'. To help chart time, the Tiv even employed terms equivalent in their own language to 'first sleep' and 'second sleep'. So, too, from the Woolwa Indians of Central America and Surinamese Maroons on the northern coast of South America to the Asante and Fante in West Africa, the dominant pattern of sleep has been biphasic (Ekirch, 2015b, 2016).

How much sleep?

Of the proper length of sleep, European medical books from the fifteenth to the eighteenth centuries frequently recommended 7–8 hours for most individuals, commencing between 9 p.m. and 10 p.m. Exceptions, necessitating an extra hour or more, included labourers, porters, and seamen. Seasonal adjustments were minor. Some writers advocated an extra hour's rest during long winter nights. Though adequate rest was deemed essential for bodily health, authorities widely criticized excessive sleep, a source not only of idleness and sin but also ill health, including poor digestion, weak blood, and troubled spirits. Popular aphorisms echoed the advice of medical texts—hence the saying, 'Custom takes seven, laziness nine, and wickedness eleven' (Dannenfeldt, 1986; Ekirch, 2005)—as did diaries, though personal curfews proved elastic. As in other traditional cultures, bedtime often depended upon the existence of things to do, whether domestic chores or the opportunity to fraternize, albeit briefly, with neighbours. An inscription over the parlour of a Danish pastor read: 'Stay til nine you are my friend, til ten, that is alright, but if you stay til 11, you are my enemy'. A parallel belief was that sleep should follow nature's course by being reserved for night-time, according to divine will, and which by its silence, darkness, and moisture was thought especially well-suited to concoction. Napping during the day was invariably derided, a frequent motif in Dutch paintings (Ekirch, 2005).

Precautions and rituals

Early modern families took numerous measures to preserve the tranquillity and safety of their slumber, which inspired a popular typology more nuanced than that employed today. Such expressions as 'dog', 'cat', or 'hare' sleep referred to rest that was light and anxious. Coveted, instead, was sleep both deep and continuous, or 'soft' and 'calm'. 'Quiet sleep', stressed an early text, 'although it is short, bears more usefulness', a conclusion that conforms to modern research attributing, in large measure, the number of times persons awaken in the night to whether they feel rested in the morning (Ekirch, 2005). Once limited to pallets of straw on earthen floors, beds featuring flock mattresses, blankets, and pillows were the most expensive pieces of furniture in middle-class European households, and as such, among the most treasured items bequeathed in wills. Normally, they were shared—other than married couples—usually by siblings and servants or a mix of both. Besides avoiding the cost and space that additional beds necessitated, bedmates afforded greater warmth and a welcome sense of security. Terrified of the devil, a white labourer, 'many nights, rather than lay alone', went to bed instead 'with black persons' at the Pennsylvania farm where he worked. Very different, and far less prevalent, was the attitude of Philippe d'Orléans, brother of Louis XIV of France. His wife, a duchess, confided to a friend, 'When His Grace slept in my bed, I had to lie so close to the edge that I sometimes fell out of bed in my sleep, for His Grace did not like to be touched; and if perchance I happened to stretch a foot in my sleep and to touch him, he would wake me up and scold me for half an hour' (Ekirch, 2005; Emich, 2003; Handley, 2013).

To promote sleep, families utilized magical amulets, spells, and prayers. A seventeenth-century English verse requested relief 'from sudden death, fire and theeves, stormes, tempests, and all affrigtments'. Germans frequently imbibed a Schlafdrincke (sleeping drink) at bedtime. The continental traveller Fynes Moryson insisted that they refused 'to suffer any man to goe to bed' sober (however effective alcoholic beverages may have been in the short term, they typically made for a restless night) (Ekirch, 2005). Alternatively, powders, ointments, and plasters were applied externally, with the temples and nostrils recommended for the quickest results. Otherwise, there was no shortage of potions and pills. Popular among the upper ranks was laudanum, a soporific made from opium and diluted alcohol (Dannenfeldt, 1986; Ekirch, 2015a).

Sleep quality in the past

Notwithstanding such measures, the quality of human sleep before the Industrial Revolution, to judge from diaries and letters, was poor. For more than a few, disturbed slumber, described as 'restless', 'troubled', or 'frighted', was chronic—one of the greatest 'miseries in the life of man', thought the Elizabethan poet Nicholas Breton. Today, it is difficult to appreciate the environmental vexations that plagued pre-industrial life, particularly the impact of adverse weather, aggravated all the more by draughty windows, ill-fitted doors, and leaky roofs. Lice, fleas, and bedbugs were common enough, as was the putrid stench of chamber pots. 'Some make the chimnie chamber pot to smel lyke filthy sinke', complained a sixteenth-century Englishman (Ekirch, 2005). Worst of all in this pre-analgesic age was sickness. Colds invariably disrupted sleep, as did symptoms associated with cluster headaches, ulcers, and gout, all of which intensified at night, along with asthma, whose victims sometimes slept upright in chairs to help open their airways. For a toothache, a Massachusetts clergyman at bedtime smeared a mixture of cow dung and hog fat on his face. 'Despicable as it seems', he wrote in his diary, 'it gave me relief' (Ekirch, 2005).

Fears, both real and imaginary, disrupted sleep. At no time following the birth of Christ until the era bounded by the late Middle Ages and the Industrial Revolution did nights appear so fraught with danger. Darkness invited the worst elements in man, nature, and the cosmos, from witches and thieves to the greatest scourge of all, the devastation wrought by fire, especially in tightly packed cities and towns teeming with wooden houses and thatched roofs (Brunt & Steger, 2008; Ekirch, 2005). According to a popular French saying, 'Night is no man's friend', and never were individuals more vulnerable than when asleep. 'Our thoughts troubled and vexed when they are retired from labour to ease', observed the writer Thomas Nashe. A diary kept by the Connecticut colonist Hannah Heaton recounts nocturnal battles with Satan, who reputedly never slept, resulting in frequent loss of rest. If anything, cries of the night watch in towns and cities, designed to calm fears as well as proclaim the hour, proved more annoying than soothing. In an early eighteenth-century Danish play, a servant moans, 'Every hour of the night they waken people out of their sleep by shouting to them that they hope they are sleeping well' (Ekirch, 2005).

Bereft of bedding, or even, on occasion, shelter, the poor suffered most. 'To lie at the star' (*coucher à l'enseigne de l'estoile*) was a French expression for the fate of numerous paupers. A Bolognese curate asked, 'Whether due to sleeping on a bed fouler than a rubbish heap, or not being able to cover oneself, who can explain how much harm is done?' It is small wonder that employers and masters complained of the lethargy of workers, among them servants and American slaves. 'Deadened slowness' was the characterization of a sixteenth-century observer in England. Large portions of the labouring population almost certainly suffered from sleep deprivation. Rather than consisting of two segments of tranquil slumber, their sleep was vulnerable to intermittent disruption—a sequence of 'brief arousals' that made daily life all the more arduous in a harsh and punishing age.

Despite the advice of both physicians and popular lore, many members of the working poor may have felt more rested when retiring to bed than when rising at dawn (Ekirch, 2001, 2005).

Nor were pre-industrial peoples immune to sleep disorders. Medical knowledge of these was naturally superficial. Of foremost concern was the nightmare, also known as the incubus or night hag, which even provoked the early interest of classical writers. The principal symptom in the midst of sleep was a pronounced feeling of pressure upon one's chest, resulting in breathlessness and an inability to speak. Although the ancient Greeks cited organic causes for these frightening sensations, the Church in the Middle Ages blamed demonic attacks (Figure 18.1), an explanation that long enjoyed widespread acceptance, notwithstanding very different diagnoses, among them overeating and epilepsy, contained in the writings of early modern physicians (Dannenfeldt, 1986; Ekirch, 2005, 2015a).

Instances of somnambulism, a disorder that figured prominently in Shakespeare's *Macbeth*, were reported as early as the twelfth century. In the thirteenth century, the *Questions de Maître Laurent* noted, 'It happens that many men get up at night while asleep, take up weapons or staffs, or get on horseback'. Dramatic occurrences of sleep violence also sparked attention, including in the 1300s several murders in southern France. More interested than physicians in such episodes were courts tasked with weighing personal culpability during a state of unconsciousness. In 1312, the canon *Si furiosus* observed, 'If a madman, a child, or a sleeper mutilates or kills a man, he incurs no penalty for this', a view echoed by the sixteenth-century Spanish scholar Diego de Covarrubias, who wrote

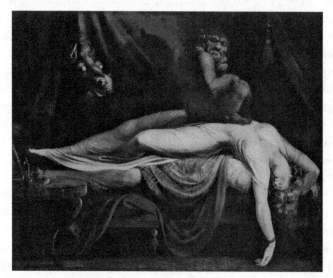

Fig. 18.1 John Henry Fuseli, *The Nightmare*.

of sleepers prone to violence, 'Such a one lacks understanding and reason and is like a madman' (Ekirch, 2015a; MacLehose, 2013).

Far more common was the malady of insomnia, sometimes referred to as 'watching' to signify either an inability or a disinclination to sleep. Instances of sleep-onset insomnia, based upon medical writings, were commonplace, whether attributable to indigestion, anxiety, or napping during the daytime. Middle-of-the night insomnia, by sharp contrast, the most common variety today in many western countries, was thought entirely normal. Rather than a reason for concern, the interval of 'watching' between first and second sleep only figured in texts as an occasion for conceiving children, ingesting medicine, or turning from one's right side to assist digestion. Fitful sleep, whether caused by sickness, bugs, or inclement weather, was not confused with wakefulness naturally arising from segmented slumber. It bears noting that not until the turn of the nineteenth century and sleep's consolidation did physicians view nocturnal awakenings as an illness requiring medication (Ekirch, 2005, 2015b).

Modern sleep

The origins of the seamless sleep to which individuals aspire today, if not always success-fully, lay in the Industrial Revolution, owing to both technological and cultural change. A greater sensitivity to time and to the heightened importance of efficiency and product-ivity transformed sleep for many into a necessary evil best confined to a single interval—'stealing a march, so to speak, on the day and on one's fellow human beings who are enjoying that second sleep', as a London writer counselled ('Imaginary Chats with an Articled Clerk', 1891). On both sides of the Atlantic, 'early rising' movements steadily grew in popularity, with parents instructed to encourage children at an early age to arise after 'their first sleep'. At the same time, the dissemination of artificial illumination within homes and businesses as well as on public streets—first gas, followed in the late 1800s by electric lighting—profoundly affected the sleep–wake cycle of men and women entering the modern age. Further, the prevalence of artificial lighting led to later bedtimes and sleep that was deeper, compressed, and more capable of being taken in a single interval. Although the transition during the 1800s was prolonged and erratic, occurring first in urban areas, by the early twentieth century, sleep that had been segmented, with a prov-enance as old as humankind, gradually became consolidated throughout much of North America and Europe—a product of modernity, not the primeval past (Ekirch, 2015b).

Summary

- Sleep is not a biological constant but a universal necessity that has varied over time and space.
- The predominant form of pre-industrial sleep in western history was segmented: two intervals at night bridged by up to an hour or so of wakefulness.
- The quality of pre-industrial sleep in western households was poor, owing chiefly to illness, environmental vexations, and anxiety for both real and imaginary reasons.

References

Brunt, L. & Steger, B. 2008. *Worlds of Sleep.* 1st ed. Berlin: Frank & Timme.

Dannenfeldt, K. H. 1986. Sleep: theory and practice in the late Renaissance. *Journal of the History of Medicine and Allied Sciences,* **41**(4), pp. 415–41.

Ekirch, A. R. 2001. Sleep we have lost: pre-industrial slumber in the British Isles. *American Historical Review,* **105**(2), pp. 343–87.

Ekirch, A. R. 2005. *At Day's Close: Night in Times Past.* 1st ed. New York: W.W. Norton.

Ekirch, A. R. 2015a. Sleep medicine in the Middle Ages and the Renaissance. In: Chokroverty, S. & Billiard, S. eds. *Sleep Medicine: a comprehensive guide to its development, clinical milestones, and advances in treatment.* 1st ed. New York: Springer Science, pp. 63–7.

Ekirch, A. R. 2015b. The modernization of western sleep: or, does insomnia have a history? *Past & Present,* **226**(1), pp. 149–92.

Ekirch, A .R. 2016. Segmented sleep in preindustrial societies. *Sleep,* **39**(3), pp. 715–16.

Emich, B. 2003. Zwischen disziplinierung und distinktion: der schlaf in der frühen neuzeit. *Werkstatt Geschichte,* **34**, pp. 53–75.

Garnier, G. 2013. *L'oubli des Peines: une histoire du sommeil (1700-1850).* 1st ed. Rennes: Presses Universitaires de Rennes.

Handley, S. 2013. Sociable sleeping in early modern England, 1660-1760. *History,* **98**(329), pp. 79–104.

'Imaginary Chats with an Articled Clerk'. 1891. *Law Notes: a Monthly Magazine for Students and Practitioners,* **X**, p. 279.

MacLehose, W. 2013. Sleepwalking, violence and desire in the Middle Ages. *Culture, Medicine, and Psychiatry,* **37**(4), p. 624.

Chapter 19

The sociology of sleep

Robert Meadows, Simon J. Williams, Jonathan
Gabe, Catherine Coveney, and Sara Arber

Introduction

Over the past decade, sociological studies have convincingly demonstrated that sleep is a
socially, culturally, and historically variable phenomenon. How we sleep, when we sleep,
where we sleep, and what meaning and value we accord sleep, let alone with whom we
sleep, vary around the world, both past and present, within and between cultures and
within different segments of society. This chapter outlines two interrelated strands of recent sociological work: how (1) sleep is a 'practice', which is 'done' and 'negotiated' with
others, and (2) the problems and prospects surrounding the medicalization of sleep. The
concluding section summarises the importance of sociological studies of sleep for public
health.

Sleep is a 'practice', which is 'done' and 'negotiated' with others

An underlying assumption of the sociology of sleep is that sleep is not simply a private, biological matter; rather, it is embedded within social interactions and everyday
life. Viewing sleep as a 'practice', which is 'done' and 'negotiated' with others, shifts the
emphasis towards rich understanding of the *patterning* of everyday, micro practices of
sleep. Through this lens, sociological studies of sleep have made visible—for example—
previously hidden components of the relationship between caregiving across the life
course and sleep. Research with heterosexual couples illustrates the lack of explicit discussion between partners about who provides care for children at night (Venn et al., 2008).
Within couples, it is almost tacitly assumed that women should get up in the night to
deal with, for example, nappy changing or settling anxious children, and this continues
even when women return to employment or full-time education. These night-time roles
are not restricted to the direct provision of care, such as attending to the physical needs
of children, but also relate to women's engagement in the emotional labour of worrying
about and anticipating the night-time needs of their family members. Bianchera & Arber
(2007) also highlight how caregiving for partners and older relatives can impact on sleep
long after their actual caregiving has stopped. Caregivers can get into the habit of 'light'
sleeping and listening out, and can become haunted by distressing images of caring.

Sleep is further patterned according to factors which include education, employment status, social class, and marital status (Figure 19.1; Arber & Meadows 2011). Within contemporary western societies, those with no qualifications report the poorest sleep quality and longest sleep latency, as well as greater problems with sleep maintenance. Unemployed people report poorer sleep than those who are employed. Among employed individuals, those in semi-routine and routine occupations report the poorest sleep. People's own definitions and normative expectations regarding 'ideal', 'adequate', or 'enough' sleep are also likely to be patterned according to sociological or socio-demographic factors such as gender, class, occupation, and education, as are their responses to disturbed sleep.

The sociology of sleep aims to elucidate how these (micro) 'practices' and 'negotiations' relate to, and are shaped by, wider 'macro-level' patterns and structures. For Hale & Hale (2009: 361), these patterns suggest that 'people who have more opportunities available to them,

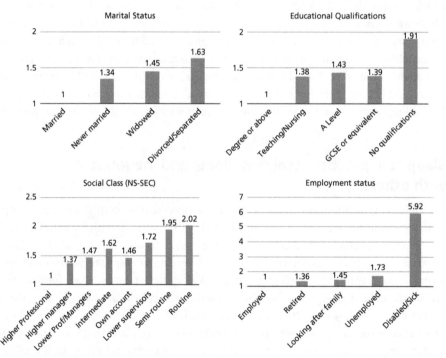

Fig. 19.1 Odds ratios of reporting poor sleep quality with socio-demographic and socio-economic variables (age and sex adjusted).

Adapted from Arber S and Meadows R. 'The Social and Health Patterning of Sleep Quality and Duration'. In: McFall SL and Garrington C (eds). (2011) *Early findings from the first wave of the UK's household longitudinal study*. Colchester: Institute for Social and Economic Research, University of Essex. ©University of Essex, 2011. https://www.understandingsociety.ac.uk/d/23/Understanding-Society-Early-Findings.pdf?1355226993, accessed 01 Apr. 2017. ©University of Essex, 2011. Data comes from the early release of Understanding Society (Wave 1). Data were collected in 2009 from a representative sample of 21717 households in Britain with a response rate of 59%. The total number of respondents in the presented analysis is circa 17000.The dependent variable is dichotomised so that those who rate their sleep as 'very good' or 'fairly good' are coded 0 and those who rate their sleep as 'fairly bad' or 'very bad' are recoded as 1. In each graph, the first category is the reference category (and therefore has odds of 1).

who have more control over their life projects—that is, people who have a distinct track record of self-governance and purpose—are those who have more optimal sleep durations and better quality sleep overall'. For Hislop & Arber (2006), sleep is embedded within four temporal dynamics: (i) biological or physical ageing, (ii) institutional structures, (iii) relational structures, and (iv) biographical transitions. In *biological or physiological ageing*, physiological changes that occur with age, which include increasing frailty, reduction in strength, impairment, increasing levels of chronic illness, and for women, the menopause, can all impact on sleep. Older people also *expect* their sleep to deteriorate with age, in part because of the widespread narratives and discourses of decline which accompany ageing. *Institutional structures*, such as engagement in paid work or education, have a complex relationship with sleep (Figure 19.1), with unemployed individuals reporting the poorest sleep and a gradient existing within occupation categories of those employed. Large-scale institutional structural changes, such as those witnessed in times of economic downturn, can strongly influence sleep through increased material and structural disadvantage and crowded households. *Relational structures* such as family contact and family support interact to influence sleep. For individuals with 'strained' family relationships, the likelihood of experiencing troubled sleep increases with more frequent family contact. Finally, *biographical transitions* are associated with life events and other transitions, such as marriage, parenthood, retirement, divorce, and widowhood, all of which may impact on sleep. As Meadows & Arber (2015) show in their analysis of 37,255 adults, while marriage appears to generally 'protect' individuals from poor sleep (Figure 19.1), the *quality* of the marriage is also important. Those who are 'married with medium/high relationship distress' report poorer sleep than both people who are 'single' and those 'cohabiting with low relationship distress'.

These four temporal dynamics intersect with *gender*. Biomedical studies of sleep tend to identify and explain differences between men and women's sleep in terms of physiology and hormones. Yet, this view misses a vital determinant: within contemporary societies there remain a set of social and cultural assumptions of what it is to be a 'man' or a 'woman' which carry with them ideas of appropriate social roles, behaviours, and attitudes. This is part of the reason why women's sleep is more likely than men's to be disturbed by caregiving and why the link between divorce, sleep, and health is stronger for women than for men (Meadows & Arber, 2015). In one of the few empirical studies to consider gendered expectations surrounding sleep and sleep disturbance, Venn (2007) found that while women were embarrassed about their snoring, men tended to discuss snoring openly and be unapologetic about it. The 'problem' of snoring was often left to the female partner, whose sleep was disrupted, to deal with rather than the snorer. Venn argues that the strategies women develop to cope with their partners' snoring are in line with normative expectations of femininity and of women being adaptive and passive. These strategies, which include prodding (but not waking) their partner, passivity, and (occasionally) re-location, can prolong their sleep disturbance rather than alleviate it.

Seen in this way, the (neuro)biological effects remain of key concern, but sleep is not simply reduced to it; rather, sociology opens up significant new opportunities for exploring the dynamic interrelations between social and biological factors regarding sleep and sleep disruption across the life course. Researching sleep in the context of people's everyday lives requires the use of both more standardized or objective measures such as polysomnography and watch actigraphy, but also interviews, focus groups, and audio sleep diaries. A *relational* or *dyadic* focus is also called for given the interdependences between couples' sleep and between the sleep of caregivers and care-recipients.

Medicalizing sleep? Problems and prospects

Medicalization, simply stated, involves the 'making medical' of some hitherto 'non-medical' matter (Conrad 2007). This in turn may occur to differing degrees, at differing levels, with the potential for de-medicalization over time too. Contrary to popular assumptions, however, medicalization is not necessarily or solely a doctor-driven process. Nor does it involve any inbuilt assumptions of over-medicalization or value judgements as to whether the medicalization of something is a 'good' or 'bad' thing.

As we know, sleep medicine is a relatively new sub-speciality within medicine, developing over the latter part of the twentieth century, particularly in the USA. It can be considered a multidisciplinary cross-speciality area involving a broad range of medical professionals that include respiratory specialists, neurologists, psychiatrists, and general practitioners, to name but a few. This reflects the wide range of 'sleep disorders' that are now clinically recognized and can be medically treated, from respiratory conditions such as obstructive sleep apnoea, to neurological disorders such as narcolepsy and restless legs syndrome, and circadian rhythm disorders such as 'jet lag syndrome' and 'shift work disorder'. However, the provision of clinical sleep services and access to sleep medicine experts remains patchy, in the UK at least, with sleep medicine sitting on the fringe of the healthcare system.

Sleep, then, can be considered a complex, if not contradictory, case of medicalization—a more or less medicalized matter, depending on which particular dimensions of sleep we are looking at. Five key issues, nevertheless, are important to address here.

The first concerns the fact that, despite the growth of sleep medicine in recent decades and the supposed 'epidemic' of sleep disorders in our midst, many sleep problems never reach the doctor's surgery. Those that do, sleep experts claim, may still go undiagnosed and untreated owing to doctors' lack of basic training in sleep medicine. It is not simply a case of a need for better public education or improved sleep 'literacy' however, important as that is. Rather, as recent sociological studies attest, it is also due to the fact that sleep is a *moral* matter, including what might be termed moral and temporal 'hierarchies of resort' as to 'if' and 'when' seeing a doctor is legitimate depending on the particular sleep problem in question. Thus, while narcolepsy, for instance, may be seen as a sleep problem requiring medical attention, sleeplessness or insomnia may not, except as a last resort when all other options have failed.

A second closely related issue concerns the role of *pharmaceuticals* in the medicalization of sleep. Pharmaceuticals are a key part of the medicalization of sleep, with approximately 10 million prescriptions for hypnotics dispensed in the community in the UK, and approximately 60 million in the USA, each year. On the one hand, we witness campaigns for wider access to sleep medications, such as sodium oxybate for those with narcolepsy. On the other hand, a series of counter-trends may also be noted in the UK today, which, if not quite amounting to the de-pharmaceuticalization of sleep(lessness), nevertheless suggest an increasing emphasis on other first-line non-pharmacological interventions such as good sleep hygiene and cognitive-behavioural therapies, resources permitting, and lifestyle changes for problems such as insomnia. Sleep medicines are highly moralized matters, particularly prescription hypnotics, which are commonly regarded as a 'last resort'—for 'deserving' if not 'desperate', yet 'responsible', patients—when all else fails (Gabe et al., 2016). Sleep, then, is a *partially medicalized* yet a *thoroughly moralized* matter, including perhaps moral *reluctance*, if not *resistance*, to any further medicalization of sleep matters in the future, however well-intentioned this may be. It is not just a case of the *pharmaceuticalization* or *depharmaceuticalization* of sleep problems today, however, but the wider reported uses of wakefulness-promoting drugs—amongst the otherwise healthy—for lifestyle or enhancement purposes. Sleep in these ways, then, is not simply being medicalized, or even pharmaceuticalized, but *customized* too perhaps in the 24/7 society, from the workplace nap to wakefulness-promoting drugs (Williams et al., 2013).

A third key issue concerns the role of the *media*. A variety of roles may spring to mind in this regard, including both negative and positive media reporting. On the one hand, the media may actively challenge or criticize certain aspects of the medicalization of sleep, as recent media coverage of research suggesting that hypnotics increase the risk of premature death demonstrates. On the other hand, the media may facilitate, if not amplify, processes of medicalization in popular culture through the framing of sleep problems in particular ways, including the potential for further inflating public anxiety through a focus on the risks of poor sleep for public health and safety. However, audiences do not simply passively absorb these messages but interact with them in complex ways to challenge, reject, or extend them within the context of their everyday lives. To the extent moreover, as Kroll-Smith (2003) shows, that the boundaries between medicine and popular culture are increasingly porous, then the potential exists, through resort to the 'rhetorical authority of medicine', for the media to contribute to turning somatic states such as 'excessive daytime sleepiness' into proto- or quasi-disorders in their own right, independently of institutional medicine—a potential made all the more likely given the multiple online opportunities to self-rate, if not self-diagnose, how 'excessively' sleepy we all are in the information age.

A fourth closely related matter concerns the role of *new digital technologies* in the medicalization of sleep, both now and in the future. It is no longer simply a matter of accessing medical information online, important as that still is, but of new digital apps and smart devices to help us monitor, measure, and manage our sleep ourselves, if not become our very own sleep experts, far beyond the scope of the doctor's surgery or the sleep clinic (Williams et al., 2015). Through the use of these technologies, people not only acquire new knowledge about their sleep, but also access information and advice on how they might improve it, which may bring many significant benefits for medicine and public health, particularly in the age of so-called 'big data'. However, there is great potential for further inflating public anxiety, if not new 'epidemics' of the 'chronorexic' kind (Van den Bulck, 2015), as we dutifully, if not obsessively, check our body data and sleep metrics, day and night. Increasing emphasis on 'gamification' in health applications– that is, the use of 'gaming' elements to motivate people in 'non-game' contexts—may also give rise to sleep becoming a competition, scored and shared with others, which in turn flags further issues surrounding both the potential benefits for public health and possibilities for inflated anxiety.

A fifth key issue concerns not simply the medicalization, but the *'healthicization'*, of sleep today. Whilst medicalization denotes the transformation of sleep into a medical problem through the language of disorder, healthicization emphasizes the importance of sleep for health, if not happiness and wellbeing. Healthicization then, once again, is more a moral than a medical matter, exemplified through good sleep hygiene and 'sleep wise' lifestyles.

As for the broader *politics of sleep* (Williams, 2011), the key point to stress perhaps is this: *downstream* measures of the medicalized kind, however beneficial, can only achieve so much when the ultimate causes or drivers of many sleep problems and inequalities today lie *upstream* in the wider workings of society (Figure 19.1). Sociology then, in keeping with public health, has much to contribute to these upstream and downstream agendas, in the interests of a better, if not a well-slept, society.

Conclusions

A sociological approach to sleep, as this chapter attests, sheds valuable new light on relations between sleep and society. A number of conclusions may be drawn here. First, sleep occurs in a social context, whether public or private, and is socially, culturally, and historically variable. Second, at the empirical level, recent sociological research has shown that sleep (and its meaning) is influenced by numerous social factors across the life course, as well as by transitions, such as marriage/cohabitation, parenthood, caregiving, and widowhood. This, moreover, includes the importance of considering how gender impacts on sleep, and the nature of power in negotiations about sleep. Third, medicating sleep is a highly moralized issue within contemporary societies, with people on the one hand, reluctant to 'give in' to sleeping medication, feeling that they *should* be able to manage problems such as sleeplessness or insomnia themselves without recourse to doctors and prescription sleeping pills, and on the other, those with diagnosed sleep disorders campaigning for wider access to medications they believe will be beneficial to them. Sleep, therefore, can be considered a complex, if not contradictory, case of medicalization; a more or less medicalized matter, depending on which particular dimensions of sleep we are considering.

These conclusions have three important implications for current and future research, policy, and practice in epidemiology and public health. First, in focusing attention on the micro/hidden aspects of everyday life, sociological research into sleep has highlighted arenas of action. For example, developing a richer understanding of the complexities of the caregiving/sleep nexus is clearly a public health priority, given that, in 2011, there were 5.78 million unpaid carers in England and Wales alone. Second, sociological studies of sleep have played a key role in highlighting how those with fewer resources and opportunities are those with poorer sleep. One response to this would be to suggest that sleep is patterned in this way because of the free choices of individual actors; however, it is difficult to justify this 'voluntary' explanation (Hale & Hale, 2009). The decisions which characterize sleep are significantly different from those regarding other health behaviours. For example, one cannot voluntarily choose one's sleep duration: 'one is either sleeping and thus not experiencing, or one is experiencing and thus not sleeping' (Hale & Hale 2009: 362). An individual's sleep behaviours are always tied to aspects of their life circumstances, such as jobs, demands of the workplace, neighbourhood environments, education, and child-rearing. To improve sleep, and in turn, health, public health should facilitate improvement in these wider spheres as a matter of *social justice*. A fairer society, in other words, might be a better-slept, if not healthier, society too. Sleep, moreover, is another vital part of the general wellbeing (GWB) as well as the gross domestic product (GDP) political agendas today, recognized or not. Third, sociology continues to highlight the complex, wider arena on which public health must reflect. Sleep, as we have shown, is more than simply a medical matter, with the boundaries between medicine, morality, and popular culture being complex and multifaceted. Public health does not exist outside of these porous boundaries.

Summary

+ Sleep occurs in a *social context* and is socially, culturally, and historically variable. Relations between the sociological and (neuro)biological dimensions of sleep are complex and variable.

+ Sleep is influenced by numerous social factors across the *life course*, as well as by *transitions*, such as marriage/cohabitation, parenthood, caregiving, and widowhood. These include the importance of how *gender* impacts on sleep, and the nature of *power in negotiations* about sleep.

+ Sleep is a complex, if not contradictory, case of medicalization—a more or less medicalized matter, depending on which particular dimensions of sleep are being considered. Sleep is also a thoroughly moralized matter which may or may not result in a visit to the doctor and the taking of sleep medicines, depending on the sleep problem in question.

+ Understanding sleep requires the use of *qualitative* as well as *quantitative* methodologies, including interviews, focus groups, and audio sleep diaries as well as other more standardized or objective measures such as watch actigraphy. A *relational* or *dyadic* focus on *couples' sleep* is also called for given that sleeping together is the norm in adult life.

+ Sociology highlights arenas for public health intervention. These include recognizing that sleep may be different from other health-related behaviours and may be better improved by targeting resources and opportunities available to individuals rather than simply targeting sleep itself.

References

Arber, S. & Meadows, R. 2011. Social and health patterning of sleep quality and duration. In: McFall, S. L. & Garrington, C. eds. *Early Findings from the First Wave of the UK's Household Longitudinal Study.* [Online]. Colchester: Institute for Social and Economic Research, University of Essex. Available from: https://www.understandingsociety.ac.uk/research/publications/findings/early

Bianchera, E. & Arber, S. 2007. Caring and sleep disruption among women in Italy. *Sociological Research Online,* **12**(5), p. 4. doi:10.5153/sro.1608

Conrad, P. 2007. *The Medicalization of Society. On the Transformation of Human Conditions into Treatable Diseases.* Johns Hopkins University Press.

Gabe, J., Coveney, C. M. & Williams, S. J. 2016. Prescriptions and proscriptions: moralising sleeping pills, *Sociology of Health and Illness,* **38**(4), pp. 627–44.

Hale, B. & Hale, L. 2009. Is justice good for your sleep? (And therefore, good for your health?). *Social Theory & Health,* **7**(4), pp. 354–70.

Hislop, J. & Arber, S. 2006. Sleep, gender, and ageing: temporal perspectives. In: Calasanti, T. M. & Slevin, K. F. eds. *Age Matters: realigning feminist thinking.* Routledge: London, pp. 225–46.

Kroll-Smith, S. 2003. Popular media and 'excessive daytime sleepiness': a study of rhetorical authority in medical sociology. *Sociology of health & illness,* **25**(6), 625–43.

Meadows, R., & Arber, S. 2015. Marital status, relationship distress, and self-rated health: what role for 'sleep problems'? *Journal of Health and Social Behavior,* **56**(3), pp. 341–55.

Van den Bulck, J. 2015. Sleep apps and the quantified self: blessing or curse? *Journal of Sleep Research,* **24**(2), pp. 121–3.

Venn, S. 2007. 'It's okay for a man to snore': the influence of gender on sleep disruption in couples. *Sociological Research Online,* **12**(5), p. 1. doi:10.5153/sro.1607

Venn, S., Arber, S., Meadows, R. & Hislop, J. 2008. The fourth shift: exploring the gendered nature of sleep disruption among couples with children. *The British Journal of Sociology,* **59**(1), pp. 79–97.

Williams, S. J. 2011. *The Politics of Sleep: governing (un) consciousness in the late modern age.* New York, NY: Palgrave Macmillan.

Williams, S. J., Coveney, C. M. & Gabe, J. 2013. Medicalisation or customisation? Sleep, enterprise and enhancement in the 24/7 society. *Social Science & Medicine,* **79**, pp. 40–47.

Williams, S. J., Coveney, C. & Meadows, R. 2015. 'M-apping'sleep? Trends and transformations in the digital age. *Sociology of Health & Illness,* **37**(7), pp. 1039–54.

Chapter 20

Sleep and shift work

John Axelsson, Mikael Sallinen, Tina Sundelin, and Göran Kecklund

Introduction

Increasing demands for available emergency and health services, constant energy supply, and the flexibility to do things such as travel and eat out at all hours of the day have resulted in the development of a so-called 24/7 society. Those whose work schedules differ from the conventional 9-to-5 are called 'shift workers', typically working during nights or weekends, or on rotating 8- or 12-hour shifts across the 24-hour cycle. About 25%–30% of the workforce in the USA and Europe have atypical schedules, and in Europe about 19% of the working population work nights at least once per month.

Shift work is particularly common in transportation and in emergency/health services, which include many safety-focused professions such as healthcare workers, police officers, fire fighters, pilots, and power plant operators. Many of these workers are more or less 'forced' to work shifts, as there are few opportunities for day jobs in these professions. Reports show that up to 80% of shift workers would prefer to work days.

Sleep patterns and disturbances in shift work

The amount of sleep a shift worker obtains is determined by a number of factors, including timing of shifts and the person's ability, need, opportunity, and motivation to sleep. Figure 20.1 illustrates how the timing of shifts affects sleep (Sallinen et al., 2003). The scheduling can also often require the worker to sleep during sub-optimal hours in relation to their circadian rhythm.

Sleep is most compromised by early-morning and night shifts, as they overlap with the normal human sleep period. Early-morning shifts, starting at 06:00 or earlier, generally curtail sleep by about 2 hours. Sleep prior to morning shifts is thus often inadequate and characterized by difficulties in waking up. To compensate for insufficient sleep, many shift workers take a nap in the afternoon after the early-morning shift.

Prior to the first night shift, about 50% take an afternoon or evening nap. Consequently, the other 50% stay awake for about 24 hours before the end of their first night shift. Daytime sleep between successive night shifts is usually reduced to about 4–5 hours. This is inadequate for most individuals, in particular since many workers are already sleep-deprived after the first shift. To compensate, about a third of the workers nap between successive night shifts.

Despite reducing sleep duration, rest periods shorter than 12 hours between two shifts are common in many shift combinations (Sallinen et al., 2003). The widespread evening–morning shift combination, with 8–10 hours off between shifts, curtails sleep drastically (Vedaa et al., 2016). The timing of the rest period may further affect sleep duration. For example, to get at least 6 hours of sleep during a 12-hour break, the break should ideally start between 20:00 and 00:00.

Consecutive shifts often cause an accumulation of sleep loss, with five consecutive night shifts resulting in up to 10 hours of lost sleep. Workers with consecutive early morning shifts show similar patterns. The degree of sleep loss is also dependent on the individual's capacity and potential to alter their circadian rhythm. For example, delaying the rhythm is beneficial while working night shifts. Exceptional circumstances, such as oil-rig work, may facilitate daytime sleep since there are few social demands and morning light exposure can be avoided.

The direction and speed of shift rotation are also important shift characteristics. It has been proposed that the best option is a shift system that rotates fast forward, i.e. in the direction morning-, evening- and night-shift with only one to three consecutive nights (Härmä, 2006). A common adjustment is to replace 8-hour shifts with 12-hour shifts. This does not dramatically affect sleep, most likely because it makes the shift schedule more regular and prevents the occurrence of rest periods shorter than 11 hours, thus enabling the worker to recover better between shifts (Figure 20.1).

Permanent night workers sleep somewhat more than their rotating counterparts in association with night shifts, but no such difference can be observed when considering the whole shift cycle (Folkard, 2008). However, permanent night workers are a select group of people, making it difficult to compare their results with those of other groups.

Napping strategies are important for maximizing sleep. It is beneficial to gain as much sleep as possible prior to early-morning and night shifts, to sleep for 1–2 hours close to the beginning of the night shift, and to recover sufficiently between shift periods (Härmä,

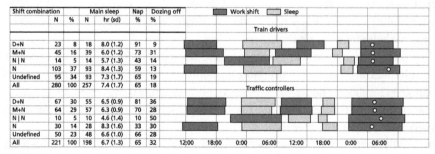

Fig. 20.1 The average sleep–wake rhythm of train drivers and railway traffic controllers in various shift combinations. D = Day shift, N = night shift, M = morning shift. White dots inside the night shifts stand for the mean timing of dozing-off at work.

Reproduced with permission from Sallinen M, Härmä M, Mutanen P, et al. Sleep-wake rhythm in an irregular shift system. *Journal of Sleep Research*, 2003; 12: 103–12. Copyright © 2003 Journal of Sleep Research

2006). The number of days needed to completely recover depends on a variety of individual and shift-system-related components.

Large individual differences exist in shift-work tolerance. While some shift workers have severe sleep–wake disturbances, others may work for decades without notable problems. Factors explaining these differences include sleep need, tolerance to sleep loss, the ability to sleep at irregular times, and diurnal type. Shift-related sleep disturbances usually ease or disappear after ceasing shift work.

Sleepiness

Fatigue and sleepiness have been widely studied in shift-work research since reduced alertness and impaired performance are two major consequences of insufficient sleep. Sleepiness is usually lowest during evening shifts, moderately increased during morning shifts, and highest during night shifts.

Sleepiness during operational shift work can be assessed through physiological measures, such as eye movements and electroencephalogram (EEG)-density. A pioneering study on train drivers showed a clear increase in physiological sleepiness during the night shift, despite incidents of falling asleep being rare. Studies on truck drivers have had similar results. Sleepiness can also become so severe that workers fall asleep during night shifts. A study measuring EEG signals on control-room operators found that 20% of the shift workers dozed off during night work.

Intervention studies show decreased levels of sleepiness when the shift schedule changes from a slow backward-rotating system to a rapid forward-rotating system (Härmä, 2006). Permanent night workers may be less sleepy than rotating shift workers because the permanent system facilitates circadian adaptation to night work. While it has been estimated that less than 5% of permanent night workers actually show a complete circadian adaptation to night work, the best compromise is likely for night workers to adapt their rhythms partially.

Other shift characteristics that increase on-shift sleepiness are quick returns (e.g. Sallinen et al., 2003). Working long shifts is also related to sleepiness. One intervention study reduced the weekly working hours of medical interns from 80 hours to 65, and the maximum shift length from 30 hours to 16, resulting in a drastic reduction in physiological sleepiness and attentional lapses (Lockley et al., 2004). Laboratory studies on cumulative sleep restriction suggest that sleepiness should accumulate over shifts. However, surprisingly few field studies show this pattern. More common is a peak of sleepiness on the first night shift followed by a gradual decline across consecutive nights.

Operational performance and safety

Few studies have looked at real work performance during shift work. Some indicate that train drivers' physiological sleepiness during night shifts coincides with observed errors. Also, one study on gas-plant operators found a clear peak in reading errors during night shifts. In another, reducing weekly working hours for interns in intensive care units decreased serious medical errors by 30%. However, several other studies showed no significant increase in errors during night shifts. The lack of robust effects on real work performance during night shifts could be due to lower work demands and fewer possibilities for making mistakes. However, it is difficult to obtain good measures of real work performance in many occupations, and studies have instead used performance tests as a proxy. The most widely used tests measure sustained attention through simple reaction time. The results are somewhat inconsistent, but in general, extended reaction times are more prevalent at the end of a night shift. One study indicates that shift work leads to a general impairment of cognition, and that it takes at least 5 years after ceasing shift work before the effects are reversed.

Night work increases the risk for accidents and injuries, probably owing to severe sleepiness. It has been estimated that the risk for an accident is 30% higher during night shifts and 18% higher during evening shifts than throughout morning shifts. The increased risk during evening shifts is somewhat surprising, considering the lower levels of sleepiness associated with these shifts. However, there is epidemiological support for a 50% increase in the risk of injuries during the evening shift. It is likely that the elevated safety risk during evening shifts is related to factors other than sleepiness—for example, work tasks, staffing levels, or duration of the shift. A review of major industrial disasters, including the Chernobyl and Three Mile Island nuclear accidents and the *Exxon Valdez* oil spill, proposed difficult shift systems as a contributing factor.

It is hard to tease out the independent contribution of particular shift characteristics for accident risk, but shift length, type of shift system, and consecutive night shifts may all play a part. Many studies show that both long shifts and long working weeks increase the risk for accidents. Accident risk may also increase across successive shifts, particularly during the night. One study estimated that the accident risk is 36% higher on the fourth night shift than on the first. Other studies have failed to find a distinct pattern relating shift systems to accidents, and it is unclear whether permanent night work has a higher accident risk than rotating shift systems.

There is an increased risk of motor vehicle accidents when driving home after a night shift. Several studies have revealed physiological and subjective sleepiness, as well as poor driving, in workers after a night shift. In addition, people with shift work, multiple jobs, and other unusual work schedules have an increased risk of being involved in road traffic accidents in general.

Health consequences of shift work

Shift work is associated with a wide range of health problems (Kecklund & Axelsson, 2016). The most prominent ones are disturbed sleep, cardiovascular and gastrointestinal diseases, and metabolic disturbances such as obesity and metabolic syndrome. There may also be a link between shift work and cancer. Other possible health-related consequences are diabetes, childbirth problems, and overall mortality (Table 20.1).

Table 20.1 Shift work and health risks compared to day work

	Risk ratio	Evidence grading
Transient insomnia and short sleep	1–2	+++
fatigue and accidents	1–2	+++
cardiovascular disease & stroke	1.2	++
metabolic syndrome	1.6–1.7	++
obesity	1–2	++
gastrointestinal disease	2–4	+
General poor health	2–3.2	++
prostate cancer	1.0–1.2	+
breast cancer	1.0–1.2	+
type 2 diabetes	1.1–1.4	+
rheumatoid arthritis	1.3	+
Long-term sleep disorders	2.8	+
preterm birth	1–2	+
low birth weight	1.0–1.6	+
mortality	1.0–1.3	+

compared to day work, +++ = strong evidence, ++ = moderate evidence, + = limited evidence, (+) = insufficient evidence.

A relative risk of 1 is the same as the general population, while a relative risk of 2 indicate that the risk is twice as high.

Reproduced courtesy of the author.

Shift work, particularly morning and night shifts, leads to acute sleep disturbances. In addition, shift workers may have an increased risk for developing chronic sleep disturbances. Shift work disorder (SWD) is a sleep disorder caused by the conflict between a person's working schedule and their endogenous sleep–wake cycle (American Academy of Sleep Medicine, 2014). The main symptom is excessive sleepiness during work or the commute to/from work, or insomnia during daytime sleep. The prevalence of SWD in shift workers has been estimated at around 32%, with 9% having more severe levels. While the majority of shift workers have severely shortened day sleep, it is likely that many workers see this as a natural part of their working life, leading to under-reporting of sleep/wake complaints.

Many studies have investigated how shift work affects cardiovascular disease (CVD). While several negative findings have been reported, some show an increase of 30%–40%, for both men and women. The risk may increase with longer exposure to shift work, but the extent of this effect is unclear. Shift workers are, however, more likely to have a CVD profile—that is, higher rates of ventricular premature beats, greater diastolic blood pressure, and subclinical atherosclerosis. Shift work may also be particularly harmful for workers with high systolic blood pressure.

The epidemiological evidence of a link between shift work and CVD is restricted owing to several study limitations. There is also an ongoing debate about whether lifestyle-related risk behaviours are confounders (factors not related to shift work) or mediators (factors caused by shift work). For example, while shift workers are more likely to start smoking, smoking is also more common in shift workers prior to their commencing shift work.

The altered sleep and eating patterns in shift workers lead to a circadian disruption of many hormones. Few shift workers adapt their circadian rhythms fully to night work, and many have poor blood lipid profiles. While night workers often adapt their circadian rhythms gradually across successive night shifts, there are large individual differences in their ability to re-adapt to diurnal living. Studies indicate that endocrine and metabolic diseases are twice as common in shift workers as in day workers, and that shift workers often have worse markers of insulin resistance. Experimental studies show that altered sleep patterns, similar to those in shift workers, impair glucose tolerance. There may also be a slightly increased prevalence of diabetes among shift workers. The fact that shift workers with developing problems may quit this kind of work is a possible explanation for the lack of more severe outcomes. This so-called 'healthy worker effect' is supported by the knowledge that shift workers with diabetes or at risk for diabetes are more likely to leave their shift work within 2–4 years. Whether shift work is related to weight gain, increased BMI, and a poorer waist-to-hip ratio is still being debated. To what degree shift work is related to developing a worse metabolic profile has rendered a lot of recent attention. The strongest evidence concern that shift workers have an increased risk for increased body weight/BMI, risk for becoming overweight and an impaired glucose tolerance.

Gastrointestinal disorders are more common in shift workers than in day workers. Peptic ulcer is a well-known problem among many shift workers. Other common complaints are constipation and diarrhoea related to night shifts, indicating that the main problems are night work and possibly night eating.

A large number of studies have attempted to answer the question of whether shift work is a risk factor for cancer. Four recent meta-analyses indicate that the cancer risk increases about 5%–9% for every 5 years of shift work, or about 12%–20% after 20–30 years of shift work. However, one of these studies also concluded that the exposure data is poor, the effects are small, and bias may be behind the many studies showing borderline effects (Ijaz et al., 2013). The studies have very mixed results and mostly focus on breast and prostate cancer. The debate of whether there is an increased risk will only be resolved once studies have better data on shift work exposure and shift schedule characteristics, two factors relevant for all epidemiological studies concerning shift work.

The few studies investigating whether shift workers are more frequently on sick leave have conflicting results. Since naturally occurring short sleep increases susceptibility to the common cold, shift workers may be more vulnerable if exposed to contagious viruses. Shift work may also increase the risk for developing rheumatoid arthritis and multiple sclerosis. However, we still know very little about how shift work affects immune functioning, or whether such effects are related to an increased risk for developing chronic inflammatory and autoimmune diseases.

Several early studies suggested that shift work is linked to low birth weight, preterm birth, spontaneous abortion, miscarriage, and irregular menstruation. More recent work shows a risk ratio of 1:3 for preterm delivery and a non-significant risk increase for low birth weight. It is thus still prudent to advise against long working hours and shift work, particularly late in pregnancy.

In a classical study on shift work and mortality, no significant effect was found. But a reanalysis of the same data showed that ex-shift workers have a 20% increased mortality risk. However, this pattern is not very robust. Several studies show a similar trend, while others report no increase in mortality. Still, the fact that shift work is related to diseases with severe outcomes indicates that it would also be related to overall mortality.

Mechanisms: why the problems occur

The main reason for reduced alertness during the night and short day sleep in shift workers is the misalignment between the circadian system, working hours, and sleep (Kecklund & Axelsson, 2016). Long waking periods, often more than 20 hours, particularly affect alertness and performance during the first night shift. Owing to interference of the circadian system, day sleep after night work is about 2–3 hours shorter than normal night sleep, resulting in more sleepiness during the following waking period.

The mechanisms by which shift work may cause health problems have been less explored, but likely include circadian disruption, insufficient sleep, behavioural disturbances, and work/non-work conflicts. A central problem with circadian misalignment, insufficient sleep, and irregular eating habits—all common among shift workers—is that they lead to metabolic disturbances. Eating during the wrong circadian phase seems related to worse lipid profiles and impaired glucose tolerance. Male shift workers under the age of 40 years already have accelerated processes of atherosclerosis, suggesting that shift work appears to contribute to negative health consequences. The proposed increased risk for cancer may be related to reduced levels of melatonin and/or increased light exposure at night. Other mechanisms that may be involved are those resulting from shifting sleep to the daytime, with a desynchronization (i.e. mis-match) of sleep-regulated hormones (e.g. growth hormone, prolactin, testosterone), hormones largely regulated by the circadian system (e.g. cortisol, melatonin), and hormones regulated by both sleep and the circadian system (e.g. thyrotropin). For example, it has been shown that intolerant shift workers have lower testosterone levels than their tolerant colleagues. There is a clear need for further studies on the individual differences in vulnerability to shift work.

Interventions and countermeasures against sleepiness and disturbed sleep

Several strategies, such as napping, caffeine, medication, and bright-light exposure, have been proposed as effective countermeasures against sleepiness and performance decrements, either directly via alertness-enhancing effects or indirectly via adaptation to night work or improved sleep.

Organizational interventions can include a variety of improvements to the work situation/environment, such as better shift schedules, sleep facilities, napping opportunities, less noise, and programmes for improving lifestyle factors such as smoking, exercising, and alcohol habits. Tolerance may be influenced by several different aspects of the shift system, such as the order and speed of rotation, shift length, number of consecutive night shifts, timing of shifts, and length of time off between shifts. Unfortunately, rather few studies have looked closer at these shift characteristics. In a systematic review of the performance and physiological aspects of shift-work systems, it was concluded that the rotation of the shift system should be forward-rotating rather than backwards-rotating in order to avoid recovery periods of less than 11 hours between shifts, but there was a lack of evidence for effects of most other aspects of shift work (Driscoll, 2007).

Among the individual-level countermeasures, melatonin, hypnotics, napping, bright light, and avoidance of daylight can be used to treat circadian sleep rhythm disorders, including SWD (Bjorvatn & Pallesen, 2009), but also to improve adaptation to longer periods with night shifts. One approach is the use of bright light to partially adapt to night work, causing the circadian 'low' to occur after, rather than during, the night shift and commute home. While bright light and melatonin are well tolerated in the short term, there is a lack of information regarding more long-term effects and possible drug interactions (Bjorvatn & Pallesen, 2009).

The most common countermeasure to fight sleepiness is to sleep, either before or during the night shift. Napping is a cheap, natural, and efficient way to improve sleepiness and performance during shift work. Napping seems to be particularly valuable in extended work shifts and in shift combinations where a night shift is preceded by a morning shift on the same day. However, napping is not always feasible in operational settings, and one drawback is sleep inertia, which may last for a considerable time upon awakening. One way to limit sleep inertia is by taking short naps (20–30 minutes) either before or during the first half of the night shift. Laboratory findings have also shown that caffeine can reduce inertia resulting from later naps.

The most common pharmacological countermeasure in shift workers is caffeine, which has strong alerting properties that may last for many hours. Although most studies on caffeine have been carried out in the lab, a few confirm its positive effects in operational settings. Note that one should avoid caffeine later during the night shift as this can disturb the subsequent sleep period.

Other pharmacological stimulants include amphetamines, modafinil, and armodafinil. While amphetamines can enhance alertness and performance, they have also been related to disturbed sleep, hypersomnia, adverse cardiovascular effects, and the development of drug tolerance, and are hence not optimal for regular use in shift workers. Modafinil and armodafinil have been tested in SWD and can improve alertness and performance during night shifts and on the commute home, without compromising sleep. These were field studies, including follow-up periods of 3 months without any obvious health consequences, possibly with the exclusion of headaches.

Hypnotics have also been used to improve sleep in shift workers, based on the idea that improved sleep will result in less sleepiness. However, the effects are somewhat inconsistent and their usage is limited as they may cause unwanted rebound insomnia and adverse withdrawal effects.

In real-life situations, workers can combine several countermeasures to improve their on-shift alertness. For example, a 1- to 2-hour nap before the night shift combined with caffeine at the beginning of the shift has been shown to improve sleepiness and performance at the end of the shift.

Summary

- Those with different work schedules than the conventional 9-to-5 one are called 'shift workers', typically working during nights or weekends, or on rotating 8- or 12-hour shifts across the 24-hour cycle.

- The amount of sleep a shift worker obtains is determined by a number of factors, including timing of shifts and the person's ability, need, opportunity, and motivation to sleep.

- Sleep is most compromised by early morning and night shifts. Naps in the afternoon are taken to compensate both for insufficient sleep after an early morning shift and in preparation of night shifts.

- Reduced alertness and impaired performance, due to fatigue and sleepiness, are two major consequences of insufficient sleep, highest in night shift-workers.

- Night work increases the risk for accidents and injuries, for road traffic accidents when driving home after a night shift, and for errors at work.

- Shift work can increase the risk to develop a wide range, including cardio-metabolic disturbances.

- Effective strategies to counteract sleepiness and performance decrements include napping, caffeine, medication, and bright-light exposure.

- Organizational interventions can include a variety of improvements to the work situation/environment, such as more sleep friendly shift schedules, screening and treatment of sleep disorders, sleep facilities, napping opportunities, less noise, and programmes for improving lifestyle factors such as smoking, exercising, and alcohol habits.

- Tolerance may be influenced by several different aspects of the shift system, such as the order and speed of rotation, shift length, number of consecutive night shifts, timing of shifts, and length of time off between shifts.

References

American Academy of Sleep Medicine. 2014. *International Classification of Sleep Disorders*. 3rd ed. (ICSD-3). Westchester, IL: American Academy of Sleep Medicine.

Bjorvatn, B. & Pallesen, S. 2009. A practical approach to circadian rhythm sleep disorders. *Sleep Medicine Reviews*, **13**, pp. 47–60.

Driscoll, T., Grunstein, R. R. & Rogers, N. L. 2007. A systematic review of the neurobehavioural and physiological effects of shiftwork systems. *Sleep Medicine Reviews*, **11**, pp. 179–94.

Folkard S. 2008. Do permanent night workers show circadian adjustment? A review based on the endogenous melatonin rhythm. *Chronobiology International*, **25**, pp. 215–24.

Kecklund G & Axelsson J. 2016. Health consequences of shift work and insufficient sleep. *BMJ*, **355**, i5210. doi: 10.1136/bmj.i5210

Härmä, M., Tarja, H., Irja, K., Mikael, S., Jussi, V., Anne, B. & Pertti, M. 2006. A controlled intervention study of the effects of a very rapidly forward rotating shift system on sleep-wakefulness and well-being among young and elderly shift workers. *International Journal of Psychophysiology*, **59**, pp. 70–79.

Ijaz, S., Verbeek, J., Seidler, A., Lindbohm, M.L., Ojajärvi, A., Orsini, N., Costa, G. & Neuvonen, K. 2013. Night-shift work and breast cancer—a systematic review and meta-analysis. *Scandinavian Journal of Work, Environment & Health*, **39**, pp. 431–47.

Lockley, S. W., Cronin, J. W., Evans, E. E., Cade, B.E., Lee, C. J., Landrigan, C. P., Rothschild, J. M., Katz, J. T., Lilly, C. M., Stone, P. H., Aeschbach, D., Czeisler, C. A.; Harvard Work Hours, Health and Safety Group. 2004. Effect of reducing interns' weekly work hours on sleep and attentional failures. *New England Journal of Medicine*, **351**, pp. 1829–37.

Sallinen, M., Härmä, M., Mutanen, P., Ranta, R., Virkkala, J. & Müller, K. 2003. Sleep-wake rhythm in an irregular shift system. *Journal of Sleep Research*, **12**, pp. 103–12.

Vedaa, O., Harris, A., Bjorvatn, B., Waage, S., Sivertsen, B., Tucker, P. & Pallesen, S. 2016. Systematic review of the relationship between quick returns in rotating shift work and health-related outcomes. *Ergonomics*, **59**, pp. 1–14.

Chapter 21

Drowsy driving

Pierre Philip, Stephanie Bioulac, Patricia Sagaspe, and Jean-Arthur Micoulaud-Franchi

Introduction

Traffic accidents are an increasing cause of death and injury in the world, initially in western societies but now more and more in developing countries. Major countries have launched road safety campaigns in recent decades to decrease mortality and morbidity on their roads. Alcohol and excessive speed have been highlighted in past years as major killers, and the health status of drivers has started receiving attention as a cause of accidents. Sleepiness at the wheel is clearly associated with an increased risk of accidents (Connor et al., 2002), but the respective causes (behaviours versus sleep disorders) deserve further explorations (Philip et al., 2010). Extended or nocturnal driving is associated with accidents, but few reports have differentiated fatigue, which is usually seen as a consequence of driving time, from sleepiness due to reduced sleep, extended time awake, and/or being awake at the circadian trough (Connor et al., 2002; Lee et al., 2016). Many studies have looked at the respective role of sleep disorders in the occurrence of traffic accidents. Sleep apnoea syndrome is associated with traffic accidents (Ellen et al., 2006), but other diseases such as insomnia and narcolepsy are also responsible for traffic accidents (Philip et al., 2010).

Although both the European Union and the United States have launched public campaigns to make their citizens aware of the risk of drowsy driving (e.g. the US National Sleep Foundation 'Drive Alert–Arrive Alive' campaign, and the 'wake up bus' in Europe), a major problem remains in identifying patients or behaviours at risk for traffic accidents and the best way to reduce this risk by appropriate countermeasures. In this review we present an update on the relationship between extrinsic and intrinsic sleep disorders, drug intake and traffic accidents, the present state of knowledge, and which major studies are needed to improve patient safety.

Prevalence and associated risks

Rest/activity patterns

Behavioural changes affecting the sleep–wake pattern help to explain sleep-related accidents. Driving is frequently associated with extensive wakefulness, which induces sleepiness at the wheel. By studying large populations of drivers, we demonstrated that long-distance driving is very frequently associated with sleep curtailment. Extensive wakefulness is also associated with nocturnal driving, which alters driving performances and induces inappropriate highway line crossings. These inappropriate line crossings are strong predictors of accident risk (Philip et al., 2013).

Sleep deprivation affects not only the general population of automobile drivers, but also many professional drivers worldwide. A study on professional truck drivers (Mitler et al., 1997) demonstrated a mean duration of sleep of 4.78 hours per day over a 5-day period. Fifty-six per cent of drivers presented at least 6 non-continuous minutes of electroencephalographic (EEG)-recorded sleep while driving. The vast majority of these micro-sleep episodes occurred during the late night and early morning. Interestingly, the episodes of sleep at the wheel were not always associated with accidents, showing that actual sleep at the wheel in trained professionals does not mean accidents in 100% of cases. A possible explanation could be that automatic behaviours allow drivers to remain on the road when they sleep lightly for very brief periods (Mitler et al., 1997). Nevertheless, sleep restriction is a dangerous behaviour and involves a significant driving risk for most drivers.

Shift work is also dangerous for driving. One recent real driving study (Lee et al., 2016) showed that participants tested after daytime work and after a night shift had a significantly higher rate of lane excursions, blink duration, and slow eye movements during post-nightshift drives than during post-sleep drives. This performance decrement may be due to the circadian phase, but also to the cumulative effect of work load and sleep pressure. Time on task is also an additive risk, and we showed that extensive nocturnal driving dramatically worsens driving performance. Eight hours of nocturnal driving increased 6-fold the number of inappropriate highway line crossings compared with a 2-hour nocturnal driving session (at 3–5 a.m.) (Figure 21.1). These results suggest that fatigue related to driving duration is amplified at night, so maximal driving duration should be shorter at night than during the day.

Sleep duration, work duration, time on task, and shift work schedules are key factors in behavioural sleepiness at the wheel.

Sleep disorders

Many drivers are also sleep disorder patients, and a significant number of traffic accidents can be attributed to medical conditions. Of all sleep disorders, obstructive sleep apnoea syndrome is possibly the most studied pathological process with regard to traffic accidents. Indeed, several studies in the past 20 years have shown a clear relationship between sleep disorders and traffic accidents.

In a meta-analysis (Ellen et al., 2006) on sleep apnoea and driving risk, 23 of 27 studies and 18 of 19 studies with control groups found a statistically significant increased risk, with many of the studies finding a 2- or 3-fold increased risk. Clearly apnoeic subjects have a higher accident risk than controls, but the severity of the disease (as measured by the apnoea–hypopnoea index (AHI)) does not explain the driving risk. Indeed, the best predictive symptom for risk of sleep-related accidents is still a matter of debate. AHI

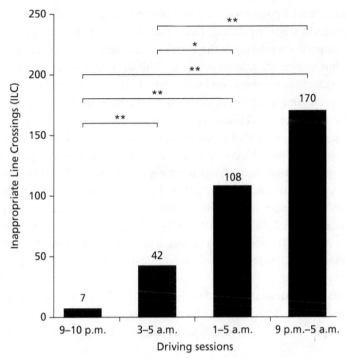

Fig. 21.1 Cumulative number of inappropriate line crossings (ILC) in subjects in the last hour of the three nocturnal driving sessions (short, intermediate, and long duration of driving), as well as ILC for reference drive (9–10 p.m. of long drive).

Reproduced with permission from Sagaspe P, Taillard J, Åkerstedt T, Bayon V, Espié S, Chaumet G, et al. Extended Driving Impairs Nocturnal Driving Performances. *PLoS ONE*, Volume 3, Issue 10, e3493. Copyright © 2008 Sagaspe et al.

is a non-linear predictor of accident risk, but one could question whether sleepiness is not an even better risk predictor because this symptom refers to behavioural (i.e. sleep deprivation) and organic factors (i.e. sleep fragmentation). Surprisingly, excessive day-time sleepiness per se, as measured by the Epworth Sleepiness scale (ESS), has not been associated with accident risk in apnoeic patients (Ellen et al., 2006). This finding could be explained by the fact that the majority of questions in the ESS refer to the ability to fall asleep in monotonous conditions, while the driving risk pertains more to the difficulty in remaining awake (Lloberes et al., 2000).

Sleep apnoea is not the only disease responsible for excessive daytime sleepiness. Narcolepsy is a major disorder responsible for excessive daytime sleepiness and it has also been studied as a risk factor for traffic accidents. Narcoleptic patients present a higher risk of sleep-related accidents than do apnoeic subjects (Philip et al., 2010). This could be explained by the fact that untreated narcoleptic or idiopathic hypersomnia patients have worse MWT (maintenance of wakefulness test) sleep latencies than OSAS (obstructive sleep apnoea syndrome) patients (Philip et al., 2013).

Apart from central hypersomnia, mental disorders can be associated with daytime sleepiness. A recent study on ADHD (attention deficit hyperactivity disorder) patients showed that a significant number of these patients also presented an altered level of alertness in addition to their attentional problems. This drug-free-patient study, which used driving simulator measurements combined with electrophysiological measures, showed that subjects presenting sleep latencies under 19 minutes displayed significantly worse driving performances than did the other patients and controls.

These findings were confirmed by an epidemiological study (Philip et al., 2015) performed on French highway drivers. In total, 36,140 drivers answered a questionnaire exploring driving risks, sleep complaints, sleepiness at the wheel, ADHD symptoms (Adult ADHD Self-Report Scale), and distraction at the wheel. Drivers with ADHD symptoms reported significantly more sleep-related (adjusted OR = 1.4, CI 1.21–1.60), $p < 0.0001$) and inattention-related (adjusted OR 0.9, CI 1.71–2.14; $p < 0.0001$) near misses than those with no ADHD symptoms. The fraction of near misses attributable to severe sleepiness at the wheel was 4.24% for drivers with no ADHD symptoms versus 10.35% for those with ADHD symptoms.

These results clearly show the links between attention, distraction, and sleepiness at the wheel, so it is therefore important to consider driving impairment as a multimodal concept where sleepiness and attentional disorder can co-exist in the same subject.

Drugs

Another classical source of driving impairment is licit drugs used by physicians to treat their patients, or self-prescription by patients themselves. Even if many publications have shown associations between central nervous system drugs and risk of accidents, very few studies show a link between sleep-related accidents and drug intake. An increased risk of being responsible for a road traffic accident was found in users of prescribed medicines defined as presenting a level 2 (be very careful) or level 3 (danger: do not drive) risk of driving impairment according to the French medication classification system (Orriols et al., 2010). The fraction of road traffic accidents attributable to level 2 and 3 medicine use was 3.3% (2.7%–3.9%) (Orriols et al., 2010). Hypnotics with long half-lives (medium- and long-term BSD and histaminics) induce a risk of accident when subjects drive in the morning. Indirect factors such as the type of drugs responsible for traffic accidents (i.e. hypnotics and benzodiazepines) suggest that sleepiness could be the major cause of drug-related accidents, but further evidence is needed.

Evaluation of risk in patients with sleepiness while driving

Many physicians with sleepy patients look for simple questions to evaluate their fitness to drive. Studies have shown that asking a subject about excessive sleepiness while driving may better predict which individuals with sleep-disordered breathing are at greatest risk of accidents than asking about overall sleepiness (Philip et al., 2010). Moreover, self-reported sleepiness at the wheel is significantly more prevalent than OSAS. It is therefore reasonable to consider that behavioural sleepiness (i.e. sleep deprivation) is a more frequent cause of sleepiness at the wheel than sleep disorders (e.g. OSAS). For these reasons, a thorough clinical interview can usefully evaluate patients' driving risks in the vast majority of cases. However, this strategy relies on a truthful, subjective assessment by the driver talking to the physician. Deceit cannot be excluded, especially in drivers dependent on their driving licence for their job.

However, it remains very important to question patients about sleepiness at the wheel when clinicians have to determine their medical fitness to drive. Indeed, sleepiness at the wheel is the consequence of many different sleep disorders combined, or not, with various behavioural factors (e.g. sleep deprivation, shift work), which are independent major risk factors for motor vehicle accidents (Connor et al., 2002) (Figure 21.2). We suggest asking the following question to evaluate the driving risk: 'In the last 12 months have you experienced at least one episode of severe sleepiness at the wheel that made driving difficult or forced you to stop the car?'

Of course there is always a risk of under-reporting of sleepiness at the wheel, especially in professional drivers, and objective measures can help to complement the clinical evaluation. Studies have investigated the relationship between objective measurement of sleepiness (MSLT (multiple sleep latency test) or MWT scores) and driving performance. We showed that the MWT (four trials of 40 minutes each) is a suitable clinical tool for assessing fitness to drive in patients with hypersomnias of central origin (narcolepsy or idiopathic hypersomnia) as well as in OSAS patients (Philip et al., 2013). It seems reasonable to consider that patients with an MWT sleep latency of < 19 minutes are unsafe to drive.

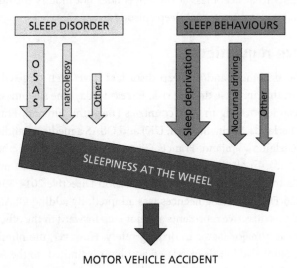

Fig. 21.2 Sleepiness at the wheel as the common final pathway in evaluating the risk of motor vehicle accidents.
Reproduced courtesy of Prof Pierre Philip.

Physicians should combine objective measures (MWT scores) and clinical evaluation (self-report of sleepiness at the wheel) to provide recommendations about fitness to drive in these sleepy patients. Further data are needed to understand the predictive value of the MWT on accident risk in large cohorts of apnoeic and narcoleptic patients.

Impact of treatment and measures to counter accident risk

Several studies investigating the impact of continuous positive airway pressure (CPAP) or uvulopalatopharyngoplasty on traffic accidents have confirmed that they are associated with a reduction in motor vehicle accidents due to OSAS.

Even if modafinil improves on-road driving ability in narcoleptic or idiopathic hypersomnia patients, epidemiological evidence questions the real beneficial effect of hypersomnia treatments on accident risk. Health authorities should require systematic driving evaluations to measure the impact of alerting treatments on driving risk.

Coffee and naps are very efficient at combating sleepiness at the wheel (Taillard et al., 2012). We have shown that subjects should select specific countermeasures according to their age or individual physiology. Indeed, a cup of coffee containing 200 mg of caffeine significantly improves performance in both young (20–25 years) and middle-aged (40–50 years) participants on night-time highway driving performances, whereas a 30-minute nap is more efficient in younger drivers than in middle-aged drivers. Continuous nocturnal blue-light exposure could be used to fight nocturnal sleepiness at the wheel in blue light-tolerant drivers. Night coffee intake or blue-light exposure delivered in the early evening to limit nocturnal sleepiness at the wheel does not modify the quality, quantity, or timing of the subsequent nocturnal sleep episodes.

Driving licence regulations

Excessive daytime sleepiness and/or sleep disorders have been targeted by experts as medical conditions that increase driving risk. Excessive daytime sleepiness is considered a medical handicap for driving in nine countries (Belgium, Finland, France, Germany, Hungary, the Netherlands, Spain, Sweden, UK) and OSAS a medical handicap for driving in ten countries (Belgium, Finland, France, Germany, Hungary, the Netherlands, Spain, Sweden, UK, Poland). In all these European countries a patient with untreated OSAS is considered unfit to drive. Recently, the Commission Directive 2014/85/EU amending Directive 2006/126/EC on driving licences was adopted. By adding OSAS to the Annex of fitness to drive, this directive represents a major step forward in the official recognition of sleep disorders as a major factor in driving safety. However, the number of patients with OSAS who are involved in sleep-related accidents is limited, so the AHI should not be considered as a single parameter when evaluating driving risk. As mentioned earlier, sleepiness at the wheel is a much more pertinent symptom that covers behavioural and sleep disorder factors with regard to traffic accidents.

Medico-legal authorizations to drive once a patient is diagnosed with a sleep disorder are provided by a certificate issued by a general practitioner or specialist (pulmonologist or neurologist) in eight countries (Belgium, Finland, France, Germany, Hungary, Spain, UK, Poland). This certificate is based on a patient's clinical improvement and therapeutic compliance, but in two countries of the aforementioned countries the final decision regarding fitness to drive is based on the patient's self-evaluation.

Non-professional and professional drivers differ in terms of medical evaluations. The frequency and type of evaluation differ dramatically. Because professional drivers are highly motivated to keep their driving licence, this can affect their self-reporting of symptoms.

Several states in the United States require physicians to report whether a professional driver is affected by a sleep disorder. Such a reporting requirement can have dramatic consequences for the driver's continued employment. The 1991 US Department of Transportation Federal Highway Administration Recommendations refer to a 1988 conference on neurological disorders and commercial drivers that recommended that anyone diagnosed with narcolepsy should be disqualified from driving professionally. This restrictive attitude regarding clinical conditions and driving fitness is not currently adopted in Europe.

As recommended by the task force of the American College of Chest Physicians, apnoeic professional drivers are subject to more permissive regulations than narcoleptic drivers and can go back to work after appropriate treatment. In Europe, driving regulations are similar to US recommendations for apnoeic commercial drivers, but with minor differences in terms of period of evaluation (e.g. 1 year in France).

Finally, whereas some countries consider sleepiness while driving as the major problem regarding driver safety, only France requires an objective quantification of alertness (the maintenance of wakefulness test) when evaluating fitness to drive. This specific position has been adopted on account of the frequent combination of sleep disorders and poor sleep hygiene in professional drivers. To ensure the legal protection of drivers and physicians, French experts consider it mandatory to demonstrate objectively that patients respond to treatment before allowing them to drive again. In the event of a sleep-related accident in treated drivers, physicians cannot be sued for insufficient efficacy of treatment and patients cannot be prosecuted for misreporting the beneficial effects of treatments. It seems reasonable, based on available evidence, to consider that patients presenting mean sleep latencies of < 19 minutes on the maintenance of wakefulness test present a major risk for sleep-related traffic accidents.

Future considerations

Although much has already been done in this field, many questions remain unanswered. At the diagnostic level there is still no simple objective measure for quantifying the risk to our patients, unlike for other accident risk factors (e.g. using a breathalyzer for alcohol testing). Ideally, we need a 'somnotest' to quantify the driving risk, but up to now driving simulators or EEG measures have provided only indirect and variable estimations of the driving risk and are obviously not suitable for use outside the clinic or laboratory. Connected car technologies may represent the future in terms of evaluating drivers' behaviour.

Treatments other than CPAP, uvulopalatopharyngoplasty, and orthodontic treatment could provide an interesting alternative in the prevention of accidents, but there are still no long-term data on the impact of alertness substances on the driving risk of patients, and oral appliances have received little attention in this field.

Studying the impact of extensive driving in treated and untreated patients is another key factor on the research agenda because of the high prevalence of sleep-disordered breathing in professional drivers. More studies are needed to better define the phenotype of apnoeic individuals involved in traffic accidents. Whereas only a limited number of patients with sleep-disordered breathing fall victim to a sleep-related accident, there is an urgent need to track these patients and develop special evaluations plus driving recommendations (e.g. no nocturnal driving) for them.

New pharmacological countermeasures should be tested and inter-individual response rates to these countermeasures need to be defined. Moreover, road safety campaigns on the risks of acute/chronic sleep deprivation and drowsy driving need to be released in every country. Finally, the effectiveness of naps and coffee as countermeasures should be promoted to reduce the risk of accidents.

Summary

◆ Evaluation of fitness to drive in drowsy drivers should not be reduced to evaluating the severity of sleep disorders.

◆ Evaluating sleep behaviour is essential in the evaluation of fitness to drive.

◆ Sleepiness at the wheel has to be systematically evaluated to ascertain the risk of drowsy driving.

◆ Sleepiness at the wheel can be evaluated by asking the following: 'In the last 12 months, have you experienced at least one episode of severe sleepiness at the wheel that made driving difficult or forced you to stop the car?'

◆ In specific cases (i.e. professional drivers), sleepiness at the wheel can be objectively evaluated by means of the maintenance of wakefulness test (MWT).

References

Connor, J., Norton, R., Ameratunga, S., Robinson, E., Civil, I., Dunn, R., Bailey, J. & Jackson, R. 2002. Driver sleepiness and risk of serious injury to car occupants: population based case control study. *British Medical Journal*, **324**(7346), p. 1125.

Ellen, R. L., Marshall, S. C., Palayew, M., Molnar, F. J., Wilson, K. G. & Man-Son-Hing, M. 2006. Systematic review of motor vehicle crash risk in persons with sleep apnea. *Journal of Clinical Sleep Medicine*, **2**(2), pp. 193–200.

Lee, M. L., Howard, M. E., Horrey, W.J., Liang, Y., Anderson, C., Shreeve, M.S., O'Brien, C.S. & Czeisler, C.A. 2016. High risk of near-crash driving events following night-shift work. *Proceedings of the National Academy of Sciences of the United States of America*, **113**(1), pp. 176–81.

Lloberes, P., Levy, G., Descals, C., Sampol, G., Roca, A., Sagales, T. & de la Calzada, M.D. 2000. Self-reported sleepiness while driving as a risk factor for traffic accidents in patients with obstructive sleep apnoea syndrome and in non-apnoeic snorers. *Respiratory Medicine*, **94**(10), pp. 971–6.

Mitler, M. M., Miller, J. C., Lipsitz, J. J., Walsh, J. K. & Wylie, C. D. 1997. The sleep of long-haul truck drivers. *New England Journal of Medicine*, **337**(11), pp. 755–61.

Orriols, L., Delorme, B., Gadegbeku, B., Tricotel, A., Contrand, B., Laumon, B., Salmi, L. R., Lagarde, E.; CESIR research group. Prescription medicines and the risk of road traffic crashes: a French registry-based study. *PLoS Medicine*, **7**(11), e1000366.

Philip, P., Chaufton, C., Taillard, J., Sagaspe, P., Léger, D., Raimondi, M., Vakulin, A. & Capelli, A. 2013. Maintenance of Wakefulness Test scores and driving performance in sleep disorder patients and controls. *International Journal of Psychophysiology*, **89**(2), pp. 195–202.

Philip, P., Micoulaud-Franchi, J. A., Lagarde, E., Taillard, J., Canel, A., Sagaspe, P. & Bioulac, S. 2015. Attention deficit hyperactivity disorder symptoms, sleepiness and accidental risk in 36140 regularly registered highway drivers. *PLoS One*, **10**(9), e0138004.

Philip, P., Sagaspe, P., Lagarde, E., Leger, D., Ohayon, M. M., Bioulac, B., Boussuge, J. & Taillard, J. 2010. Sleep disorders and accidental risk in a large group of regular registered highway drivers. *Sleep Medicine*, **11**(10), pp. 973–9.

Taillard, J., Capelli, A., Sagaspe, P., Anund, A., Akerstedt, T. & Philip, P. 2012. In-car nocturnal blue light exposure improves motorway driving: a randomized controlled trial. *PLoS One*, **7**(10), e46750.

Chapter 22

Sleep, work hours, and medical performance

Glenn Rosenbluth and Christopher P. Landrigan

Introduction

Illness respects no clock or schedule. Parents may be awakened at any hour by their sick children, mothers may labour for 24 hours straight, and emergencies happen at every hour of the day and night. At every one of these hours, there are doctors, nurses, and other healthcare providers awake and ready to provide care. While a growing number of industries in the twenty-first century function 24 hours per day, it is particularly critical that doctors and nurses are available at all hours of the day and night.

This work ethos has long been part of our image of the prototypical, idealized doctor. Television and pop culture abound with representations of solo general practitioners who provide all of the medical care for small towns, obstetricians on call for deliveries day and night, and trauma surgeons available to provide life-saving surgical care at all hours. These characters are often utterly exhausted, yet able to recover at a moment's notice when called. A 'good' doctor rallies, and never allows the need for sleep to interfere with the provision of care. Consequently, sleep deprivation and prolonged wakefulness have come to represent badges of honour, rather than red flags that might warn patients and society of potential hazards.

Only recently have the dangers of working long hours in medicine been studied and discussed, and this low rumbling about long hours has not had a dramatic impact on the provision of care. Despite some increased scrutiny and modest increases in the regulation of their work hours, US-based physicians in training continue to routinely work shifts of up to 28 hours in duration, and up to 80 hours per week (or sometimes more), while trained physicians continue to be unregulated, with respect to both consecutive and cumulative weekly hours. In many quarters, there is little recognition that long work hours can pose serious hazards to physicians and their patients.

Sleep physiology, sleep deprivation, and physician performance

All humans, including doctors, must have adequate sleep to achieve alertness and optimal performance. The timing and amount of sleep are largely driven by two underlying physiological systems: endogenous circadian rhythms—the near 24-hour biological clock—and the sleep homeostat, a system that drives sleepiness the longer one is awake, regardless of the time of day. The endogenous circadian rhythms establish near-24-hour cycles of temperature fluctuation, hormonal secretion (including melatonin and cortisol), and varying levels of neurobehavioural function. Concurrently, the sleep homeostat regulates the timing and duration of sleep and wakefulness in a delicate balance necessary to provide optimal alertness and performance. Even small decreases in sleep can lead to measurable deterioration in cognitive performance, often with no self-awareness of these deficits.

Adding to these two physiological controls is a third process—sleep inertia—which impairs alertness and cognitive function in the minutes and hours immediately after awakening. Anyone who has ever been awakened suddenly from a deep sleep and needed a few seconds before thinking clearly has experienced sleep inertia. Immediate reversal from sleep to wakefulness is rarely met with an immediate return to optimal cognitive function. Individuals emerging from sleep may have a basic conversation before they are completely awake, then fall back asleep and be unable to recall the conversation in the morning. It can take 2–4 hours to become fully alert after waking.

Sleep deprivation is the lack of adequate sleep necessary to recover brain and body function, and may be acute, chronic, or acute-on-chronic. Acute sleep deprivation, as occurs when a well-rested person attempts to work an all-night shift after being awake all day, impairs many aspects of human functioning, including cognitive performance, memory, and fine motor skills, all of which may be essential in the provision of medical care. Clinical performance and vigilance have been shown to be particularly impaired, across a variety of research settings and studies (Philibert, 2005).

Chronic lower levels of sleep deficiency can also impair human performance, with effects that may manifest more insidiously because they are unexpected. After 2 weeks of getting 6 hours of nightly sleep (an amount perceived as reasonable by many), individuals on average perform at the same level as if they had been kept awake for 24 hours continuously, with cognitive performance dropping by close to 1 standard deviation (Van Dongen et al., 2003), a degree equivalent to approximately 15 IQ points.

When chronic sleep deprivation compounds acute sleep deprivation and circadian misalignment (a common phenomenon for doctors), performance is far worse than under the influence of any of these three factors alone (Anderson et al., 2012; Cohen et al., 2010). A doctor who gets a baseline of 6 hours per night, and then provides care during the middle of the night as part of a 24-hour continuous duty period, is likely to be extremely impaired.

Researchers have found that the level of impairment caused by sleep deprivation can be compared to the level caused by alcohol consumption. In one study, residents on a schedule with regular daytime work in addition to prolonged call shifts (34–36 continuous hours every four to five nights, a common schedule to this day in the United States) had similar levels of cognitive and driving performance as well-rested individuals with a blood alcohol level of 0.04%–0.05%, even while averaging 3 hours of sleep per night during these shifts; estimates of performance impairment after 24 hours of *consecutive* wakefulness are closer to that induced by a blood alcohol level of 0.10%—well above the legal driving limit for almost every nation.

Physician performance deficits due to sleep deprivation have also been quantified in clinical tasks in a variety of studies. In one of these earliest studies, interns were asked to interpret electrocardiograms under rested and sleep-deprived conditions (Friedman et al., 1971). The interns who were sleep-deprived made errors at almost twice the rate of their rested colleagues. This finding has been replicated in doctors performing non-clinical tasks as well, and is not limited to cognitive tasks.

Surgical residents who are awake all night make more errors and are less efficient at performing simulated laparoscopic surgery than residents who are rested, a finding reproduced in several studies. The effects of sleep deprivation on processes such as surgical technique have primarily been studied using simulators, though at least one field study from 1972 documented that fatigued surgeons exhibited impaired performance (Goldman et al., 1972). Even modest disruptions in sleep—as might occur on account of awakenings from telephone calls—have been associated with decreased performance in simulated surgeries (Taffinder et al., 1998).

In real-life surgeries, one hopes the supervision provided by attending physicians would lessen the potential effects of errors by sleep-deprived doctors-in-training (assuming the attending physicians are well-rested), but while some studies have found no impact of sleep deprivation on the rates of complications or errors linked to trainee surgeons, a number have found increased errors. Some have suggested that the performance decrement may be less pronounced with experienced surgeons, though one study found that senior surgeons experienced a tripling in rates of complications in the operating room when they had less than a 6-hour opportunity to sleep while on call (Rothschild et al., 2009). It is worth noting that the broader literature on sleep deprivation does not suggest that humans learn to tolerate it over time; quite the contrary, chronic sleep deprivation compounds acute sleep deprivation, tending to worsen its effects on performance, as discussed earlier.

Field studies of sleep deprivation in medical residents have convincingly demonstrated that detrimental effects are not limited to the laboratory, and in fact have real and measurable impacts on patients and the doctors themselves. In one of the very few randomized controlled trials on the topic, researchers demonstrated that ICU staff working traditional 30-hour shifts made 36% more serious medical errors and five times as many serious diagnostic errors as colleagues working shifts limited to 16 consecutive hours (Landrigan et al., 2004). Other studies by this group have reported a variety of related outcomes, including a 7-fold increase in self-reported fatigue-related medical errors, and a 4-fold increase in self-reported errors that led to a patient death after a working shift of > 24 continuous hours. The impact of these errors is not limited to patients—interns working > 24 hours are more than twice as likely to be involved in a car accident when driving home after work, and have a 61% increased chance of suffering a percutaneous injury at work.

Taken *en masse*, the body of literature on physician sleep deprivation has provided a fairly consistent global message: sleep deprivation, both acute and chronic, has important detrimental effects on physician performance. Faced with overwhelming data suggesting physician impairment, and an absence of data in support of prolonged wakefulness, we must ask the question, 'Why do we allow doctors to work such long hours?' Truck drivers in the United States are limited to 14 consecutive hours of work, and only 11 of those duty hours can include actual driving. Pilots are limited to 8 hours of flying in a 24-hour period, and that depends on them having at least an 8-hour period of rest. One can't help but wonder whether stricter regulations would exist for physicians if every medical error were as obvious as a truck or plane crash, or if the doctor's life, rather than the patient's, were at risk with every error.

Approaches to limiting physician work hours

Regulations

In the United States, physician duty hours were not a subject of national discourse, let alone regulation, until 1984 (some might argue that they still aren't). It was in 1984 that a woman named Libby Zion died in New York. Her family attributed her death at least partly to sleep deprivation on the part of the resident physician caring for her. Subsequently, New York State limited hours for physicians in training to no more than 80 hours per week. From the passage of the 'Libby Zion Law' in 1989 until 2003, New York's regulations were the most stringent in the United States.

In the ensuing years, data on the detrimental effects of sleep deprivation in medical trainees began to accumulate. Beginning in 2003, the Accreditation Council for Graduate Medical Education (ACGME) implemented the first set of duty hour requirements common to all accredited training programmes in the United States. These requirements limited the number of hours worked by trainees to a maximum of 30 consecutive hours and 80 total hours per week, and mandated that trainees have at least one day off in seven. Of note, despite several attempts to pass federal laws, duty hour requirements have never been mandated, but rather left to self-regulation via the ACGME.

By contrast, most physicians in Europe are subject to the European Working Time Directive (EWTD), which limits junior doctors, senior doctors, and nurses to a maximum of 48 hours per week, and limits all shift work to a maximum of 13 hours' continuous duty. In the UK in particular, doctors' weekly work hours (averaged over a 6-month period) have been gradually reduced from a 72-hour weekly limit in 2004, to a 56-hour limit, to the current 48-hour limit, which was implemented in August 2009. These limits are based on a 6-month average, and include an option for individuals to opt out of the weekly (but not the shift) limits. Implementation of an EWTD-compliant roster has been shown to improve patient safety (Cappuccio et al., 2009).

In 2009, the US National Academy of Medicine (formerly the Institute of Medicine) formed the Committee on Optimizing Graduate Medical Trainee (Resident) Hours and Work Schedules to Improve Patient Safety, which recommended further limitations on physician duty hours. Among the major recommendations at that time were that physicians-in-training be limited to: a maximum of 16 hours of consecutive work if no rest-periods were provided, or 30 hours if given a 5-hour undisturbed nap period; breaks of 10 hours after a day shift, 12 hours after a night shift, and 14 hours after an extended duty shift; and a maximum of four consecutive night shifts, to be followed by a 48-hour duty-free period. Absent legal standing, and without the provision of additional financial or workforce resources, these recommendations were adapted somewhat by the ACGME in 2011, and revised again in 2017. The current (2017) guidelines apply a narrower set of restrictions, which include allowing residents to work up to 28 hours and include a guideline that residents should (rather than 'must') have at least 8 hours off between shifts. Physicians in the United States who have completed training are not subject to any specific regulations limiting work hours.

Until recently, studies of schedules which limit shift work to < 16 hours demonstrated a relatively consistent pattern of improvements in trainee education as well as in measures of patient safety and quality. More recently, however, some studies of shift changes in response to duty hour guidelines have revealed concerns among physician trainees about increased rates of errors. Most field studies of the implications of shorter shifts have relied on self-reports and perceptions rather than chart audits and real-time error tracking. In addition, adaptations to duty hour requirements have been highly variable, resulting in schedules which may not be physiologically desirable.

In the largest study to date of these new duty hour limits, the FIRST (Flexibility in Duty Hour Requirements for Surgical Trainees) trial compared surgical outcomes in patients cared for by trainees working under current limitations (maximum shift length of 28 hours) to outcomes in those cared for by trainees who did not have a maximum shift length (Bilimoria et al., 2016). Using large administrative datasets, researchers found no differences in mortality or severe surgical complications after implementation of the duty hour limitations. An important limitation of this study is that surgery trainees are generally directly supervised during surgical procedures, and therefore mistakes likely to cause postoperative death or serious complications (the primary study outcomes) might be caught and corrected by better-rested senior physicians before impacting patients. Less impactful medical errors were not measured. As physician sleep time was not tracked and schedules were not standardized, it is not possible to make any conclusions about the impact of acute and/or chronic sleep deprivation based on this study. Trainees in the intervention group which allowed longer shift lengths self-reported their own health as poorer than those who worked the limited schedule. Additional trials which robustly measure outcome, process, and balancing measures will be needed before we fully understand the potential impacts of physician duty hour limitations.

Reactions to limitations

In the United States as well as Europe, attempts to adapt physician schedules in consideration of the data on sleep-related safety outcomes have been met with new concerns about other unintended safety consequences. The most commonly cited concerns are that increased transitions of care between providers working shorter shifts may lead to errors, and fewer educational opportunities in shorter shifts might lead to a generation of physicians who are less well-trained than their predecessors. The concern about transitions of care has some foundation in the fact that, until recently, most physicians were not trained to provide handoffs. Newer data suggest, however, that providing handoff training can actually reduce medical errors (Starmer et al., 2014). Furthermore, the lack of difference in surgical outcomes in the FIRST trial suggests that concern over the increased number of handoffs can be mitigated (Bilimoria et al., 2016).

New assessment tools may be required to adequately determine the second concern—educational opportunities. European physicians who train with schedules that limit shift length and cumulative hours are generally considered no less competent than US physicians, although the structure of medical training varies in both sequence and duration. In 2010, the UK government commissioned a report on the impact of the EWTD on physician training which identified challenges and areas for further study and monitoring. Similar investigations and oversight will be needed in the United States. If studies demonstrate that US physicians are less well-trained with duty hour restrictions, accrediting bodies will need to reassess the current structure and process of training. Assessment-based advancement, the ACGME's 'Milestones Project', and entrustable professional activities all provide useful frameworks for rethinking physician training, and the era of time-based training may itself be time-limited.

A further challenge inherent in addressing sleep deprivation is that humans cannot be forced to sleep. As regulations have been imposed, the natural assumption was that if physicians worked shorter shifts and were granted more time away from work, they would sleep more. Research has shown that work hour limits are an important starting point, but they don't guarantee good sleep. Schedules designed with attention to sleep and circadian science likely reduce sleep deprivation and improve performance. Poorly designed schedules, however, even with short shifts and fewer total work hours, have the potential to result in lower quality sleep and therefore to worsen performance. These effects may also be impacted by other factors, including handoff processes, supervision, desire for personal and family time, and time needed to read and/or study.

The shifting landscape

Patient safety has received more attention and resources in the past 15 years than at any time in history, and it is likely that scrutiny will continue to increase. One downstream effect is that patients, advocacy groups, and regulatory agencies have begun to demand higher levels of physician presence in hospitals at night. Although the focus has been on trainee duty hours, many US teaching hospitals have addressed this demand by increasing faculty presence in supervisory roles, and many community hospitals have hired additional providers as hospitalists and/or 'nocturnists'. In all likelihood, this increased senior physician presence at night provides a substantial benefit for patients—even a sleepy doctor is probably better than no doctor. However, most senior physicians have not adapted their shift and sleep schedules the way nurses have, and are therefore highly susceptible to the dangers of sleep disruption and deprivation described earlier (see 'Sleep physiology, sleep deprivation, and physician performance').

Ambulatory physicians are not immune to changing expectations. In our 24-hour on-demand society, text-messaging, email, and electronic health records with patient-portals all contribute to a system in which doctors may feel as if they are actually on-call 24/7. As patients have more access to information, more avenues of contact, and higher service expectations, doctors increasingly face the conflicting demands of physiological needs for sleep and patient expectations of accessibility. Attempts to reduce panel sizes or otherwise compensate lead to conflicts of interest: physicians in many countries operate under a business model in which they must earn their salaries by seeing patients. A doctor who chooses to work only a half-day following a night with many calls may be subject to a lower income. A surgeon who chooses to do three operations in a day rather than five may feel the pain of a 40% drop in income. Any new limitations on physician duty hours must acknowledge these realities.

The provision of high-quality medical care has always depended on physicians adapting their practices to reflect the best evidence. An abundance of research now demonstrates that despite best intentions, the long hours worked by physicians may result in sub-optimal care delivery. In this era of increased attending to patient safety and outcomes, new models of medical care may be needed, perhaps requiring disruptive changes to existing healthcare systems in many countries. Physicians will need to embrace, and ideally lead, these changes in order to continue to best serve their patients.

Summary

- Physicians in many settings work extended duty shifts, up to or exceeding 24 hours, often with little opportunity for rest.

- Normal timing and amount of sleep are driven by two underlying physiological systems: endogenous circadian rhythms and the sleep homeostat. These two systems regulate the timing and amount of sleep in all humans.

- Sleep deprivation is the lack of adequate sleep necessary to recover brain and body function. Chronic lower levels of sleep deficiency can impair physician performance. Physicians experiencing sleep deprivation show impairments in both cognitive and procedural skills.

- Interventions limiting physicians to shifts of < 16 hours' duration are associated with a decrease in medical errors, including a decrease in diagnostic errors.

- Physicians in Europe are currently subject to a work hour limit of 48 hours per week. Physicians in the United States who have completed training are not currently subject to any work hour limits, and those in training are limited to 80 hours per week.

- As we evolve to a 24-hour on-demand society, physicians will need to develop new strategies for providing care and service to patients safely.

◆ Adaptations to physician work hour limits cannot be a one-size-fits-all. Physicians and specialty societies should purposefully design schedules that take into account sleep physiology, patient safety, and physician wellness.

References

Anderson, C., Sullivan, J. P., Flynn-Evans, E. E., Cade, B. E., Czeisler, C. A. & Lockley, S. W. 2012. Deterioration of neurobehavioral performance in resident physicians during repeated exposure to extended duration work shifts. *Sleep*, **35**(8), pp. 1137–46.

Bilimoria, K. Y., Chung, J. W., Hedges, L. V., Dahlke, A. R., Love, R., Cohen, M. E., Hoyt, D. B., Yang, A. D., Tarpley, J. L., Mellinger, J. D., Mahvi, D. M., Kelz, R.R., Ko, C. Y., Odell, D. D., Stulberg, J. J. & Lewis, F. R. 2016. National cluster-randomized trial of duty-hour flexibility in surgical training. *New England Journal of Medicine*, **374**(8), pp. 713–27.

Cappuccio, F. P., Bakewell, A., Taggart, F. M., Ward, G., Ji, C., Sullivan, J. P., Edmunds, M., Pounder, R., Landrigan, C. P., Lockley, S. W., Peile, E.; Warwick EWTD Working Group. 2009. Implementing a 48 h EWTD-compliant rota for junior doctors in the UK does not compromise patients' safety: assessor-blind pilot comparison. *Quarterly Journal of Medicine*, **102**(4), pp. 271–82.

Cohen, D. A., Wang, W., Wyatt, J. K., Kronauer, R. E., Dijk, D. J., Czeisler, C. A. & Klerman, E. B. 2010. Uncovering residual effects of chronic sleep loss on human performance. *Science Translational Medicine*, **2**(14), p. 14ra13.

Friedman, R. C., Bigger, J. T. & Kornfeld, D. S. 1971. The intern and sleep loss. *New England Journal of Medicine*, **285**(4), pp. 201–3.

Goldman, L. I., McDonough, M. T. & Rosemond, G. P. 1972. Stresses affecting surgical performance and learning. I. Correlation of heart rate, electrocardiogram, and operation simultaneously recorded on videotapes. *Journal of Surgical Research*, **12**(2), pp. 83–6.

Landrigan, C. P., Rothschild, J. M., Cronin, J. W., Kaushal, R., Burdick, E., Katz, J. T., Lilly, C. M., Stone, P. H., Lockley, S. W., Bates, D. W. & Czeisler, C. A. 2004. Effect of reducing interns' work hours on serious medical errors in intensive care units. *New England Journal of Medicine*, **351**(18), pp. 1838–48.

Philibert, I. 2005. Sleep loss and performance in residents and nonphysicians: a meta-analytic examination. *Sleep*, **28**(11), pp. 1392–402.

Rothschild, J. M., Keohane, C. A., Rogers, S., Gardner, R., Lipsitz, S. R., Salzberg, C. A., Yu, T., Yoon, C. S., Williams, D. H., Wien, M. F., Czeisler, C. A., Bates, D. W. & Landrigan, C. P. 2009. Risks of complications by attending physicians after performing nighttime procedures. *Journal of the American Medical Association*, **302**(14), pp. 1565–72.

Starmer AJ, Spector ND, Srivastava R, et al. 2014. Changes in medical errors after implementation of a handoff program. *New England Journal of Medicine*, **371**(19):1803–12.

Taffinder, N. J., McManus, I. C., Gul, Y., Russell, R. C. & Darzi, A. 1998. Effect of sleep deprivation on surgeons' dexterity on laparoscopy simulator. *Lancet*, **352**(9135), p. 1191.

Van Dongen, H. P., Maislin, G., Mullington, J. M. & Dinges, D. F. 2003. The cumulative cost of additional wakefulness: dose-response effects on neurobehavioral functions and sleep physiology from chronic sleep restriction and total sleep deprivation. *Sleep*, **26**(2), pp. 117–26.

Chapter 23

The built environment and sleep

Jose G. Cedeño Laurent, Joseph G. Allen,
and John D. Spengler

Introduction

In 2008, the world population achieved a major milestone: more than 50% of its population had migrated to urban settings. This movement has already resulted in unprecedented growth in the size and complexity of our cities, and this trend will continue—by 2050, 80% of the world population will be living in cities. As societies become more urban, the proportion of time spent indoors increases, with individuals often spending up to 90% of their time in indoor spaces. About a third of this time is spent in our bedrooms, which represent the single space where we spend the most time throughout our lives. Given that the reason for being there is good sleep, and sleep is a cornerstone of good health, we should be paying attention to ensuring that the proper environmental conditions for sleep are provided. To date, we have underestimated the importance of the sleep environment in our lives. In fact, humans have always preferred indoor environments for protection against weather and other dangers, especially while sleeping. Modern structures are designed to meet basic physiological needs, with a focus on comfort, aesthetics, and social/work functionality. Designing our indoor spaces to promote health, including healthy sleep, is a relatively new concept. In the following chapter, we discuss the role of different environmental variables on our sleep and how vulnerable populations are currently suffering from a systematic injustice that expose them to more deleterious conditions. Our goal is to start a conversation among health professionals, architects, urban planners, engineers, and innovators to learn how we can coordinate the interaction between the environmental and behavioural factors that influence sleep (Figure 23.1). Although there is still much to learn about how the environmental conditions where we sleep shape our health, both at an individual and societal level, recent interest in this field is leading to innovations and better design solutions that address current and future issues of the built environment where we live and sleep.

Lighting and sleep

Light is the strongest environmental cue for synchronizing human circadian rhythms. Before Edison's promotion of the widespread use of electric lighting, human exposure to light was almost entirely limited to the natural light–dark cycles for millennia. We

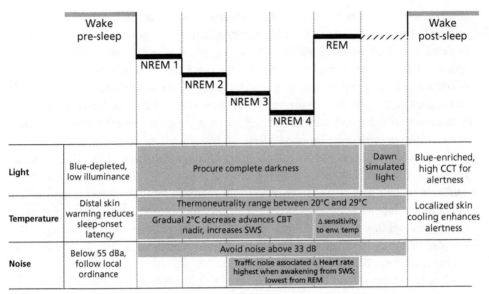

Fig. 23.1 Summary of environmental factors for optimizing the sleep environment.
Reproduced courtesy of the authors.

are only just beginning to understand the consequences of this lighting revolution. In recent decades, research has provided evidence of the deleterious effects of light exposure at night in humans and other species. In our built environment, lighting standards have historically been focused on visual performance, comfort, aesthetics, and safety, primarily for daytime functioning. The status quo in buildings is to comply with a minimum illumination level at task surfaces, in hallways, and in other spaces, often installing fixtures that disregard light quality in favour of meeting energy-saving targets. The relatively recent discovery of the 'non-visual' effects of light on human circadian rhythms and a range of other neuro-endocrine and neurobehavioural responses is transforming the application of new lighting systems. Current technology now allows the use of light sources that can mimic the natural daily variation in the sun's intensity and spectrum. Such systems can now cater to our physiological needs, ensuring proper circadian rhythm synchronization and, at the same time, enhancing our cognition while awake. The general principle is to ensure exposure to a distinct and stable 24-hour light–dark cycle each day, with daylight or high-intensity blue-enriched electric light in the day and sleep in darkness at night. In the evening prior to sleep, decreasing the light intensity and short-wavelength content will reduce the alerting effects of light and calm the brain, making it easier to fall asleep and increasing the amount of deep sleep.

The effects of light exposure on sleep and cognitive effects have two main mechanistic pathways: (i) a range of short-term acute effects, for example directly influencing alertness and cortical activity at all times of day, and inhibiting melatonin production at night; and (ii) a longer-term effect through exposure to more stable light–dark cycles, leading to better alignment of circadian rhythms. Laboratory studies have characterized in detail how light intensity, wavelength, timing, pattern, and duration affect these responses. Field studies, however, involve higher variability in results owing to the lack of control of factors that directly or indirectly affect measures of alertness, productivity, and cognition. Despite these challenges, the positive effects of lighting interventions have been shown in office and schools settings, corroborating the laboratory-based studies. For example, improvement in mood, alertness, concentration, and sleep quality was reported by office workers when working under blue-enriched white light (17,000 K) as compared to standard fluorescent lights (4,000 K) (Viola et al., 2008). Similarly, multiple studies in schools have shown improvements in cognitive throughput and concentration under higher intensity blue-enriched white light (fluorescent and LED) when compared to standard lighting conditions. These benefits were apparent even when tested on the first day following installation, demonstrating acute benefits of lighting in a real-world setting (Keis et al., 2014).

All light sources should be considered when assessing effects on sleep. Smartphones and the use of other mobile electronic devices near bedtime are emerging as substantial contributors to the circadian disrupting effects in our built environment. In a survey conducted by the National Sleep Foundation, nine out of ten participants reported using electronic devices immediately before bedtime. Using highly interactive devices increased the difficulty in falling asleep and increased the propensity to report unrefreshing sleep (Gradisar et al., 2013). To counteract these effects, software programs such as 'f.lux' modify the light spectrum of a computer's monitor based on the sunset and sunrise times of the geographical location where the computer is registered. Other large electronic device manufacturers such as Apple and Amazon have adopted similar software in their operating systems, recognizing the importance of reducing the exposure to blue-enriched light from electronic devices at night.

Besides advancing the development of new lighting technologies, making building professionals aware of the biological effects of lighting will be one of the critical steps for creating an environment where sleep is a priority. The use of a metric to characterize the non-visual responses of light will be a key step to achieving greater awareness. The development of a weighting function that reflects the spectral sensitivity of circadian responses (λ_{max} 480 nm) has been proposed as an equivalent of the existing luminosity function, which estimates the photopic sensitivity of the human eye (λ_{max} 555 nm). Different properties such as illuminance (measured in lux) are derived from this existing weighting function and have facilitated the implementation of visual comfort and performance standards. Therefore, just as the photopic lux estimates how well-lit an area is (visual function), an analogous *melanopic* lux can measure the alerting and circadian entraining effects of lighting in a space (non-visual function) (Lucas et al., 2014). Such a metric will expand the existing guidelines, lighting standards, and verification methods to ensure that appropriate light schemes are implemented for optimal health and wellbeing.

Thermal environment and sleep

Temperature is another strong environmental factor that affects sleep. Sleep requires a loss of heat and therefore temperature is vital when creating a better sleeping environment. Similar to our history of altering light exposure patterns after Edison's promotion of electric light, the invention of the first modern air conditioning system by Willis Carrier, in 1902, forever altered our relationship with the built environment.

Thermoregulation is controlled by a homeostatic and a circadian system. The homeostatic system controls our responses to thermal environmental stimuli by balancing two thermal compartments: one that produces heat (i.e. the homeothermic core, characterized by the core body temperature (CBT)), and one that regulates the heat exchange with the environment (i.e. the poikilothermic shell, characterized by skin temperature). To keep our CBT close to 37°C, the homeostatic control orchestrates a set of autonomic responses that start with changes in the vasomotor tone of distal skin regions (i.e. hands and feet), and are followed by other thermoeffector functions (e.g. sweating or shivering). Furthermore, the temperature thresholds that activate such thermoeffectors follow circadian oscillations originating from the suprachiasmatic nuclei—the same centre in the hypothalamus that regulates the sleep–wake cycle (Kräuchi & de Boer, 2011).

There is an intimate relationship between thermoregulation and sleep regulation. Prior to sleep, metabolic activity is diminished and the heat generated by the homeothermic core is dissipated. In controlled laboratory settings, where masking effects such as physical activity, body position, or food intake have been isolated, an endogenous decrease in CBT and an increase in distal skin temperature prior to sleep are observed. This has profound implications for the way in which we control the thermal properties of our sleep environment. Facilitating the increase in distal skin temperature promotes the down-regulation of our CBT and results in reduced sleep-onset latency. It has been observed that warmer evening temperatures lead to shorter sleep-onset latencies in seniors (Saeki et al., 2015). Likewise, therapeutic interventions focusing on localized skin warming before sleep have proven to be helpful in inducing sleep onset and reducing wakefulness among elderly study subjects and patients with sleep disorders such as insomnia and narcolepsy—bed socks work!

In addition to sleep initiation, other components of sleep architecture are affected by the built environment. Once sleep has been consolidated, the autonomic nervous system reduces the temperature thresholds required to activate sweating or shivering, increasing the propensity of awakening if room temperatures get too hot or too cold. Several chamber studies indicate that a thermoneutral condition is characterized by a temperature range of 20°C–29°C; this wide temperature range is due partly to the variability in clothing and bedding insulation, and partly to the convective and radiative thermal loads of the sleep environment. Colder overnight temperatures (close to 21°C) result in decreased total sleep time, a decrease in Stage 2 sleep duration, and an increased number of awakenings. A gradual decrease in environmental temperature of approximately 2°C advances the nadir of our CBT, however, leading to an increase in short-wave sleep (SWS). High humidity values at higher temperatures inhibit the capacity of our body to lose heat via evaporative cooling, having a stronger disruptive effect at the initial stage of a sleep period (Okamoto-Mizuno & Mizuno, 2012). While few studies have looked at the influence of airflow on maintaining adequate thermal sleep environments, personalized ventilation systems providing low-velocity airflow at the bedside have demonstrated a reduction in wakefulness in a warm humid setting (Lan et al., 2016).

Despite the technical complexity of our buildings today, and the impact of the thermal environment for sleep, remarkably little has been done to provide adequate thermal conditions for optimal sleep and sleep induction. Most existing thermal comfort standards were created to address the metabolic needs, body postures, and clothing insulation found in office settings. In fact, the American Society of Heating, Refrigerating and Air-Conditioning Engineers (ASHRAE) acknowledges in their Standard 55 (specifying the minimum set of requirements for acceptable thermal indoor environments) that adequate thermal conditions for sleep cannot be determined by their methodology. These limitations might arise from the definition of thermal comfort itself. The recent advent of 'smart' sensor technologies, thermostats, and wearable devices might change this situation, however. With the possibility of continuously measured indoor thermal parameters, as well as objective metrics of sleep efficiency, a new generation of personalized controls that dynamically respond to our physiological needs will be feasible in the near future.

Noise and sleep

Urban living is accompanied by a plethora of sounds, another new experience for humans that was relatively constant for millennia but changed dramatically at the start of the Industrial Revolution in the nineteenth and twentieth centuries. Social interactions, construction, transportation, and even nature create the complex acoustic texture of the urban soundscape. While some of these sounds might be disregarded or even considered pleasant, others are a pollutant and become a nuisance. Characterizing noise by its physical characteristics, such as intensity (usually measured as the sound pressure level in decibels, dB) or frequency, permits us to define noise exposure standards that address auditory health effects in occupational settings, most notably noise-induced hearing loss. There are also non-auditory health effects associated with noise, including cardiovascular disease and sleep disturbance. Annoyance due to noise, particularly at night time, has been associated with deleterious health effects due to sleep disturbance; the World Health Organization (WHO) estimates that sleep disturbance represents the single most important cause of disability associated with environmental noise exposure in highly urbanized societies. Moreover, the number of people exposed to average noise levels from aircrafts exceeding 55 dB in a 24-hour period (the limit published in the *WHO Guidelines for Community Noise* in 1999) is expected to increase by up to 1.6% every year (Hume et al., 2012).

Noise properties affecting sleep and health were first documented in experimental studies. Even sound pressure levels as low as 33 dB induce an arousal of the autonomic, motor, and cortical systems. Although monotonical associations between physiological arousal and stimulus intensity level (in decibels) have been found, these associations were modified by factors such as sleep deprivation, which leads to higher auditory-sensitivity thresholds. Noise sensitivity is also dependent on sleep phase; during REM (rapid eye movement) sleep, the encephalographic (EEG) activation and behavioural responses to noise are lower than during short-wave sleep (SWS), but peripheral vasoconstriction is higher (Williams et al., 1964).

Different characteristics of traffic noise have been studied on account of their disruptive potential during sleep. Latency of heart rate (HR) increase was shorter for railway noise than for road traffic and aircraft noise. This may have been due to the rate of noise level increase, which also led to higher maximum HR values. Noise stimuli that led to awakenings resulted in HR elevations for periods longer than 1 minute; these HR increases were higher when waking up from SWS than for awakenings from REM. An important finding is that cardiac arousals occur even if sleep is not totally interrupted: maximum HR increases of nine beats per minute have been registered after noise periods without awakenings (Griefahn et al., 2008).

Observational studies have been able to look at the effects of night-time noise exposure and its chronic effects on health. In addition to an increase in the proportion of light sleep and a higher propensity for wakefulness, nocturnal noise has a stronger association with cardiovascular disease than daytime noise exposure. Epidemiological findings have indicated that more nuanced factors of the built environment can affect sleep and health. Open windows, as well as orientation of the bedroom towards the road, result in increased cardiovascular and hypertension risk (Chepesiuk, 2005). Some cultural components of our environment could also be addressed to reduce the intrusion of outdoor noise into our bedrooms, although regional and cultural differences make it difficult to enforce noise regulations. For example, Switzerland has one of the strictest set of noise regulations in Europe, but still there is much room for improvement. On the one hand, it is common for landlord and tenant associations to establish strict rules during night periods and specific days of the week (e.g. 10 p.m. to 6 p.m. and Sundays), with municipalities capable of enforcing fines of up to CHF10,000 per residential offence. On the other hand, it has been estimated that 40,000 people living in Zurich experience, on average, at least one additional awakening per night due to the bell sounds from churches at night.

The future soundscape of our built environment is uncertain. Energy efficiency is promoting the development of electric cars that generate less noise. Emergency sirens from first responders may be quieter since they will not have to overcome traffic noise; maybe self-driving technologies will make them entirely disappear. Buildings and homes are being designed with enhanced acoustical dampening technologies. New acoustic challenges may arise, however; the future might be dominated by the alarms and notifications from smartphones and other unforeseen gadgets indoors, or the intermittent, low-frequency noise from wind turbines, for example. Without question, a big part of the transformation towards quieter sleep environments will require the collective consciousness to respect the neighbours' sleep time.

Socio-economic disparities and sleep

It is recognized that good sleep is the result of a complex balance between psychosocial factors, physical health, and the right environmental conditions. These factors are not always under our control, however. Therefore, having access to a space that allows the mind and body to rest should be a right, more than a privilege. Unfortunately, among the most urgent issues to solve in our built environment is the ever increasing amount of harmful environmental exposures present in low-income communities. In the United States, homes located in low-income neighbourhoods have become places where environmental risks are compounded, defeating the sheltering purpose that housing once had. Environmental inequalities in combination with other psychosocial stressors in poor communities are associated with insufficient sleep or precarious sleep hygiene, resulting in increased risk for presenting cardiovascular and other chronic diseases—such as hypertension, obesity, diabetes, obesity, and cancer—that are associated with poor sleep.

Indoor poor air quality factors, such as particulate matter concentrations, environmental tobacco smoke, allergens, and other pollutants, are more prevalent in disadvantaged neighbourhoods, and have been associated with decreases in sleep quality and duration of sleep. Ethnic groups living in these communities, particularly blacks and Hispanics, are more likely to report sleep times both below and above the recommended values by the National Sleep Foundation. Epidemiological studies show that urbanicity (a measure of the proportion of urban land use in a 1-km radius) is associated with a decrease of almost 20 minutes of sleep per day among 1-year-old infants (Bottino et al., 2012). Residents of disadvantaged communities that perceive higher levels of noise and uncleanliness, and report lower sleep quality, also declare worse self-rated physical health (Hale et al., 2013). Increased particulate matter concentrations and high short-term temperatures have been associated with decreased sleep efficiency and higher scores in the respiratory disturbance index, a measure used to quantify sleep-disordered breathing severity (Zanobetti et al., 2010).

Other environmental risk factors in housing, such as occupancy density, noise levels, and an overall housing quality, have been combined to estimate a cumulative environmental risk exposure index for the purpose of exploring chronic physiological stress in different housing settings. Higher index values are positively correlated with higher levels of stress biomarkers among children from low-income families (Evans & Marcynyszyn, 2004). In addition to the current environmental issues, climate change may impose additional challenges to the most vulnerable populations. Extreme weather events may occur with higher frequency and severity, thus aggravating the existing fuel poverty issues, where people could compromise a thermally safe environment to cover other basic needs. Meanwhile, massive blackouts during recent heatwaves have highlighted the frailty of electrical grids. It is thought that sleep quality plays an important mediating role in the risk of heat-related mortality when thermally stable environments are jeopardized.

In this chapter, we have suggested that the modern human environment has created conditions that our biology has not had time to adapt to, in an evolutionary sense. Our sleep cycles and quality evolved in a very different lighting, thermal, and noise environment to what we experience today. Technology can help transform the way we sleep, however, by enabling a finer control of our built environment. We must ensure, though, that new solutions for improving our sleep become universally accessible. It would be disappointing if revolutionary products and services are designed only with affluent customers in mind. Other disruptive technologies, such as smartphones, have proven to be successful and permeate all market sectors. We believe that the concept of the quantified self, enabled by massive data collection from wearable devices and environmental sensors, will deliver its promise to solve important issues at a societal level, such as achieving an optimal sleep environment.

Summary

+ Lighting, thermal, and acoustic conditions in our built environment exert an important influence on our sleep.

+ Light is the strongest environmental cue for synchronizing human circadian rhythms. Short-term acute effects directly influence alertness and cortical activity at all times of day, and inhibit melatonin production at night; longer-term effects manifest through exposure to more stable light–dark cycles, leading to better alignment of circadian rhythms.

+ Temperature is another strong environmental factor that affects sleep. Thermoregulation is controlled by a homeostatic and a circadian system.

+ Noise exposure is another factor affecting sleep, particularly in highly urbanized areas.

+ Good sleep is the result of a balance between psychosocial factors, physical health, and environmental conditions. In our built environment is the ever-increasing amount of harmful environmental exposures present in low-income communities.

+ The modern human environment has created conditions that our biology has not had time to adapt to, in an evolutionary sense.

References

Bottino, C. J., Rifas-Shiman, S. L., Kleinman, K. P., Oken, E., Redline, S., Gold, D., Schwartz, J., Melly, S. J., Koutrakis, P., Gillman, M. W. & Taveras, E.M., 2012. The association of urbanicity with infant sleep duration. *Health & place,* **18**(5), pp.1000–5.

Chepesiuk, R. 2005. Decibel hell: the effects of living in a noisy world. *Environmental Health Perspectives,* **113**, A34–A41.

Evans, G. W. & Marcynyszyn, L. A., 2004. Environmental justice, cumulative environmental risk, and health among low-and middle-income children in upstate New York. *American journal of public health,* **94**(11), pp.1942–4.

Gradisar, M., Wolfson, A., Harvey, A., Hale, L., Rosenberg, R. & Czeisler, C. 2013. The sleep and technology use of Americans: findings from the National Sleep Foundation's 2011 Sleep in America poll. *Journal of Clinical Sleep Medicine,* **9**, pp. 1291–9.

Griefahn, B., Brode, P., Marks, A. & Basner, M. 2008. Autonomic arousals related to traffic noise during sleep. *Sleep*, **31**, pp. 569–77.

Hale, L., Hill, T. D., Friedman, E., Nieto, F. J., Galvao, L. W., Engelman, C. D., Malecki, K. M. & Peppard, P. E., 2013. Perceived neighborhood quality, sleep quality, and health status: evidence from the Survey of the Health of Wisconsin. *Social Science & Medicine*, **79**, pp. 16–22.

Hume, K., Brink, M. & Basner, M. 2012. Effects of environmental noise on sleep. *Noise & Health*, **14**, pp. 297–302.

Keis, O., Helbig, H., Streb, J. & Hille, K. 2014. Influence of blue-enriched classroom lighting on students' cognitive performance. *Trends in Neuroscience and Education*, **3**, pp. 86–92.

Kräuchi, K. & de Boer, T. 2011. Body temperature, sleep, and hibernation. In: Kryger, M. H., Roth, T. & Dement, W. C. eds. *Principles and Practice of Sleep Medicine*. St. Louis, MO: Elsevier, pp. 323–34.

Lan, L., Lian, Z. W. & Lin, Y. B., 2016. Comfortably cool bedroom environment during the initial phase of the sleeping period delays the onset of sleep in summer. *Building and Environment*, **103**, pp. 36–43.

Lucas, R., Peirson, S., Berson, D., Brown, T., Cooper, H., Czeisler, C., Figueiro, M., Gamlin, P., Lockley, S., O'Hagan, J., Price, L., Provencio, I., Skene, D. & Brainard, G. 2014. Measuring and using light in the melanopsin age. *Trends in Neurosciences*, **37**, pp. 1–9.

Okamoto-Mizuno, K. & Mizuno, K. 2012. Effects of thermal environment on sleep and circadian rhythm. *Journal of Physiological Anthropology*, **31**, p. 14.

Saeki, K., Obayashi, K., Tone, N. & Kurumatani, N. 2015. A warmer indoor environment in the evening and shorter sleep onset latency in winter: the HEIJO-KYO study. *Physiology & Behavior*, **149**, pp. 29–34.

Viola, A., James, L., Schlangen, L. & Dijk, D. 2008. Blue-enriched white light in the workplace improves self-reported alertness, performance and sleep quality. *Scandinavian Journal of Work Environment & Health*, **34**, pp. 297–306.

Williams, H. L., Hammack, J. T., Daly, R. L., Dement, W. C. & Lubin, A. 1964. Responses to auditory stimulation, sleep loss and the EEG stages of sleep. *Electroencephalography and clinical neurophysiology*, **16**(3), pp. 269–79.

Zanobetti, A., Redline, S., Schwartz, J., Rosen, D., Patel, S., T O'Connor, G., Lebowitz, M., Coull, B. A. & Gold, D.R. 2010. Associations between PM10 with Sleep and Sleep-Disordered Breathing in Adults from Seven US Urban Areas. *American Journal of Respiratory and Critical Care Medicine*, **182**(6):819–25.

Chapter 24

Adolescent sleep and later school start times

Amy R. Wolfson and Terra Ziporyn

Introduction

Over the last 30 years, an accumulation of studies has clearly demonstrated that delaying school start times is an effective countermeasure to adolescents' chronic insufficient sleep while also enhancing students' health, safety, and academic success (Adolescent Sleep Working Group, et al., 2014). Insufficient sleep is one of the most common, arguably epidemic, and potentially reparable health challenges that adolescents face. The optimal amount of sleep for adolescents is approximately 8.5–9.5 hours nightly (Adolescent Sleep Working Group, et al., 2014). Studies from a range of countries show that, while younger children generally get enough sleep, by early adolescence, most do not; this trend continues to worsen throughout the teenage years (Iglowstein et al., 2003). Moreover, looking back over the last two decades, adolescents' nightly sleep has continued to decrease.

The National Sleep Foundation's 2006 'Sleep in America' poll showed that adolescents report sleeping 7.6 hours on school nights, even though they feel that they need an average of 8.2 hours of sleep for optimal daytime function. Only about 20% of all surveyed adolescents (sixth to twelfth graders) report an adequate amount of nightly sleep (= 9 hours per night); among high-school students (ninth to twelfth graders), the percentage decreases to 9%, suggesting that sleep deprivation is more common in older adolescents (National Sleep Foundation (NSF), 2006). In a 2015 study that examined data from 'Monitoring the Future', an annual, nationally representative cross-sectional survey of adolescents (grades 8, 10, 12) in the United States from 1991 to 2012 (n = 272,077) representing birth cohorts from 1973 to 2000, adolescents were asked how often they get 7 hours of sleep and how often they get less sleep than they should (Keyes et al., 2015). Adolescents' sleep declined over the 21 years, with the greatest change during the 1990s, with older adolescents reporting less sleep, and sleep consistently decreasing over time. Girls were less likely than boys to report getting 7 hours of sleep, as were racial/ethnic minorities, students living in urban areas, and those of low socio-economic status (SES) (Keyes et al., 2015).

Sleep needs and patterns

As observed across many countries, self-reported sleep patterns show marked changes during the course of adolescence (Iglowstein et al., 2003). Teenagers report increasingly later bedtimes, especially on weekend and vacation nights. School-night bedtimes range from 9.30 p.m. to midnight with high-school-aged adolescents (ages 14–19 years), reporting significantly later bedtimes than their early-adolescent peers (ages 10–13 years) (NSF, 2006). Rise times on school days remain relatively stable across this developmental stage largely due to school schedules (Carskadon et al., 1998). Consequently, adolescents tend to report increasingly less sleep during the week over the middle- and high-school years. Time in bed ranges from as little as 5 hours to closer to 8 hours, with older adolescents reporting less time in bed than younger adolescents (Wolfson & Carskadon, 1998). In striking contrast to self-report studies, laboratory-based research reveals that older adolescents may need the same amount, or even more, sleep than early adolescents (Carskadon, 1980).

Adolescents attempt to make up for insufficient school-night sleep by oversleeping by about 0.5–2.5 hours more on weekend nights than school nights, and this disparity increases from age 14 to age 18 years (Wolfson & Carskadon, 1998). Likewise, most adolescents typically delay going to sleep about 1–2 hours on weekend nights compared to school nights, and extend their sleep period by waking 1–4 hours later at weekends. Self-reported bedtimes characteristically range from about 10.30 p.m. to midnight or later at weekends, and weekend wake times typically range from 9 a.m. to 10 a.m. or later, with older adolescents reporting later sleep–wake schedules than younger siblings and friends.

Developmental changes to the sleep–wake regulatory system

Three key changes in sleep regulation help to explain adolescents' erratic sleep–wake schedules and inadequate sleep: (i) until age 10, many children wake up feeling fresh and energized to start the day. In contrast, by the early teen years, adolescents experience a delay in the timing of the circadian rhythms of sleep and melatonin secretion, expressed as a shift in diurnal preference from *lark* to *owl* type, resulting in difficulty falling asleep and waking up as early; (ii) adolescents undergo a change in regulatory homeostatic 'sleep drive' whereby the accumulation of sleep propensity while awake slows relative to that in younger children, making it harder to fall asleep earlier; and (iii) adolescents' sleep *needs* do not decline from pre-adolescent levels, with optimal sleep amounts ranging from 8.5 hours to 9.5 hours per night (Adolescent Sleep Working Group, et al., 2014). Realistically, this means that the average adolescent has difficulty falling asleep before about 11 p.m., and is unlikely to wake before 8 a.m., whereas their younger and less mature peers are more likely to fall asleep easily and awaken early. This pronounced sleep debt leads to school absenteeism and tardiness, daytime sleepiness, emotion regulation difficulties, and academic struggles. Undoubtedly, the biological delay in sleep onset and social pressures of the teen years combined with the need to arise early in the morning for school easily create a situation in which the adolescent chronically obtains inadequate sleep, with clear negative implications for physical and emotional wellbeing, academic performance, and other daytime behaviours and activities.

In addition to the three significant developmental changes, environmental and life-style factors interfere with adolescents getting sufficient and regular sleep. Alterations to the sleep–wake regulatory systems during puberty that cause mature adolescents to stay awake later at night facilitate wake behaviours such as binging on their favourite TV series or text-messaging a few more friends. Adolescents may also compensate for sleep loss with increased caffeine and stimulant use or drug use and abuse (Ludden & Wolfson, 2010). Other factors, including family socio-economic status, after-school employment hours, and light exposure from technology, further exacerbate and interfere with many adolescents' ability to obtain sufficient sleep or to maintain a regular sleep–wake schedule. While extracurricular activities and technology use may be more or less under adolescent control, the determination of high-school and middle-school start times is not in their hands (Adolescent Sleep Working Group, et al., 2014).

Healthy sleep with delayed school start times

Moving middle- and high-school start times later gives adolescents the opportunity to obtain an adequate amount of sleep, with positive implications for academic performance and health. In a now hallmark school transition study, researchers assessed the impact of shifting school start times 65 minutes earlier across the transition from ninth grade (8.25 a.m.) to tenth grade (7.20 a.m.) for forty 14- to 16-year-olds attending a suburban US public school (Carskadon et al., 1998). Actigraphic sleep records demonstrated that just over 60% of the ninth graders, and fewer than 50% of the tenth graders, obtained an average of 7 hours or more of sleep on school nights, and even though tenth graders awakened significantly earlier on school mornings and obtained less sleep, they did not go to sleep earlier in tenth grade than in ninth grade. In tenth grade, students' circadian melatonin rhythm was significantly later, and they also fell asleep faster in the daytime, with about 50% of the tenth-graders experiencing at least one REM sleep episode on the multiple sleep latency test (MSLT), an abnormal finding indicative of insufficient sleep (Carskadon et al., 1998).

Since the 1990s, researchers have examined the effects of high-school start times on sleepiness, sleep duration, and academic performance and shown that, while student bed-time is relatively similar, students at schools with earlier start times have shorter total sleep times, more daytime sleepiness, and poorer grades. For example, a change in high-school start times from 7.15 a.m. to 8.40 a.m. for 18,000 students in the Minneapolis School District showed (i) improved attendance rates for grades 9–11; (ii) increased enrolment; (iii) slight, but not statistically significant, improvement in grades; and (iv) nearly an hour more sleep per night, as reported by high-school students themselves (Wahlstrom, 2002). Similarly, a 3-year study of eight high schools across three states (n = 9,000) showed that 60% of those students with 8.30 a.m. or later start times obtained at least 8 hours of sleep per night and reported better academic performance, less depression, less caffeine use, and better decisions regarding substance use (Wahlstrom, 2014). Similar findings have been reported when comparing start times for middle-school pupils (seventh and eighth graders) (Wolfson et al., 2007). Furthermore, delaying school start times is a powerful counter-measure for adolescents attending school in a range of different environments and geographic locations as discussed in the special issue of Sleep Health (Troxel & Wolfson, 2017).

Additional and significant benefits of later school start times

Driving after chronic insufficient sleep or close to the circadian nadir in alertness (which can coincide with the commute to school) puts adolescents at particular risk for sleepy driver and fall-asleep-at-the-wheel crashes. Multiple studies have shown that delaying high-school start times results in substantial reductions in car accidents for adolescents. For example, Danner & Phillips (2009) showed a 16.5% decrease in accident rates for 17- and 18-year-olds in the 2 years after delaying high-school start times by 1 hour (from 7.30 a.m. to 8.30 a.m.), while the rest of the state increased by 7.8% over the same time frame. More recently, Wahlstrom (2014) demonstrated a 70% reduction in accidents in 16- to 18-year-olds when a district shifted school start times from 7.35 a.m. to 8.55 a.m. Taken together, these and other group-level studies document a disturbing association between early school start times & insufficient sleep and drowsy driving, putting both teenagers and other members of the public at risk.

RAND economists conservatively project that delaying U.S. middle and high schools to at least 8:30 a.m. would contribute at least $83 billion to the U.S. economy within a decade, based on higher graduation and reduced car crash rates alone (Hafner, 2017). Other economic analyses project that academic improvement associated with delaying start times would lead to an average increase in lifetime earnings of $17,500 per student. When offset against potential increased bus transportation costs of up to $1,950 over the student's school career, a 9:1 benefit-to-cost ratio for later start times is seen (Edwards, 2012; Jacob & Rockoff, 2011). Given that children from families with lower socio-economic status (SES) obtain less sleep and have more erratic sleep–wake schedules than peers from higher SES families (Marco et al., 2012), it is perhaps not surprising that improvements in test scores were twice as high in disadvantaged students (Edwards, 2012). Since insufficient sleep places adolescents at greater risk for behavioural disorders, academic difficulties, and physical illness, the economic benefits of later school start times are likely to be much greater.

Barriers to change

Despite well-recognized benefits of delaying bell times, most secondary schools continue to require attendance at times incompatible with healthy sleep. In the United States alone, over 85% of secondary schools begin the day before 8.30 a.m., contrary to recommendations from the American Academy of Pediatrics (AAP) and other health and educational leaders. The average start time for US high schools is 7.59 a.m., with 46.2% starting before 8 a.m., and over 10% before 7.30 a.m., meaning that wake-up and commute times are considerably earlier (National Center for Education Statistics, 2015). There is no indication that these hours are improving either in the United States (Wheaton et al., 2016) or overseas, suggesting that sleep science and empirical data studies have thus far been insufficient grounds for reform, even accounting for the translation lag that often keeps scientific discoveries from reaching the clinic, the public, or the policymaker in a timely fashion. This reluctance to embrace and implement new public health findings that require behavioural or policy changes is common in the history of public health reform. As social scientists repeatedly find, behaviours and policies rarely change solely on the basis of scientific evidence, but often, and perhaps more strongly, on the basis of emotions and values shaped by reigning social norms.

That remaining barriers to start-time change have deeper social and political roots than scientific roots is clear from the many examples of school leaders and community members who purport to 'understand the science' but who cite one or more, often interchangeable, logistical obstacles. Many of these obstacles, whether warranted or not, reflect understandable fears. Given that many aspects of community life revolve around public school hours—including childcare, sports, and other extracurricular activities, after-school jobs, teacher training, bus costs, and even traffic patterns—speculations naturally arise about how any changes to these hours, whether earlier or later, might impact them. Proposed school schedule changes lead stakeholders to extrapolate shifting classroom schedules into corresponding changes in their personal lives and budgets. The result is often vitriolic public opposition, based on the belief that the logistics and cost of change are intolerable and unjustifiable.

Fuelling this inertia are underlying attitudes towards sleep and, to some extent, teenagers. Many people still see sleep as an issue resolvable through character and individual will rather than a public health matter requiring a systemic solution. Opponents of change argue that teenagers can get enough sleep by 'going to bed earlier' or that parents should stop 'coddling' them and simply yank them out of bed or 'throw cold water on them' to ready them 'for the real world'. Others recognize the need for sleep in babies and younger children, but see sleep as a luxury for adults, with teenagers characterized as smelly, surly, lazy versions of adults. Another common response (often inaccurate) in this cohort is, 'I went to school that early, and I'm just fine'.

The past two decades have seen the accumulation of evidence confirming that this community pushback primarily reflects fear of change and failure of imagination. Virtually every obstacle held up has been proven unfounded or surmountable, as evidenced by the hundreds of districts that have delayed bell times and the many more that have never moved to such early hours at all. The fact that communities push back even when superintendents propose changing bell times to save money or to start classes even earlier also suggests that the real obstacle is change itself. Over the past two decades hundreds of schools have found feasible and affordable ways to run schools at times compatible with adolescent sleep needs and discovered that community life adjusts accordingly (Owens, 2014).

Empirical evidence notwithstanding, objections to change remain politically powerful, particularly in countries such as the United States, where school schedules are considered to be local educational decisions. Educational researchers have called the school start time issue a 'political hot potato', and school officials, even those who privately support bell-time change, know that proposing a schedule change in any direction will generate venomous pushback to the point where their jobs may be threatened. Such awareness of political complications may help explain why initial efforts to change bell times in the 1990s, often initiated by school leaders familiar with sleep research, have led to a huge reluctance, even obstructionist, scaremongering efforts to block change, including citation of overblown costs or 'poison pill' options that help teenagers at the expense of younger students and their families. Fear of political repercussions may also help explain why traditional approaches to start-time change, which assume sleep science will sway school administrators, have largely failed.

Despite these continuing challenges, the fact remains that hundreds of schools have overcome them successfully. Owens et al. (2014) have found a sufficient number of such schools, in fact, to generate a 'blueprint for change' that culls out factors necessary for success. The number one conclusion is that there is no one-size-fits-all approach to delaying bell times. Various commonalities can be found in districts that have changed successfully, however, including a supportive leader within the system, community education, consensus building among stakeholders, and adequate transition time. In addition, most bell-time change thus far has been driven by perceived school performance benefits and cost savings rather than potential health, safety, or satisfaction benefits. The report's most striking conclusion, however, is that school start-time change isn't a matter of evidence, but rather, a matter of priorities and political will.

A blueprint for change

Ensuring developmentally appropriate school hours will require reframing school start times as a fundamental matter of public health, a shift that ultimately rests on shifts in social norms about sleep itself. Without this reframing, most communities will continue to treat school hours as negotiable school budget items, leaving what amounts to a public health decision in the hands of local educators and forcing school officials to balance healthy sleep against other pressing needs such as instructional materials and teacher salaries. This political quagmire dissolves once sleep and school start times are regarded as matters of public health, and running schools at unhealthy hours becomes as inconceivable as not heating them in sub-zero temperatures or not removing asbestos from their walls.

Even with attitudinal shifts, however, policy changes are more easily accomplished in certain political and educational contexts, including that of private institutions, which are typically at greater liberty to make radical changes than are government-run schools. Thus, in the UK, several independent schools have shifted relatively easily to mid-morning class times for teenagers; the most extreme of these shifts is Surrey's Hampton Court House School, which in 2014 started running classes for older students from 1.30 p.m. to 7 p.m. In an even more extreme example, Venezuela's Hugo Chávez solved the problem of students going to school in the dark by ordering that the entire country move its clocks back by half an hour. In countries such as the United States with highly decentralized education systems, however, addressing the school start time problem beyond a piecemeal approach may require creative solutions that question assumptions about the way schools are run, including consideration of longer or shorter school days, year-round schooling, distance learning, and alternative transportation models. In most places, large-scale school start time change will also require a multi-pronged approach that goes beyond stockpiling and disseminating evidence. As in most public health reform, a diversity of players at local, state, and national levels will have to push policy and change social norms from above as well as influence behaviours and beliefs from below.

Community education and grassroots activism, together with position statements, legislation, and potentially litigation, are all likely to play a role and are already well under way. A growing number of health, education, and civic organizations have issued resolutions on sleep and school start times, including the AAP, American Medical Association (AMA), the US Centers for Disease Control and Prevention (CDC), Education Commission of the States, American Thoracic Society, Society of Pediatric Nurses, National Association of School Nurses, National Parent Teacher Association, American Academy of Sleep Medicine, Society of Behavioral Medicine, and National Education Association (Adolescent Sleep Working Group, 2014; Start School Later, 2016). These statements, most notably the AMA's and AAP's position that middle and high schools start class no earlier than 8.30 a.m., have played an enormous role in legitimizing the issue. Several US states have also recently passed school start time legislation, beginning with Maryland's 2014 passage of a bill requiring the state health department to conduct a study on student sleep needs and school start times. New Jersey passed similar legislation the following year, commissioning a study by the state education department. In 2016, Maryland enacted the Orange Ribbon Bill for Healthy School Hours, a voluntary, no-cost, incentive programme that recognized districts for implementing evidence-based school hours.

Finally, social media has changed the playing field for the research, health, and advocacy communities alike, potentially accelerating the change process. More accessible, affordable, and efficient communication tools are uniting the local advocacy groups that have arisen sporadically since the 1990s with health professionals, sleep researchers, educators, and policymakers. The emergence of the non-profit organization Start School Later, which uses social media to unite stakeholders and to serve as an information clearinghouse, signals an increasingly sustainable and deliberate approach to the issue. Health professionals and sleep scientists are increasingly seizing on this infrastructure and growing media interest in the topic, serving as expert resources, modelling and mentoring behaviours, and raising awareness via social and traditional media to reform cultural attitudes about sleep and, ultimately, shape policies compatible with healthy hours in the classroom and beyond.

Summary

◆ Early school bell times, combined with a biological delay in sleep–wake times and social pressures during puberty, make obtaining sufficient and optimally timed sleep difficult for most adolescents, potentially impacting physical and emotional wellbeing, safety, and academic performance.

◆ Delaying school start times can effectively counter chronic insufficient sleep in adolescents, as well as enhance health, safety, and school success.

◆ Empirical data have played a smaller role in influencing school hours than social and political factors such as fear of change, failure of imagination, and ignorance about sleep.

◆ Reframing school start times as a public health issue may be required to change social norms about sleep and help communities overcome obstacles that prevent sleep science from being translated into public policy.

References

Adolescent Sleep Working Group; Committee on Adolescence; Council on School Health. 2014. Policy statement: school start times for adolescents. *Pediatrics*, **134**(3), pp. 642–9.

Carskadon, M. A., Harvey, K., Duke, P., Anders, T. F., Litt, I. F. & Dement, W. C. 1980. Pubertal changes in daytime sleepiness. *Sleep*, **19**, pp. 453–60.

Carskadon, M. A., Wolfson, A. R., Acebo, C., Tzischinsky, O. & Seifer, R. 1998. Adolescent sleep patterns, circadian timing, and sleepiness at a transition to early school days. *Sleep*, **21**(8), pp. 871–81.

Danner, F. & Phillips, B. 2009. Adolescent sleep, school start times, and teen motor vehicle crashes. *Journal of Clinical Sleep Medicine*, **4**, pp. 533–5.

Edwards, F. 2012. Early to rise? The effect of daily start times on academic performance. *Economics of Education Review* **31**(6), 970–983.

Hafner, M., Stepanek, M. & Troxel, W. 2017. *Later school start times in the U.S.: an economic analysis.* [Online]. Santa Monica, CA: RAND Corporation. [Accessed 10 February 2018]. Available from: https://www.rand.org/pubs/research_reports/RR2109.html

Iglowstein, I., Jenni, O. G., Molinari, L. & Largo, R. H. 2003. Sleep duration from infancy to adolescence: reference values and generational trends. *Pediatrics*, **111**(2), pp. 302–7.

Jacob, B. A. & Rockoff, J. E. 2011. *Organizing schools to improve student achievement: start times, grade configurations, and teacher assignments* (Hamilton Report Policy Brief 2011-08). Hamilton Report. [Online]. Washington, DC: The Brookings Institution. [Accessed 1 January 2018]. Available from: https://www.brookings.edu/wp-content/uploads/2016/06/092011_organize_jacob_rockoff_brief.pdf

Keyes, K. M., Maslowsky, J., Hamilton, A. & Schulenberg, J. 2015. The great sleep recession: changes in sleep duration among US adolescents, 1991–2012. *Pediatrics*, **135**(3), pp. 460–8.

Ludden, A. & Wolfson, A. R. 2010. Understanding adolescent caffeine use: connecting use patterns with expectancies, reasons, and sleep. *Health Education and Behavior*, **37**(3), pp. 330–42.

Marco, C. A., Wolfson, A. R., Sparling, M. & Azuaje, A. 2012. Family socioeconomic status and sleep pattern of young adolescents. *Behavioral Sleep Medicine*, **10**(1), pp. 70–80.

National Center for Education Statistics. 2015. *Characteristic of Public Elementary and Secondary Schools in the United States: results from the 2016–16 National Teacher and Principal Survey.* [Online]. [Accessed 10 February 2018]. Available from: https://nces.ed.gov/pubs2017/2017071.pdf

National Sleep Foundation. 2006. Sleep in America Poll. *Teens and sleep.* [Online]. [Accessed 1 January 2018]. Available from: https://sleepfoundation.org/sleep-polls-data/sleep-in-america-poll/2006-teens-and-sleep

Owens, J., Drobnich, D., Baylor, A. & Lewin, D. 2014. School start time change: an in-depth examination of school districts in the United States. *Mind, Brain, and Education*, **8**(4), pp. 182–213.

Start School Later. 2016. *Position statements and resolutions on sleep and school start times.* [Online]. [Accessed 1 January 2018]. Available from: http://www.startschoollater.net/position-statements.html

Wahlstrom, K. 2002. Changing times: findings from the first longitudinal study of later high school start times. *NASSP Bulletin*, **86**(633), pp. 3–21.

Troxel, W. & Wolfson, A.R. eds. (2017). The intersection between sleep science and policy: introduction to the special issue on school start times. *Sleep Health*, 3(6), pp. 419–22.

Wahlstrom, K., Dretzke, B., Gordon, M., Peterson, K, Edwards, K. & Gdula, J. 2014. Examining the impact of later school start times on the health and academic performance of high school students: a multi-site study. [Online]. The University of Minnesota Digital Conservancy. [Accessed 1 January 2018]. Available from: http://conservancy.umn.edu/handle/11299/162769

Wheaton, A. G., Chapman, D. P. & Croft, J. B. 2016. School start times, sleep, behavioral, health, and academic outcomes: a review of the literature. *Journal of School Health*, **86**(5), pp. 363–81.

Wolfson, A. R. & Carskadon, M. A. 1998. Sleep schedules and daytime functioning in adolescents. *Society for Research in Child Development*, **69**(4), pp. 875–87.

Wolfson, A. R., Spaulding, N., Dandrow, C. & Baroni, E. 2007. Early versus late starting middle schools: the importance of a good night's sleep for young adolescents. *Behavioral Sleep Medicine*, **5**, pp. 194–209.

Chapter 25

Sleep, law, and public policy[a]

Clark J. Lee and Shantha M. W. Rajaratnam

Introduction

Individuals experiencing drowsiness[b] or poor sleep health[c] are hazardous to themselves and to anyone with whom they come into contact. This is particularly true for persons who operate heavy machinery in a public setting (e.g. driving a car) or whose decisions have potentially life-threatening consequences for others (e.g. a medical practitioner making a decision about a patient). Thus, drowsiness and poor sleep health in individuals have population-wide impacts which societies often feel compelled to address as a matter of law and public policy. This chapter introduces some examples of how governmental entities, multinational organizations, and non-governmental regulatory bodies around the world have used law and public policy to address some public health and safety hazards related to drowsiness and poor sleep health in individuals.

Addressing drowsiness and poor sleep health in society

Drowsiness and poor sleep health in individuals and populations

Drowsiness and poor sleep health adversely impact a person's cognitive performance (Whitney et al., 2015) and cause attentional failures (Lockley et al., 2004), which compromise personal and public health and safety (Landrigan et al., 2004). Researchers have identified numerous factors that contribute to drowsiness and poor sleep health in individuals, and general knowledge about the long-term health outcomes of healthy sleep and chronic sleep restriction is ever expanding (Buysse, 2014; Lockley et al, 2006; Luyster et al, 2012). Based on this knowledge, it is possible to identify groups within a population that are more likely to be affected by drowsiness and poor sleep health and consequently pose significant risks to personal and public health and safety. Examples of such groups include adolescents; workers in jobs requiring extended duration duty or shift-work schedules, including duty during night-time hours; and persons with sleep disorders.

Drowsiness and poor sleep health impact not only the health and safety of individuals in 'high-risk' groups within a population, but also that of others in the population. Given the multi-factorial contributors to drowsiness and poor sleep health in society, multi-faceted prevention strategies targeting high-risk individuals and entire populations are required to address the health and safety hazards posed by these societal ills. The successful development and implementation of such strategies often necessitate the involvement of governments, multinational organizations, and non-governmental regulatory bodies.

Role of government: legal and policy interventions

Governments are responsible for ensuring the health and safety of the people they govern. In fulfilling this responsibility, governments often develop and implement legal and policy interventions to address myriad health and safety issues in the populations they serve (Hodge et al., 2015). Conceptually, legal interventions and policy interventions are closely related because legal interventions are usually designed to operationalize the public policy decisions of governmental entities. Legal interventions can take numerous forms, including statutes and other legislation enacted by legislative bodies, executive orders issued by governmental chief executives, regulations promulgated and enforced by government administrative agencies, and litigation in the courts. Although policy interventions are often implemented through legal interventions, they may also be operationalized by the way governmental entities implement legal interventions.

Both legal and policy interventions may influence the behaviour of all individuals in a population, or individuals in targeted groups within a population, through direct or indirect mechanisms. Thus, law and public policy can be used to operationalize and implement both population and high-risk strategies of preventive medicine to address public health and safety issues affecting society. These strategies may involve multi-faceted, synergistic approaches that combine official government regulation of certain private, public, and occupational activities with non-regulatory approaches (e.g. public awareness and education campaigns) and private sector self-regulation.

Addressing drowsiness and poor sleep health through law and public policy

Governments, multinational organizations, and non-governmental regulatory bodies worldwide have recognized drowsiness and poor sleep health as public health and safety issues that societies need to address as a matter of public policy. Consequently, these entities have adopted legal and policy interventions to address the various health and safety impacts on individuals and populations associated with drowsiness and poor sleep health in society (Jones et al., 2013; Lee et al., 2013). Typically, these interventions target intra-personal, social, and environmental factors that contribute to drowsiness and poor sleep health in society. This section briefly introduces examples of such interventions developed for the general motoring public, workers in safety-critical jobs or occupations requiring unusual work hours or extended duration duty, and adolescent pupils.[d]

Drowsy driving prevention in the general motoring public

Drowsy driving is a hazard on roadways around the world which endangers drowsy drivers and the motorists sharing the road with them. Governments worldwide have adopted legal and policy interventions to address drowsy driving in the general motoring public and in high-risk groups for this risky driving behaviour. Several such interventions adopted in the United States are illustrative of those adopted in other countries.

Anti-drowsy driving policy and legislation

Policymakers throughout the United States have acted to address drowsy driving on American roadways. In February 2003, legislation was introduced in the US House of Representatives to encourage state efforts to educate the public and law enforcement officials on various aspects of drowsy driving and to improve police reporting of motor vehicle crashes related to drowsy driving.[1] Although not enacted into law, this proposed federal legislation has served as a model for subsequent drowsy driving legislation introduced in various US states, where most legal and policy interventions against drowsy driving in the United States have been implemented.

Several states have proposed or enacted legislation that legally prohibits drowsy driving in the general motoring public. New Jersey[2] and Arkansas[3] have enacted legislation that explicitly addresses drowsy driving in their criminal vehicular homicide laws. Other states have considered legislation that directly regulates drowsy driving in non-commercial drivers by defining drowsy driving behaviour, specifying legally prohibited conduct related to drowsy driving behaviour (*e.g.* drowsy driving resulting in serious injury or death to another person) and the legal consequences for engaging in such conduct (e.g. administrative, civil, and criminal sanctions), and identifying individuals or situations (e.g. emergency responders during catastrophic events) that are exempt from these legal prohibitions (Jones et al., 2010). Massachusetts has considered legislation relating to the role of the state's law enforcement officials and driver licensing authorities in preventing drowsy driving on public roadways.[4,5]

US states have also used legislation to reduce drowsy driving incidence on public roadways indirectly. For example, Virginia has enacted a statute prohibiting a person from driving more than 13 hours in a 24-hour period, thereby indirectly regulating drowsy driving in non-commercial drivers on Virginia roadways.[6] In addition, state graduated driver-licensing laws in the United States typically prohibit under-age novice drivers from driving at night while unsupervised by a parent or legal guardian. This legal restriction on night-time driving is designed to reduce the risk of sleep-related accidents involving teenage drivers, who are particularly susceptible to being involved in such accidents (Pack et al., 1995). Evidence of the effectiveness of such provisions in reducing motor vehicle crashes in teenage drivers has been reported (Rajaratnam et al., 2015). Furthermore, some states have taken legislative action to designate a day or week of awareness regarding drowsy driving[7] or to establish special commissions[8] to study various aspects of drowsy driving and to generate recommendations for addressing drowsy driving as a matter of state public policy.

Anti-drowsy driving litigation

In jurisdictions that have not enacted laws specifically addressing drowsy driving, courts have applied existing statutes and legal precedents to situations involving drowsy drivers.

For example, an appellate court in the US state of Maryland upheld the vehicular manslaughter conviction of a drowsy driver based on evidence that the driver behaved in a 'grossly negligent' manner when he deliberately ignored the risk of falling asleep at the wheel and continued to drive despite dozing off repeatedly and recognizing that he was extremely drowsy while driving.[9] By contrast, the High Court of Australia quashed the culpable driving (i.e. vehicular manslaughter) conviction of a driver who experienced no premonitory symptoms of drowsiness before apparently falling asleep while driving and causing a fatal crash.[10] In this case, the Court reasoned that this particular driver was not acting in a conscious or voluntary manner at the time of the fatal crash and so could not be legally required to be held criminally responsible for his conduct. After articulating the factors required to be taken into account to obtain a culpable driving conviction against a drowsy driver under Australian law, the Court concluded that these factors had not been met in this case (Tasmania Law Reform Institute, 2010).

While governments may criminally prosecute a drowsy driver whose conduct harms others, parties injured by a drowsy driver may pursue civil litigation to remedy harms they have suffered as a result of a drowsy driver's conduct. The most basic example of such litigation would be a personal injury lawsuit filed by the victim of a drowsy driving crash against the drowsy driver who caused the crash. In such a lawsuit, the victim might use tort law principles of negligence to hold the driver civilly liable for the victim's injury and to obtain compensation or other types of relief from the driver. To achieve this outcome, the victim would allege that the driver owed the victim a legal duty to operate a motor vehicle with due care, that the driver breached this duty by knowingly operating a motor vehicle while drowsy, that this breach of duty caused the victim's injuries, and that the victim suffered a loss as a result of these injuries.

If the drowsy driver was driving while in the course of his or her employment at the time of the crash, as would be the case for commercial transport drivers, an injured party may also pursue civil redress from the driver's employer. One mechanism permitting such recoveries from employers is the vicarious liability doctrine of *respondeat superior*, under which an employer is held liable for the tortious actions or omissions of its employees committed during the course, or 'within the scope', of their employment. However, because work commutes are considered to be outside an employee's scope of employment, an injured party could not use *respondeat superior* to recover from a drowsy driver's employer if the injury-causing accident occurred during the drowsy driver's commute to or from work.

An alternative mechanism for obtaining civil redress from employers of drowsy drivers would be to argue that the employer acted negligently in a way that allowed its employee to drive drowsily on a public roadway, and that the employer therefore should be held directly liable for the resultant injuries to the victim. This is the legal theory that the American comedian Tracy Morgan adopted in his recently settled lawsuit against Wal-Mart for injuries he sustained in a crash with a lorry driven by a drowsy Wal-Mart employee.[11] Theoretically, this approach allows victims of drowsy driving accidents to recover compensation from the employers of drowsy drivers even if the crash occurred during the driver's work commute. Although courts in some US states have permitted drowsy driving victims to recover from the employers of commuting drowsy drivers using this direct liability approach,[12,13] most US state courts have declined to do so (Bowen, 1996; Ingham, 2010).

Litigation arising from drowsy driving incidents can indirectly affect health and safety in society. Highly publicized prosecutions and lawsuits of drowsy drivers may deter individuals from engaging in drowsy driving behaviour. The threat of litigation may also prompt employers to develop and implement policies for their workers relating to work schedules, occupational fatigue management, and commuting after long shifts. Such responses to litigation arguably impact the health and safety of individual drivers and the motoring public in a population.

Work-related drowsiness

Workplace drowsiness is widely recognized as a significant occupational health hazard for many workers, especially those in jobs or professions requiring extended hours; shift-work schedules, including night work and rotating shifts; early morning hours; or safety-critical tasks to be performed immediately after waking (Geiger-Brown et al., 2013). When drowsy, such workers may also threaten the health and safety of others with whom they come into contact. Legal and policy interventions pertaining to hours of service (HOS), occupational health and safety (OH&S), and occupational sleep disorders screening have been adopted worldwide to address the hazards of work-related drowsiness in these groups of high-risk workers.

Hours of service regulations

HOS regulations adopted in several countries limit the number of work hours and prescribe minimum rest periods for commercial transport workers on land, sea, and air, as well as for workers in safety-critical occupations and industries such as health care (Geiger-Brown et al., 2013; Jones et al., 2013; Lee et al., 2013). Some HOS regulations also specify exceptions to the work hour restrictions and rest period requirements normally in effect. These regulations are most often adopted by government administrative agencies at a national or state level, although some jurisdictions have issued HOS regulations through legislation for certain occupations or by leaving the issue to be addressed through the normal industrial relations or collective bargaining mechanisms present in those jurisdictions (Geiger-Brown et al., 2013; Institute of Medicine (IOM), 2009).

Multinational organizations and non-governmental regulatory bodies have also adopted HOS regulations. For example, the European Working Time Directive (EWTD) requires all European Union member states to enact legal limitations on working time arrangements in all sectors of their respective economies, with some exceptions.[14] The EWTD reflects international norms on working time and represents a society-wide legal approach to addressing worker health and safety (Jones et al., 2010). Furthermore, the accrediting organization for US graduate medical education programmes has adopted HOS restrictions in its accreditation standards for US residency programmes, in part to avoid direct government regulation of HOS for resident physicians (IOM, 2009).

Occupational health and safety laws

Governments around the world have adopted OH&S laws to protect the health and safety of their working population, and some such laws address drowsiness in workers (Geiger-Brown et al., 2013; Jones et al., 2013). Some OH&S laws impose affirmative legal duties on workers and employers in certain occupations to mitigate or reduce the personal and public health and safety hazards that arise from work-related drowsiness.[15] OH&S laws may also be designed to target workers at high risk of suffering a drowsiness-related injury because of an undiagnosed sleep disorder. For example, an OH&S law could require workers in certain occupations who meet certain clinical criteria to undergo mandatory screening for and treatment of sleep disorders.[16]

Workers' compensation and disability law

Like drowsy driving, work-related drowsiness and its associated hazards can be addressed through litigation. As mentioned in 'Anti-drowsy driving litigation', employers may act to minimize drowsiness in their workers to avoid potential tort litigation with victims of drowsiness-related incidents caused by their employees. Additional motivation for employers to take such action is the threat of workers' compensation claims and disputes involving employees injured by work-related drowsiness incidents (Jones et al., 2013).

Litigation threats may also motivate employers to accommodate the needs of their employees with sleep disorders. Under the Americans with Disabilities Act of 1990 (ADA),[17] employers are prohibited from discriminating against their employees on the basis of a disability. Such discrimination includes failing to make 'reasonable accommodations to the known physical or mental limitations' of an otherwise qualified employee with a disability, unless such accommodation would impose an undue hardship on the employer's business operations. Because people with sleep disorders or other conditions causing sleep loss arguably have a disability as defined by the ADA (Jones et al., 2013), a worker with such a disorder or condition might have an ADA legal claim against an employer who fails to make reasonable accommodations in scheduling night work or extended duration duty.

School start times

Growing recognition of the adverse health and safety consequences arising from the lack of synchronization between the early school start times and circadian rhythms of adolescent pupils in many jurisdictions has spurred efforts around the world to implement later school start times for adolescents as a matter of public policy (Kelley et al., 2015). These efforts have ranged from school scheduling decisions of local school districts to proposed legislation at state and national levels mandating that schools start after a certain time for adolescent pupils. The medical and public health communities have endorsed these policies and legal interventions intended to promote good sleep health and academic performance in this vulnerable segment of the population (Adolescent Sleep Working Group et al., 2014; Wheaton et al., 2015).

Directions for future research and intervention

The legal and policy interventions discussed in this chapter have not been a panacea for every health and safety issue related to drowsiness and poor sleep health in society. Designing and implementing such interventions involve challenges such as limits on regulatory and jurisdictional authority, industry-specific demands, public awareness, and the inability of any single intervention to account for every effect and aspect of drowsiness and poor sleep health. Furthermore, the efficacy and effectiveness of such interventions on health and safety have rarely been evaluated using rigorous research methods, with some exceptions that have focused primarily on HOS regulations for certain types of workers (IOM, 2009; Mansfield & Kryger, 2015). One significant challenge has been the lack of well-established methods for conducting such evaluations, as public health law research, legal epidemiology, and policy surveillance are relatively new fields that are still developing their methodologies (Burris et al., 2010, 2016; Presley et al., 2015). As these fields continue to mature, more tools should become available to evaluate legal and policy interventions in all areas of public health so that appropriate actions can be taken by the appropriate stakeholders to maintain and improve existing interventions and to inform future interventions.

In the meantime, opportunities exist to improve current legal and policy interventions addressing drowsiness and sleep health in society. For example, policymakers might convene a multidisciplinary team of experts to review existing laws and policies; identify strengths and areas for improvement in the way they are written or implemented; and recommend follow-up actions, including possible amendments to existing law and policy based on the best sleep science and field practices available. Opportunities also exist for research to inform the development of better legal and policy interventions in order to address drowsiness and poor sleep health. For example, any legal or policy intervention aimed at addressing drowsiness which is not based on prescriptive work hour limitations would need to be accompanied by some method of assessing impairment or impairment probability due to drowsiness (Jones et al., 2010). The search for a 'breathalyzer for drowsiness' provides scientists and entrepreneurs with exciting opportunities to innovate for the benefit of society.

Summary

- Drowsiness and poor sleep health in individuals have population-wide impacts which societies often feel compelled to address as a matter of law and public policy.

- Governments, multinational organizations, and non-governmental regulatory bodies worldwide have adopted legal and policy interventions to address the various health and safety impacts on individuals and populations associated with drowsiness and poor sleep health in society.

- Given the multi-factorial contributors to drowsiness and poor sleep health in society, effective legal and policy interventions must adopt multi-faceted prevention strategies at the intra-personal, social, and environmental levels of society.

◆ More research is required to evaluate the efficacy and effectiveness of existing legal and policy interventions addressing drowsiness and poor sleep health in society and to inform future interventions.

Acknowledgements

The authors acknowledge Christopher B. Jones, LLB, PhD, lead author of the first edition of this chapter, who regrettably was unable to contribute to this chapter update.

Notes

a. The contents of this chapter should not be construed as legal advice in any way and should be used strictly for informational purposes only. Readers should consult with appropriate legal counsel for formal legal advice.

b. In this chapter, *drowsiness* is used to refer to the likelihood of falling asleep. This meaning does not extend to concepts associated with muscular exertion or to chronic fatigue syndrome. The reader should be aware that in some circumstances, including legislation or other sources of law or policy, other terms are used to describe drowsiness (*e.g.* 'sleepiness,' 'fatigue,' 'tiredness'), and specific definitions for these terms may be provided that restrict or expand the definition used in this chapter.

c. In this chapter, the term *sleep health* means 'a multidimensional pattern of sleep-wakefulness, adapted to individual, social, and environmental demands, that promotes physical and mental well-being.' Furthermore, the term *poor sleep health* means the opposite of 'good sleep health,' which is characterized by 'subjective satisfaction, appropriate timing, adequate duration, high efficiency, and sustained alertness during waking hours' (Buysse, 2014, p. 12).

d. Most of the legal and policy interventions discussed in this section come from countries that have adopted the common law legal system (*e.g.* U.S. and Australia) rather than the civil law tradition (*e.g.* Continental Europe).

Legal References

1. Maggie's Law: National Drowsy Driving Act of 2003, H.R. 968, 108th Cong. (2003).

2. 2003 N.J. Laws *c.*143, § 1 (codified as amended at N.J. STAT. ANN. § 2C:11-5(a) (2015)).

3. 2013 Ark. Acts 1296 (codified as amended at ARK. CODE ANN. § 5-10-105 (2014)).

4. S. 2072, 185th Gen. Ct., 2007-2008 Sess. (Mass. 2008), §§ 2–5, 8–9 and 12.

5. S. 2124, 184th Gen. Ct., 2005-2006 Sess. (Mass. 2005), §§ 2–5, 8–9 and 12.

6. VA. CODE ANN. § 46.2–812.

7. 2010 Fla. Laws ch. 223, § 48 (codified as amended at FLA. STAT. § 683.332 (2010)).

8. 2006 Mass. Acts ch. 428, § 26.

9. Skidmore v. State, 887 A.2d 92, 97 (Md. Ct. Spec. App. 2005).

10. Jiminez v. The Queen (1992) 173 C.L.R. 572 (Austl.).

11. Complaint, Morgan v. Wal-Mart Stores, Inc., No. 3:14-cv-04388-MAS-LHG (D.N.J. July 10, 2014).

12. Robertson v. LeMaster, 301 S.E.2d 563 (W.V. 1983).

13. Faverty v. McDonald's Restaurants of Oregon, Inc., 892 P.2d 703 (Or. App. 1995), *appeal dismissed*, 971 P.2d 407 (Or. 1998).

14. Council Directive 93/104/EC (23 Nov. 1993), 1993 O.J. (L 307) 18, *amended by* Directive 2000/34/ EC (22 June 2000), 2000 O.J. (L 195) 41, *replaced by* Directive 2003/88/EC (4 Nov. 2003), 2003 O.J. (L 299) 9.

15. National Transport Commission (Model Legislation—Heavy Vehicle Driver Fatigue) Regulations 2007, Fed. Reg. Legis. Instruments F2007L03869 (26 Sept. 2007).

16. Pub. L. No. 113-45, 127 Stat. 557 (2013).

17. Pub. L. No. 101-336, 104 Stat. 327 (1990), *amended by* ADA Amendments Act of 2008, Pub. L. No.110-325, 122 Stat. 3553 (2008) (codified as amended at 42 U.S.C. § 12101 to 12213).

References

Adolescent Sleep Working Group; Committee on Adolescence & Council on School Health. 2014. School start times for adolescents. *Pediatrics*, **134**(3), pp. 642–9.

Bowen, G. P. 1996. Wherein lies the duty? Determining employer liability for the actions of fatigued employees commuting from work. *Wayne Law Review*, **42**, pp. 2091–115.

Burris, S., Ashe, M., Levin, D., Penn, M. & Larkin, M. 2016. A transdisciplinary approach to public health law: the emerging practice of legal epidemiology. *Annual Review of Public Health*, **37**, 135–48.

Burris, S., Wagenaar, A. C., Swanson, J., Ibrahim, J. K., Wood, J. & Mello, M. M. 2010 Making the case for laws that improve health: a framework for public health law research. *Milbank Quarterly*, **88**(2), pp. 169–210.

Buysse, D. J. 2014. Sleep health: can we define it? Does it matter? *Sleep*, **37**(1), pp. 9–17.

Geiger-Brown, J. M., Lee, C. J. & Trinkoff, A. M. 2013. The role of work schedules in occupational health and safety. In: Gatchel, R. J. & Schultz, I. Z. eds. *Handbook of Occupational Health and Wellness*. New York: Springer, pp. 297–322.

Hodge, J. G., Weidenaar, K., Baker-White, A., Barraza, L., Bauerly, B. C., Corbett, A., Davis, C., Frey, L. T., Griest, M. M., Healy, C., Krueger, J., Lowrey, K. M. & Tilburg, W. 2015. Legal innovations to advance a culture of health. *The Journal of Law, Medicine & Ethics*, **43**(4), pp. 904–12.

Ingham, G. W. 2010. Another drink, another hour: using dram shop liability to determine employer liability for injuries caused by fatigued commuting employees. *George Mason Law Review*, **17**, pp. 565–92.

Institute of Medicine. 2009. *Resident Duty Hours: Enhancing Sleep, Supervision, and Safety*. Washington, DC: The National Academies Press.

Jones, C. B., Lee, C. J. & Rajaratnam, S. M. W. 2010. Sleep, law, and policy. In: Cappuccio, F. P., Miller, M. A. & Lockley, S. W. eds. *Sleep, Health, and Society: from aetiology to public health*. Oxford: Oxford University Press, pp. 417–34.

Jones, C. B., Lee, C. J. & Rajaratnam, S. M. W. 2013. Legal implications of sleep loss. In: Kushida, C. A. ed. *Encyclopedia of Sleep*. Waltham, MA: Academic Press, pp. 335–42.

Kelley, P., Lockley, S. W., Foster, R. G. & Kelley, J. 2015. Synchronizing education to adolescent biology: 'let teens sleep, start school later'. *Learning, Media and Technology*, **40**(2), pp. 210–26.

Landrigan, C. P., Rothschild, J. M., Cronin, J. W., Kaushal, R., Burdick, E., Katz, J. T., Lilly, C. M., Stone, P. H., Lockley, S. W., Bates, D. W. & Czeisler, C. A. 2004. Effect of reducing interns' work hours on serious medical errors in intensive care units. *New England Journal of Medicine*, **351**(18), pp. 1838–48.

Lee, C. J., Sanna, R. A. & Czeisler, C. A. 2013. Public policy, sleep science, and sleep medicine. In: Kushida, C. A. ed. *Encyclopedia of Sleep*. Waltham, MA: Academic Press, pp. 156–66.

Lockley, S. W., Cronin, J. W., Evans, E. E., Cade, B. E., Lee, C. J., Landrigan, C. P., Rothschild, J. M., Katz, J. T., Lilly, C. M., Stone, P. H., Aeschbach, D. & Czeisler, C. A. 2004. Effect of reducing interns' weekly work hours on sleep and attentional failures. *New England Journal of Medicine,* **351**(18), pp. 1829–37.

Lockley, S. W., Landrigan, C. P., Barger, L. K. & Czeisler, C. A. 2006. When policy meets physiology: the challenge of reducing resident work hours. *Clinical Orthopaedics and Related Research,* **449**, pp. 116–27.

Luyster, F. S., Strollo Jr., P. J., Zee, P. C. & Walsh, J. K. 2012. Sleep: a health imperative. *Sleep,* **35**(6), pp. 727–34.

Mansfield, D. & Kryger, M. 2015. Regulating danger on the highways: hours of service regulations. *Sleep Health,* **1**(4), pp. 311–13.

Pack, A. I., Pack, A. M., Rodgman, E., Cucchiara, A., Dinges, D. F. & Schwab, C. W. 1995. Characteristics of crashes attributed to the driver having fallen asleep. *Accident Analysis and Prevention,* **27**(6), pp. 769–75.

Presley, D., Reinstein, T., Webb-Barr, D. & Burris, S. 2015. Creating legal data for public health monitoring and evaluation: Delphi standards for policy surveillance. *The Journal of Law, Medicine & Ethics,* **43**(suppl.1), pp. 27–31.

Rajaratnam, S. M. W., Landrigan, C. P., Wang, W., Kaprielian, R., Moore, R. T. & Czeisler, C. A. 2015. Teen crashes declined after Massachusetts raised penalties for graduated licensing law restricting night driving. *Health Affairs,* **34**(6), pp. 963–70.

Tasmania Law Reform Institute. 2010. *Criminal Liability of Drivers Who Fall Asleep Causing Motor Vehicle Crashes Resulting in Death or Other Serious Injury: Jiminez.* [Final Report No. 13]. Hobart, Tas.: Tasmania Law Reform Institute.

Wheaton, A. G., Ferro, G. A. & Croft, J. B. 2015. School start times for middle school and high school students—United States, 2011–12 School Year. *Morbidity and Mortality Weekly Report,* **64**(30), pp. 809–13.

Whitney, P., Hinson, J. M., Jackson, M. L. & Van Dongen, H. P. A. 2015. Feedback blunting: total sleep deprivation impairs decision making that requires updating based on feedback. *Sleep,* **38**(5), pp. 745–54.

Chapter 26

Narcolepsy: Living with a sleep disorder

Matt O'Neill and Henry Nicholls

Introduction

Awareness of narcolepsy is poor, even among health professionals. Historically, people have gone undiagnosed for decades. More recently, the internet has been a powerful tool for self-diagnosis. Anyone presenting with sleepiness should be asked about signs of cataplexy, a diagnostic symptom that is often underplayed by patients.

Population perspective

There is no right time to develop narcolepsy. The onset is often hard to pinpoint, other than in reflection. It develops most commonly in adolescence or early adulthood, and in some cases in very young children and adults. The descent into a world of sleep is usually the first symptom of narcolepsy (Dauvilliers et al., 2001). The progress can be slow, almost evolutionary, and is easy to write off as a biological stage in young adults or temporary payback for some excess of youth. After a time, however, it is impossible to ignore.

The sleepy feeling is not so very different to that experienced by those without narcolepsy from time to time. The difference for the person with narcolepsy (PWN) is that it is a near-permanent state, the periods of wide-eyed clarity infrequent and fleeting. The overwhelming need to sleep begins to make the basic, daily schedule hard to adhere to, affecting education, employment, relationships, and personal safety (Ingravallo et al., 2012).

Before diagnosis, it is very common for people with narcolepsy to fight the sleepiness, imagining it to be a fleeting phenomenon. There are some tricks that help. Pinching, slapping, head-shaking, singing, and running on the spot are all tried and tested methods for battling the somnolence, though they usually only provide relief for a matter of seconds and are often as inappropriate as sleep itself. A better solution is to go to the toilet and, in the privacy of a cubicle, drift off for a minute or two. If this is not possible, as in the middle of a meeting, there may be nothing for it but to rest head in hands for a moment and close eyes as if in reflection. Without an understanding of what is happening, this experience of battling and losing to sleep is so unpleasant, so stressful, that it is time to seek help from the family doctor.

The diagnosis

Unfortunately, most doctors know little about sleep disorders in general and very little about narcolepsy in particular (Rosemberg & Kim, 2014). Failure to diagnose narcolepsy is very common (Morrish et al., 2004). There are so many possible explanations for too much sleep that many people with narcolepsy will need to fight to be taken seriously, or present the doctor with other symptoms that turn out to be linked to the pathological sleep.

In terms of securing a diagnosis, the most important of these is cataplexy, a state of muscle paralysis triggered by emotions, most commonly laughter, but also by others such as surprise, happiness, sporting elation, orgasm, anger, and grief, sometimes even by particular odours (Overeem et al., 2011). Cataplexy affects the majority of people with narcolepsy, its onset usually occurring alongside or shortly after the first signs of sleepiness. At first, cataplexy manifests as a momentary collapse and recovery of muscles, around the mouth, the neck, the shoulders, the chest, and behind the knees. As with the sleepiness, these first few moments of weakness are noteworthy but not much more. They are easy to conceal. Within a month or two, however, the cataplexy has usually progressed such that an attack will cause the head to fall, chin onto chest, arms flopping to the sides and knees buckling. By the time the person with narcolepsy is falling to the ground in a crumpled heap, it is clear that this is more than just 'feeling weak with laughter'.

Other signs and symptoms

There are other symptoms too, ones that usually begin to show themselves after the sleepiness and the cataplexy. There are fabulous dreams, so cinematic and so visual that they far outshine the most exciting, creative dreams of those without narcolepsy. On the downside, sleep paralysis is very common, affecting many of those with narcolepsy. The experience of waking but being unable to move will often be accompanied by terrifying hallucinations on the way into and out of sleep, hyper-real visions in which a malevolent presence—a witch, the devil, a murderer, a rapist—has entered the bedroom and often climbs onto the sleeper (Cheyne et al., 1999). The struggle to fight the paralysis with the aim of taking on the intruder can last from a few seconds to many minutes. For many people with narcolepsy, it can be the most frightening experience they will ever know. Such experiences are much more likely to occur if the sleeper is lying on his or her back. A touch from a bed partner can be enough to break the paralysis and banish the intruder, but often the vision returns immediately on falling back to sleep. But no amount of repetition dulls the intense, heart-thumping, sweating stress of these profoundly distressing visitors.

These parasomnias—the dreaming, the sleep paralysis, and the hallucinations—may explain the profound irony that most people with narcolepsy have sleep that is so fractured that they also suffer a form of insomnia (Plazzi et al., 2008). This troubled nighttime sleep may help account for the first and best-known symptom of narcolepsy: the irresistable need to sleep during the day.

How to adapt to a lifelong condition

With several symptoms—the sleepiness, cataplexy, sleep paralysis, hypnagogic hallucin-ations, and insomnia—there is a greater chance of an accurate diagnosis. The internet is a great help too, allowing people to make sense of their symptoms far earlier than was possible in the past. A diagnosis, when it comes, is often met with mixed feelings. There is the relief of finally having an explanation for the disabling sleepiness, the perplexing cataplexy, and the horrifying parasomnias. As yet, however, there is no way of repairing the brain damage that underlies narcolepsy, so being diagnosed with this condition even-tually leads to the realization that this is a defining and lifelong condition.

For those fortunate enough to have a tolerant, accommodating employer, regular work remains a possibility. A short nap of just 5 or 10 minutes may, for some, be sufficient to provide some immediate relief from the oppression. It is important to recognize, though, that narcolepsy is a spectrum disorder and that napping strategies do not work effectively for those at the upper end of the spectrum. Sadly, narcolepsy is still seen by many as lazi-ness rather than the profoundly disabling condition that it undoubtedly is. Under these circumstances, the stress of trying to function profitably can lead many to seek refuge in self-employment. While this gives the person with narcolepsy the freedom to sleep as ne-cessary without prejudice, it can contribute to a growing sense of isolation that many feel in the years after diagnosis.

Sleep, by definition, is an absence of consciousness, so too much sleep during the day can lead to a feeling that you've missed out on social interactions. In addition, those PWN with cataplexy learn to avoid the social, humorous situations most likely to trigger a collapse. People often report difficulties with memory. Subtle changes in metabolism mean that many PWN put on weight (Poli et al., 2009), adding to a lack of self-esteem, a risk of depression, and, in rare cases, suicidal thoughts.

Narcolepsy in children

Narcolepsy can be particularly damaging for young children. In 2009 and 2010, the wide-spread use of Pandemrix—a vaccine produced by GlaxoSmithKline to protect against a perceived swine flu pandemic—was associated with caused a significant increase in the incidence of narcolepsy among the young children targeted with vaccination (Nohynek et al., 2012). With all the difficulties faced by adults, plus an increased prevalence of pre-cocious puberty (Poli et al., 2013), the challenges that this can pose for children are im-mense and could have lifelong consequences unless their needs are properly addressed.

Drugs can help

In spite of these difficulties, there are several drugs that may be able to control the worst of the symptoms. For the sleepiness, doctors are likely to prescribe a stimulant such as modafinil, Ritalin, or Dexedrine. A small dose of a tricyclic antidepressant, such as clomipramine, imipramine, or protriptyline, or the serotonin-noradrenaline reuptake in-hibitor venlafaxine can help control cataplexy, sleep paralysis, and hallucinations. Sodium oxybate (Xyrem) is used in the United States and elsewhere to improve both sleepiness and cataplexy, but it is not currently widely available through the National Health Service in the UK. Interestingly, what works for one person with narcolepsy might do nothing for another, and most people end up experimenting with a range of different medications in different doses until they come up with a cocktail that works.

With time, medication, and exposure to others with narcolepsy, the person with narcolepsy generally gets used to those symptoms that remain and learns to manage them. What is important here is that to simply state that with medication and 'lifestyle' changes, people with narcolepsy either will, may, or can live either a normal or near-normal life is a fallacy. We are talking about individuals, not statistics, and even within the small field of global experts, there can be a tendency to highlight the relative positives and ignore the many negative aspects of the condition.

This is particularly relevant when it comes to driving. Even within an urban setting, the ability to drive, to be 'somewhere' by a means and time of one's own choosing is extremely important to people with narcolepsy, regardless of age at diagnosis. When judging an individual's ability to drive, the clinician must also consider the socio-economic impact of not being able to drive. For the provisional licence holder this could be the difference between attending college or university and leading a fulfilling independent life—or not. For an adult with late-onset narcolepsy, any withdrawal of a licence can transfer to loss of work, income, and also status within the family group. Outside of major cities and robust transport systems, the impact of being unable to drive means so much more than the driving element itself.

Narcolepsy and the law

It is crucial that those with narcolepsy declare their condition to the relevant authorities (the Driving and Vehicle Licensing Agency (DVLA) in the UK) and go through the proper procedures with respect to a licence. Even if their symptoms are well controlled by medication and a licence is granted, the individual must maintain constant vigilance for signs of sleepiness. In this respect, people with narcolepsy are no different from any other road users, except for one simple truth. Those with narcolepsy understand their condition, tend to take sleep more seriously, and are very aware of their limitations and the need to take rests where appropriate. It is easy to assume that people with narcolepsy are involved in more accidents than those without this sleep disorder, but further studies are required into specific causality data retaining to narcolepsy and driving.

Summary

◆ Narcolepsy is a profoundly disabling neurological disorder that affects around 1 in 2,500 people.

◆ In addition to excessive daytime sleepiness, people with narcolepsy often suffer from cataplexy, sleep paralysis, hypnagogic hallucinations, and disrupted night-time sleep.

- Awareness of these symptoms is low. Currently, the mean delay between onset of symptoms and diagnosis is between 10 and 20 years.

- Narcolepsy can have devastating consequences, resulting in isolation, low self-esteem, depression, and sometimes suicide.

References

Cheyne, J. A., Rueffer, S. D. & Newby-Clark, I. R. 1999. Hypnagogic and hypnopompic hallucinations during sleep paralysis: neurological and cultural construction of the night-mare. *Consciousness and Cognition*, **8**, pp. 319–37.

Dauvilliers, Y., Montplaisir, J., Molinari, N., Carlander, B., Ondze, B., Besset, A. & Billiard, M. 2001. Age at onset of narcolepsy in two large populations of patients in France and Quebec. *Neurology*, **57**, pp. 2029–33.

Ingravallo, F., Gnucci, V., Pizza, F., Vignatelli, L., Govi, A., Dormi, A., Pelotti, S., Cicognani, A., Dauvilliers, Y. & Plazzi, G. 2012. The burden of narcolepsy with cataplexy: how disease history and clinical features influence socio-economic outcomes. *Sleep Medicine*, **13**, pp. 1293–300.

Morrish, E., King, M. A., Smith, I. E. & Shneerson, J. M. 2004. Factors associated with a delay in the diagnosis of narcolepsy. *Sleep Medicine*, **5**, pp. 37–41.

Nohynek, H., Jokinen, J., Partinen, M., Vaarala, O., Kirjavainen, T., Sundman, J., Himanen, S. L., Hublin, C., Julkunen, I., Olsén, P., Saarenpää-Heikkilä, O. & Kilpi, T. 2012. AS03 adjuvanted AH1N1 vaccine associated with an abrupt increase in the incidence of childhood narcolepsy in Finland. *PLoS One*, **7**(3), e33536.

Overeem, S., van Nues, S. J., van der Zande, W. L., Donjacour, C. E., van Mierlo, P. & Lammers, G. J. 2011. The clinical features of cataplexy: a questionnaire study in narcolepsy patients with and without hypocretin-1 deficiency. *Sleep Medicine*, **12**, pp. 12–18.

Plazzi, G., Serra, L. & Ferri, R. 2008. Nocturnal aspects of narcolepsy with cataplexy. *Sleep Medicine Reviews*, **12**, pp. 109–28.

Poli, F., Pizza, F., Mignot, E., Ferri, R., Pagotto, U., Taheri, S., Finotti, E., Bernardi, F., Pirazzoli, P., Cicognani, A., Balsamo, A., Nobili, L., Bruni, O. & Plazzi, G. 2013. High prevalence of precocious puberty and obesity in childhood narcolepsy with cataplexy. *Sleep*, **36**, pp. 175–81.

Poli, F., Plazzi, G., Di Dalmazi, G., Ribichini, D., Vicennati, V., Pizza, F., Mignot, E., Montagna, P., Pasquali, R. & Pagotto, U. 2009. Body mass index-independent metabolic alterations in narcolepsy with cataplexy. *Sleep*, **32**, pp. 1491–7.

Rosenberg, R. & Kim, A.Y. 2014. The AWAKEN survey: knowledge of narcolepsy among physicians and the general population. *Postgraduate Medicine*, **126**, pp. 78–86.

Index